Surgical Management of Knee Arthritis

Ajit J. Deshmukh · Bujar H. Shabani
Wenzel Waldstein · Julius K. Oni
Editors

Savyasachi C. Thakkar
Editor-in-Chief

Surgical Management of Knee Arthritis

Advances in Technique and Technology

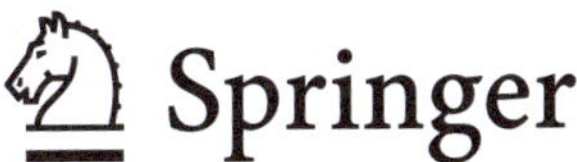
Springer

Editors
Ajit J. Deshmukh
Department of Orthopedic Surgery
Hospital For Joint Diseases
New York, NY, USA

Bujar H. Shabani
University Clinical Center of Kosovo
Pristina, Kosovo

Wenzel Waldstein
Orthopedic Clinic Paulinenhilfe
Diakonie Klinikum
Stuttgart, Germany

Julius K. Oni
Department of Orthopedic Surgery
Johns Hopkins Bayview Medical Center
Baltimore, MD, USA

Editor-in-Cheif
Savyasachi C. Thakkar
Department of Orthopedic Surgery
Johns Hopkins University
Baltimore, MD, USA

ISBN 978-3-031-47931-1   ISBN 978-3-031-47929-8   (eBook)
https://doi.org/10.1007/978-3-031-47929-8

This Springer imprint is published by the registered company Springer Nature Switzerland AG
The registered company address is: Gewerbestrasse 11, 6330 Cham, Switzerland

Paper in this product is recyclable

I dedicate this work to my mentors Dr. Jose A. Rodriguez and Dr. Rajeev Arora for teaching me the art, craft, and ethics of orthopedic surgery. I would like to thank my parents, Drs. Jayant and Asha Deshmukh, my wife Somali and kids Shivani and Aryan for their encouragement and unwavering support.

Ajit J. Deshmukh

In memory of my beloved father, Hilmi Shabani, whose voice still guides me!

Bujar H. Shabani

I dedicate this book to my wonderful parents, Dr. Julius K. Oni and Mrs. Taiwo A. Oni, for their sacrifice, unwavering love, and guidance. To the memory of Mr. Larry Cowan, who saw greatness in me when few did. To Mr. Idowu Adewakun and Mr. Bunmi Akindebe, for their love and invaluable support when I needed it most. And finally, to my amazing wife, Mrs. Temi Oni, and children, Kike and Kemi, for their relentless patience, love, and inspiration.

Julius K. Oni

I would like to dedicate this book to my parents Mrs. Heena C. Thakkar and Dr. C.J. Thakkar for their dedicated upbringing and commitment towards excellence in life. I would also like to dedicate the book to my wife Dr. Rashmi S. Thakkar and to my children Sahuri and Shaarav who have provided me with untiring support, love, and patience. Without these individuals, I would not be where I am today!

Savyasachi C. Thakkar

Preface

This is an exciting time to train and practice as a knee reconstruction surgeon! The orthopedic community is avidly debating technical and technological innovations that aim to restore native function for the arthritic knee. Alignment paradigms are shifting towards more functional concepts. There is now an incredible array of knee implant designs and matching technology to assist in placing these implants. Artificial Intelligence is making a foray into orthopedics and surgeons must bridge the gap between their training and experience alongside the digital transformation in the operating room.

Ironically, my co-editors and I decided to present this new and emerging information by means of this book instead of a digital alternative. The idea of this book was conceived during the European Knee Society Traveling Fellowship in 2019 when I had the opportunity to visit various centers specializing in knee surgery. My co-fellows and I quickly realized that there was no unifying manuscript that could provide a framework to understand current ideas. Co-fellows became co-editors as we entered the COVID-19 pandemic and reached out to several experts that have graced us with their chapters. The book comprises of two underlying themes—techniques and technologies. Technological advances, whether it is related to implants, robotics and navigation are covered in detail throughout the book. Techniques—which are an amalgamation of technology and surgical experience is where the true magic happens!

It is our hope that the readers of this book will receive a comprehensive framework to base their clinical decisions in caring for patients with knee arthritis. This book would not have been possible without the tremendous contributions of masters in knee surgery with a passion for teaching. On behalf of the editors and the authors, we hope that you enjoy reading this book and apply the techniques towards the care of your patients.

New York, NY, USA
Pristina, Kosovo
Stuttgart, Germany
Baltimore, MD, USA
Baltimore, MD, USA

Ajit J. Deshmukh MD
Bujar H. Shabani MD-PhD
Wenzel Waldstein
Julius K. Oni MD
Savyasachi C. Thakkar MD

Acknowledgments

The creation of this book has been a collective effort of several professionals. We would like to thank all the masters of knee surgery that have provided us with their invaluable time and efforts to describe their techniques. This book was written during the COVID-19 pandemic which was a tumultuous and challenging time for everyone.

The book would not have been possible without the oversight and planning provided by Mr. Kristopher Spring and Mr. Janakiraman Ganesan. Both have provided us with invaluable resources to help complete the book.

Finally, and most importantly, we would like to thank our families for providing us with undying support and motivation to see this endeavor past the finish line.

Contents

Kinematics of the Native and Arthritic Knee

Alexis Jorgensen, Niraj Kalore, Ryan Scully, and Gregory J. Golladay

Knee kinematics is the study of motion patterns of native or prosthetic knees. In kinematics, the geometry of moving surfaces is utilized to predict motion patterns. The native knee provides satisfactory function in daily activities and in higher demand activities such as running, climbing, or kneeling. Contemporary artificial knees provide satisfactory function in the basic functions of walking and stair climbing, yet are unsatisfactory in stair descent, deep squatting, and running. Multiple studies have confirmed the inadequacies of current knee designs. About 20% of patients continue to be unsatisfied with their total knee arthroplasty (TKA), mainly due to inadequate pain relief and unsatisfactory function [1]. Recent advances in perioperative optimization, multimodal pain management, regional anesthesia, and surgical techniques have reduced complications and improved patient experience but have failed to close the gap in patient satisfaction.

Historically, improved understanding of knee kinematics has led to improvements in prosthetic knee designs, which in some cases have improved outcomes. Despite multiple improvements over the years, the contemporary prosthetic knee designs fail to replicate native knee kinematics. For example, various TKA designs demonstrate condylar liftoff through range of motion [2], paradoxical rollback [3], and significant understuffing of the patellofemoral joint [4] in comparison to native knees. Gait mechanics have been found to be significantly altered following TKA as well [5]. Deviations from normal knee kinematics may contribute to patient dissatisfaction. Optimizing prosthetic knee kinematics to closely resemble native knee kinematics may improve patient satisfaction.

Methods of Studying Knee Kinematics

Cadaveric studies improve understanding of knee geometry that is used to predict knee kinematics: for example, the study of cadaveric femoral condyles to determine the axes of sagittal plane motion through the femoral condyles. This led to one of the early models of knee kinematics—the idea of an instant center of motion [6].

Cross-sectional imaging studies like CT and MRI can provide information about the bone, implant, or cartilage surfaces. This data is very accurate but fails to capture motion or function. It is challenging to reproduce weight-bearing and functional activities in cross-sectional imaging.

A. Jorgensen · N. Kalore (✉) · G. J. Golladay
Virginia Commonwealth University Medical Center, Richmond, VA, USA
e-mail: Alexis.Jorgensen@vcuhealth.org;
niraj.kalore@vcuhealth.org;
gregory.golladay@vcuhealth.org

R. Scully
University of California, Los Angeles, Santa Monica, CA, USA
e-mail: rscully@mednet.ucla.edu

Recently, dynamic 3D MRI knee kinematic models have been investigated, which demonstrate significantly different measurements from the traditional static data [7].

Motion analyses capture motion patterns of native or prosthetic knees in vivo. Marker placement on the skin, in the prosthetic components or inside the bone yields information regarding the gross angular movements of the knee [8]. Dynamic uniplanar or biplanar fluoroscopy has discovered nuances of native knee function like femoral rollback and screw-home mechanism and identified flaws in prosthetic function like condylar liftoff and paradoxical roll-forward.

These various methods yield important data on the movement and load transmissions through the knee joint that have helped shape arthroplasty design and technique. Here, we will review the kinematics of native and arthritic knees through range of motion and during various activity states—such as walking, stair climbing, and deep squatting. Then, we will review the different total knee arthroplasty designs and the key changes in knee kinematics in these same activity states.

Native Knee Kinematics

Native Knee Anatomy

The native knee is not a simple hinge joint. Instead, it possesses six degrees of freedom—three rotations (internal-external, flexion-extension, varus-valgus) and three translations (anterior-posterior, proximal-distal, medial-lateral). The native knee has different geometry in each of its three articular compartments. This along with the surrounding soft tissues drive both normal and abnormal kinematics. The medial compartment is highly congruent with its oval, concave tibial plateau and large femoral condyle. The lateral compartment is less congruent—consisting of a convex, more circular tibial plateau and relatively smaller lateral femoral condyle (see Fig. 1.1).

The center of contact between the femoral condyles and tibial plateau shifts throughout the range of motion due to the shape of the femoral condyles. The medial femoral condyle remains relatively stationary because of the high congruity of the compartment, while the lateral femoral condyle rolls posteriorly on the tibia. This phenomenon is known as posterior rollback. As the knee goes from flexion to full extension, a "screw-home mechanism" occurs. As the knee is taken from about 30 degrees of flexion to full extension the tibia exhibits external rotation, increasing the tension in the cruciate ligaments and locking the joint, allowing for weight-bearing during gait.

The third compartment is the patellofemoral joint. The posterior surface of the patella contains convex facets that articulate with the concavity of the femoral trochlea. Given the relative incongruity of the patellofemoral joint, soft tissue stabilizers are essential for stability. The medial patellofemoral ligament is the primary restraint to the lateral translation of the patella. The retinaculum is a key stabilizing structure particularly

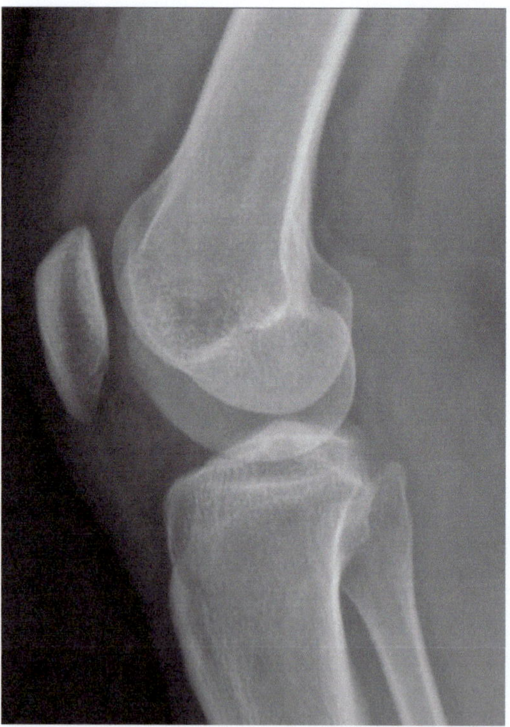

Fig. 1.1 Lateral radiograph of nonarthritic knee to illustrate differences in sagittal geometry of medial and lateral compartments

up to 30 degrees of knee flexion. The patellofemoral joint is a sliding articulation driven by the active contraction of the quadriceps muscles. As the knee is brought through its full range of motion, the points of articulation between the patella and the femur change as well as joint reactive forces. At full extension, there is minimal contact between the patella and the femur. In 30 degrees of flexion, the joint reactive forces are evenly distributed between the femoral condyles. In deep flexion, between 90 and 120°, the patella spans the intercondylar notch with only the far medial and lateral portions of the patella contacting the femur [9].

Native Knee Kinematics in Walking, Stair Climbing, and Deep Squatting

The gait cycle consists of a stance and swing phase for each limb. During initial contact, as the heel strikes, the knee is fully extended but then begins to flex to approximately 15°, stabilized in part by the eccentric quadriceps activity, to absorb energy as the foot flattens onto the ground. Throughout much of the stance phase, a varus adduction moment is present, causing up to 75% of the joint reactive forces to occur in the medial compartment [10]. During the swing phase, the knee flexes further, up to a maximum of 60°, allowing for adequate foot clearance. The swing phase completes as the knee is extended, bringing the tibia perpendicular to the ground and the swing foot returns to the ground.

During stair ascent, the knee attains greater degrees of flexion, up to 98° as a person progresses from the stance to the swing phase of the stair gait. Stair climbing kinematics are affected by various factors in healthy patients including height [11]. Since the functional demands of stair climbing are unique from level ground walking, the ease and efficiency of stair ascent can be a marker of functional outcomes following total knee arthroplasty.

In deep squatting, joint contact forces are even greater than stair ascent, up to 37 N/kg compared to 25 N/kg. Deep knee flexion is achieved with

maximal internal rotation of the tibia and posterior subluxation of the lateral femoral condyle. Maximum deep flexion can be as high as 140° and is limited in part by thigh-calf contact in healthy patients [12].

Arthritic Knee Kinematics

Altered Anatomy of Arthritic Knee

Normally, 60% of the total joint load is carried through the medial compartment and the rest through the lateral compartment. This load distribution is determined by the articular geometry, ligament tension, and the mechanical axis of the limb. Changes in these factors can cause overloading of one or more of the knee compartments and contribute to accelerated wear. Impaired proprioception in osteoarthritis contributes to abnormal loading of the joint and accelerated wear [13].

In a varus knee, the medial compartment is overloaded with the adduction moment even greater during the stance phase of gait. Conversely, in a valgus knee, the lateral compartment experiences increased joint reactive forces with a reduction in the adduction moment during gait. Interestingly, in a valgus knee, the medial compartment carries most of the joint load until the valgus deformity is severe, approximately 15° or more [10]. Figure 1.2 illustrates these concepts.

Ligament insufficiency also affects wear patterns. For example, in an anterior cruciate ligament-deficient knee more wear is noted in the posterior half of the medial tibial plateau, which is consistent with anterior tibial subluxation and increased posterior tibiofemoral contact [14].

Arthritic Knee Kinematics in Walking, Stair Climbing, and Deep Squatting

Due to changes in articular geometry, mechanical axes, and/or ligament integrity, the kinematics of arthritic knee in movements such as walking,

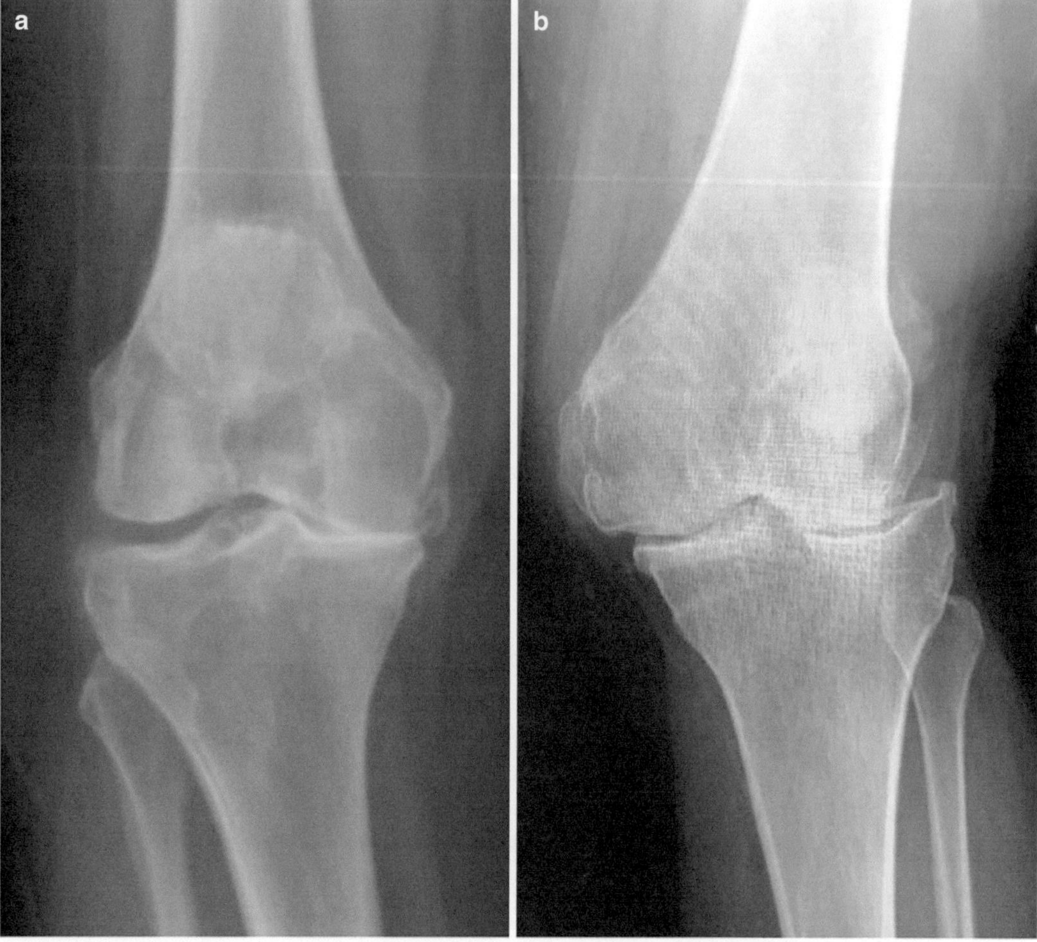

Fig. 1.2 Standing anteroposterior radiograph of a (**a**) right knee showing varus deformity due to cartilage loss in the medial compartment resulting in overloading of the medial compartment with weight-bearing and (**b**) left knee showing valgus deformity due to cartilage and bone loss in lateral compartment resulting in overloading of the lateral compartment with weight-bearing

stair climbing, and deep squatting are altered. During walking, there is an increased knee adduction moment and decreased mid-stance knee flexion moment [15, 16]. During stair climbing, arthritic knees have a decreased knee flexion moment with compensatory increase in hip flexion [17]. Additionally, there is a delay in quadricep activation during stair ascent compared to healthy individuals [17]. Finally, patients with osteoarthritis begin to lose full range of motion, making deep flexion activities such as squatting difficult to perform, contributing to higher self-reports of disability [18].

Total Knee Arthroplasty Kinematics

Total knee arthroplasty improves the abnormal kinematics in an arthritic knee to a varying degree. During knee arthroplasty, prominent osteophytes tenting ligaments are removed, tight ligaments are partially or completely released, and the collapsed joint space is restored. These interventions correct deformity and reduce ligament tension leading to a symmetric distribution of joint reaction forces. This improves knee kinematics, but the improvements fall short of restoring nonarthritic knee kinematics [19]. There is significant variation in the kinematic improvements with each knee arthroplasty design. Here, we will review arthroplasty designs and highlight key kinematics changes during daily activities.

Cruciate Retaining

Cruciate retaining (CR) implants were first designed in the 1990s based on the premise that preserving the posterior cruciate ligament (PCL) would contribute to flexion stability and help recreate the natural femoral rollback. The approach is bone conserving and retention of the PCL can provide proprioceptive feedback. Generally, CR implants include a relatively flat polyethylene insert (Fig. 1.3). Cruciate retaining designs, however, demonstrate inconsistent and paradoxical rollback. Specifically, CR TKAs have shown anterior femoral translation through 30–60 degrees of flexion in both walking and non-weight-bearing activities [20]. Erratic axial rotation profiles have also been demonstrated during gait [21]. In terms of stair-climbing kinematics with CR implants, mid-flexion anterior-posterior stability has been consistently demonstrated [22]. But CR knees have reduced internal rotation compared to an unaffected knee during stair ascent [23]. If posterior condylar offset is not reestablished, range of motion, particularly flexion, can be reduced, and stability negatively impacted, making activities such as stair climbing and squatting more difficult [21].

Posterior Stabilized

The posterior stabilized (PS) design has a tibial post and cam mechanism, which acts in place of the PCL to help control flexion during range of motion. Generally, the polyethylene is more congruent (Fig. 1.4). Posterior stabilized implants more consistently demonstrate femoral rollback particularly during mid-flexion compared to cruciate retaining designs [24]. In kinematic analysis of stair climbing, patients with posterior stabilized implants reach greater degrees of flexion compared to those with cruciate retaining designs. The increase in flexion is likely attributed to the greater posterior translation of the femur in the PS design [22]. This has not proven to make a clinically significant difference in terms of functional outcomes, however.

Overall, both the cruciate retaining and posterior stabilized knee designs have nonconforming articular surfaces. They demonstrate equal patient-reported outcomes and survival rates [25–29]. However, both designs show abnormalities in knee kinematics like reduced femoral rollback or even paradoxical anterior femoral motion and reversed axial rotation. These kinematic abnormalities may adversely affect patient satisfaction. For example, paradoxical anterior translation of the femur may potentially reduce the moment arm of the quadriceps muscles and compromise the effectiveness of the knee-extensor mechanism.

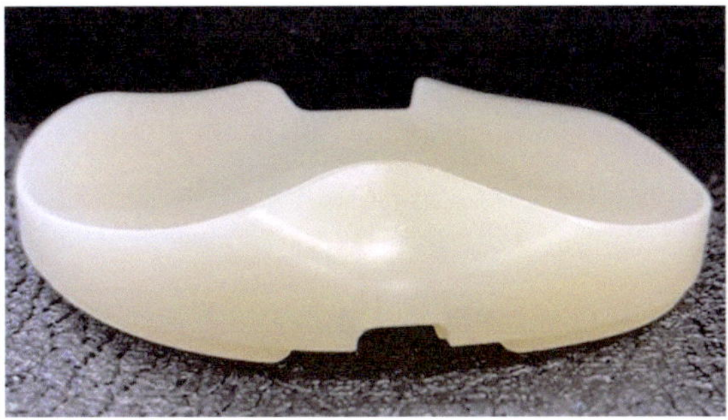
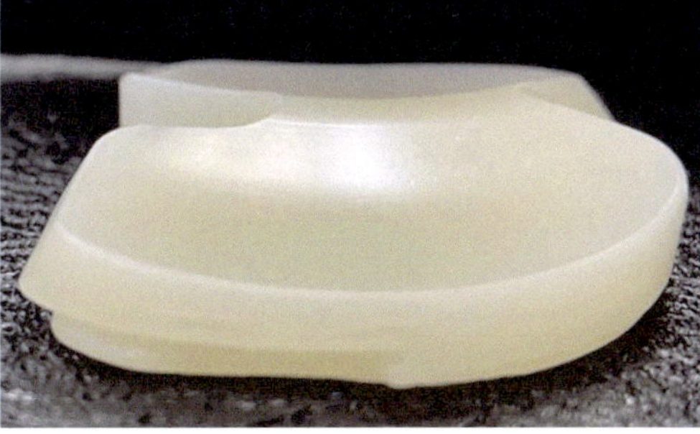

Fig. 1.3 Cruciate retaining polyethylene insert showing relatively flat articulating surface (Source: Krumme J, Kankaria R, Vallem M, Cyrus J, Sculco P, Golladay G, Kalore N. Comparative Analysis of Contemporary Fixed Tibial Inserts: A Systematic Review and Network Meta-analysis of Randomized Controlled Trials. Orthop Rev (Pavia). 2022;14(4):35502. https://doi.org/10.52965/001c.35502. eCollection 2022. PMID: 35769654)

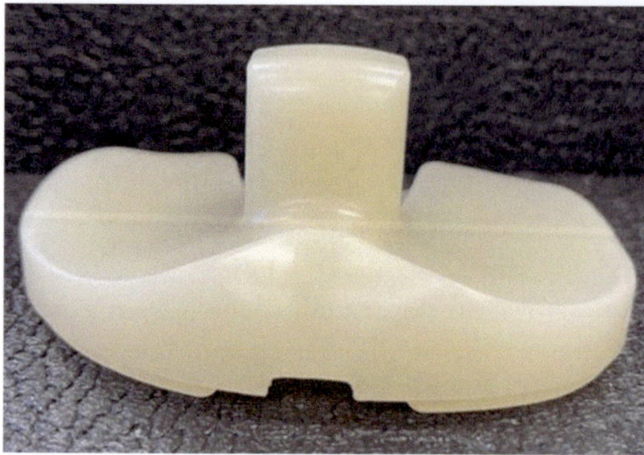
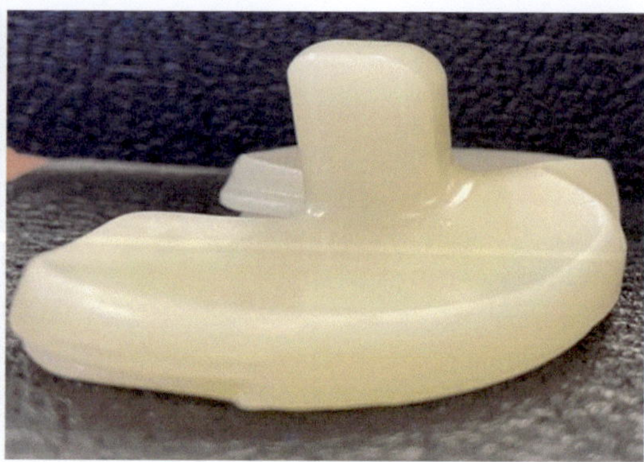

Fig. 1.4 Posterior stabilized polyethylene tibial insert showing tibial post and relatively more congruent articular surface (Source: Krumme J, Kankaria R, Vallem M, Cyrus J, Sculco P, Golladay G, Kalore N. Comparative Analysis of Contemporary Fixed Tibial Inserts: A Systematic Review and Network Meta-analysis of Randomized Controlled Trials. Orthop Rev (Pavia). 2022;14(4):35502. https://doi.org/10.52965/001c.35502. eCollection 2022. PMID: 35769654)

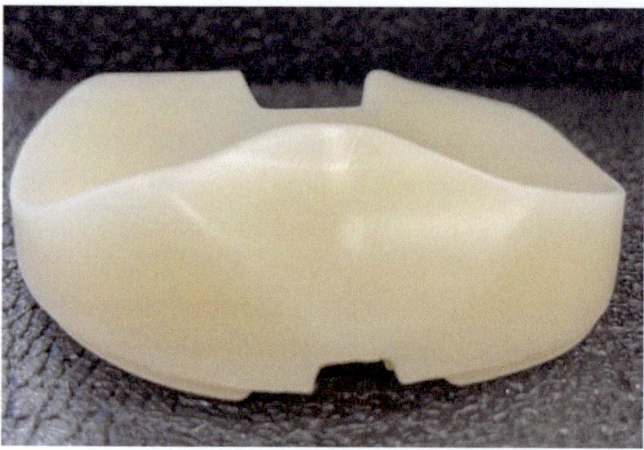
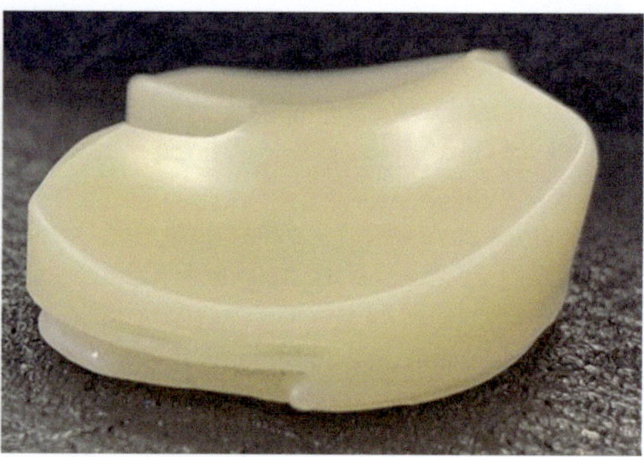

Fig. 1.5 Medial pivot polyethylene insert showing a highly conforming medial articular surface and a relatively flat lateral articular surface (Source: Krumme J, Kankaria R, Vallem M, Cyrus J, Sculco P, Golladay G, Kalore N. Comparative Analysis of Contemporary Fixed Tibial Inserts: A Systematic Review and Network Meta-analysis of Randomized Controlled Trials. Orthop Rev (Pavia). 2022;14(4):35502. https://doi.org/10.52965/001c.35502. eCollection 2022. PMID: 35769654)

Medial Pivot

Medial pivot (MP) or stabilized design mimics the differing geometry of medial and lateral compartments of the native knee. This is accomplished by a spherical medial femoral component together with a tibial bearing that is highly conforming on the medial side and relatively flat on the lateral side (Fig. 1.5). This highly conforming design lets the femur pivot about the medial compartment and permits greater anteriorposterior translation during flexion, similar to the native knee. Recent studies using single-plane X-ray fluoroscopy have shown that MS knees demonstrate minimal anterior-posterior translation of the medial femoral condyle, consistent rollback of the lateral femoral condyle, and little or no paradoxical anterior translation of the femur with knee flexion.

Anterior Stabilized

The anterior stabilized (AS) or ultracongruent design has a deeper, more conforming geometry to provide cruciate sacrificing stability without a post (Fig. 1.6). The anterior lip reduces paradoxical roll-forward in deep flexion but can result in

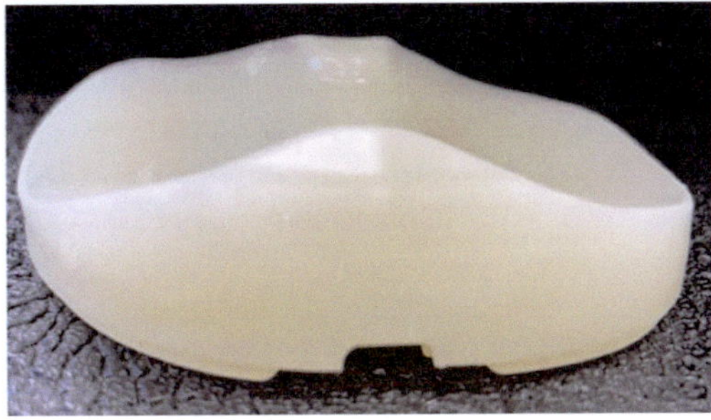

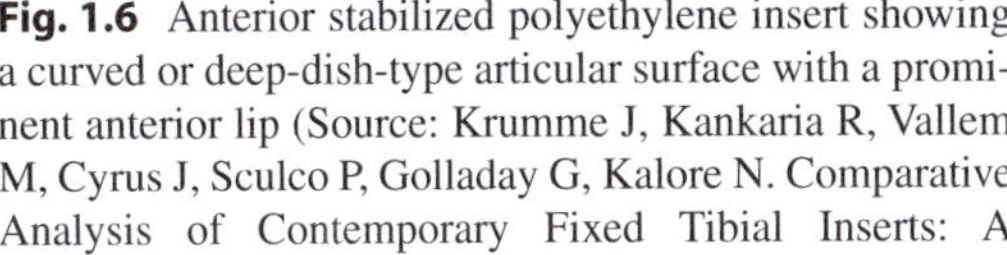

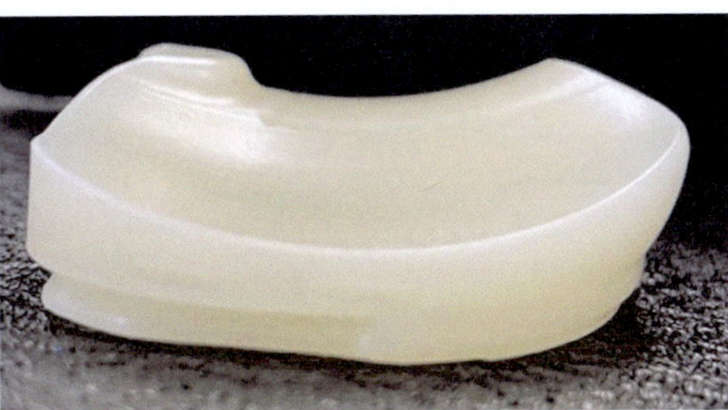

Fig. 1.6 Anterior stabilized polyethylene insert showing a curved or deep-dish-type articular surface with a prominent anterior lip (Source: Krumme J, Kankaria R, Vallem M, Cyrus J, Sculco P, Golladay G, Kalore N. Comparative Analysis of Contemporary Fixed Tibial Inserts: A Systematic Review and Network Meta-analysis of Randomized Controlled Trials. Orthop Rev (Pavia). 2022;14(4):35502. https://doi.org/10.52965/001c.35502. eCollection 2022. PMID: 35769654)

higher medial and patellofemoral contact pressure and wear. Despite these concerns, no significant differences have been noted between AS and traditional CR or PS outcomes in most clinical studies [30, 31]. Jang et al. reported no significant difference in clinical scores or dynamic stability in a prospective randomized study of patients receiving bilateral TKA with an AS TKA and PS TKA [32].

Bicruciate Retaining

The bicruciate retaining (BR) TKA is a fairly new implant design aimed to more closely mimic normal knee kinematics by retaining both the ACL and PCL. With both cruciates intact, the BR TKA implants have preserved femoral rollback during range of motion. In the anterior to posterior dimension, laxity is not significantly different from the native knee [33] but tibia internal rotation is reduced. During gait, a BR implant exhibits less extension than a native knee. In a prospective trial comparing stair climbing ability among TKA types, a significantly higher proportion of patients, approximately 90%, with BR TKA were able to ascend stairs one step at a time compared to patients with CR and PS implants [34]. Although the kinematics of BR may more closely resemble normal knee kinematics, there still is a sparsity of data supporting superior functional outcomes.

Mobile-Bearing Total Knee Arthroplasty

The mobile-bearing (rotating platform) total knee arthroplasty allows the tibial insert to rotate on the highly polished tibial tray during knee range of motion. Bearing conformity affects both the kinematics and contact stress. Low conformity designs permit sliding or translation while increased conformity decreases contact stress.

Compared to fixed bearing, the mobile bearing offers less constraint and therefore may transmit less force at the bone-implant interface, resulting in the potential for decreased tibial component loosening, improved polyethylene wear characteristics, and more natural kinematics. These theoretical advantages have not been convincingly demonstrated in the literature. Multiple comparative studies have shown no difference between mobile- and fixed-bearing designs with regard to loosening and wear [35–37]. With regard to kinematics, femorotibial axial rotation and range of motion are similar in fixed- and mobile-bearing knees [38, 39]. Another proposed advantage of the mobile-bearing designs is self-alignment. Self-alignment may allow for increased forgiveness with intra-operative technical errors or intended deviations from preferred component alignment to optimize sizing and or fixation. While in vivo kinematic data has supported the notion of self-alignment [38, 40], the clinical relevance of this remains unknown.

Hasegawa et al. performed staged bilateral TKA in 25 patients with each patient receiving a mobile-bearing and a fixed-bearing TKA [41]. At a mean follow-up of 3 years, there were no significant differences in radiographic or clinical outcomes and no patient preference for a particular design. In a similar study with a mean follow-up of 13.2 years, Kim et al. reported that 85% of patients did not have a preference for either mobile- or fixed-bearing designs [42]. Several other studies have shown no significant difference in clinical or radiographic outcomes between fixed-bearing and mobile-bearing designs [42–47].

Disadvantages of the mobile-bearing TKA include increased cost [48] and the potential for bearing dislocation or spinout. Overall, mobile-bearing TKA seems to be equivalent to fixed-bearing TKA with regard to clinical and radiographic outcomes. The specific indications and clinical benefits remain unclear.

Varus-Valgus Constraint

The varus-valgus constrained (VVC) or unliked constrained TKA is utilized for primary and revision arthroplasty. Design features include a taller and often wider tibial post and deeper femoral box compared to the posterior stabilized knee. A tibial stem extension can be used to transmit increased forces away from the joint line to protect the fixation. Most VVC implants allow for 2–3 degrees of coronal plane motion and 2 degrees of axial rotation [49].

Semi-constrained PS system reproducibly exhibited a mild external rotation with smooth posterior rolling back of the femoral condyles during deep knee bending, similar to that of the standard PS TKAs. Furthermore, post-cam engagement occurred in a relatively early phase of flexion, which contributed to the reproducible femoral rollback [50].

Sadhwani et al. reported positive clinical and radiographic outcomes at an average 3-year follow-up for a progressive constraint design with a trapezoidal femoral box allowing more constraint in extension and less in flexion [51]. The varus-valgus motion for this design is 1–4° and 2–7

degrees of internal-external rotation during flexion. A recent meta-analysis estimates that the revision rate for VVC knees is 9% at 12 years and 28% at 20 years, emphasizing the importance of judicious use of VVC implants in primary cases [52].

Rotating Hinge

The rotating hinge knee (RHK) is a highly constrained prosthesis used for complex revision and oncologic reconstruction. The femoral and tibial components are linked by an axle. Initial designs were uniplanar, did not permit rotation, and had high rates of failure from aseptic loosening [49]. Contemporary hinge designs allow rotation and have improved survivorship, with an estimated 4.5% revision rate for aseptic loosening at 10 years [53].

Table 1.1 summarizes sagittal plane motion and transverse tibial rotation in native knee and different knee designs.

Table 1.1 Summary of sagittal plane motion and transverse tibial rotation in native knee and different knee designs

	Sagittal plane motion	Transverse rotation of tibia in deep flexion
Native knee	Femoral rollback guided by PCL	Internal rotation (medial pivot)
CR	Paradoxical roll-forward	External rotation
PS	Rollback controlled by cam-post mechanism	External rotation
AS	Reduced roll-forward due to anterior lip	External rotation
MP	Femoral rollback	Internal rotation (medial pivot)
BCR	Femoral rollback guided by PCL	Internal rotation (medial pivot)
Mobile bearing	Femoral rollback guided by PCL in CR mobile bearing	Rotation permitted at tibial insert-baseplate interface
Semi-constrained	Similar to PS knees	
Rotating hinge	Uniaxial rotation without translation	Rotation permitted at tibial insert-baseplate interface

References

1. Kahlenberg CA, et al. Patient satisfaction after total knee replacement: a systematic review. HSS J. 2018;14(2):192–201.
2. Dennis DA, et al. Femoral condylar lift-off in vivo in total knee arthroplasty. J Bone Joint Surg Br. 2001;83(1):33–9.
3. Ploegmakers MJ, et al. Physical examination and in vivo kinematics in two posterior cruciate ligament retaining total knee arthroplasty designs. Knee. 2010;17(3):204–9.
4. Rivière C, et al. Differences in trochlear parameters between native and prosthetic kinematically or mechanically aligned knees. Orthop Traumatol Surg Res. 2018;104(2):165–70.
5. Hatfield GL, et al. The effect of total knee arthroplasty on knee joint kinematics and kinetics during gait. J Arthroplasty. 2011;26(2):309–18.
6. Smith PN, Refshauge KM, Scarvell JM. Development of the concepts of knee kinematics. Arch Phys Med Rehabil. 2003;84(12):1895–902.
7. d'Entremont AG, et al. Do dynamic-based MR knee kinematics methods produce the same results as static methods? Magn Reson Med. 2013;69(6):1634–44.
8. Freeman MA, Pinskerova V. The movement of the knee studied by magnetic resonance imaging. Clin Orthop Relat Res. 2003;(410):35–43.
9. Loudon JK. Biomechanics and pathomechanics of the patellofemoral joint. Int J Sports Phys Ther. 2016;11(6):820–30.
10. Scott CE, Nutton RW, Biant LC. Lateral compartment osteoarthritis of the knee: biomechanics and surgical management of end-stage disease. Bone Joint J. 2013;95-B(4):436–44.
11. Protopapadaki A, et al. Hip, knee, ankle kinematics and kinetics during stair ascent and descent in healthy young individuals. Clin Biomech (Bristol, Avon). 2007;22(2):203–10.
12. Smith SM, et al. Tibiofemoral joint contact forces and knee kinematics during squatting. Gait Posture. 2008;27(3):376–86.
13. Cammarata ML, Dhaher YY. Associations between frontal plane joint stiffness and proprioceptive acuity in knee osteoarthritis. Arthritis Care Res (Hoboken). 2012;64(5):735–43.
14. Harman MK, et al. Wear patterns on tibial plateaus from varus and valgus osteoarthritic knees. Clin Orthop Relat Res. 1998;(352):149–158.
15. Favre J, et al. Baseline ambulatory knee kinematics are associated with changes in cartilage thickness in osteoarthritic patients over 5 years. J Biomech. 2016;49(9):1859–64.
16. Astephen JL, et al. Gait and neuromuscular pattern changes are associated with differences in knee osteoarthritis severity levels. J Biomech. 2008;41(4):868–76.
17. Iijima H, et al. Biomechanical characteristics of stair ambulation in patients with knee OA: a systematic review with meta-analysis toward a better definition of clinical hallmarks. Gait Posture. 2018;62:191–201.
18. Steultjens MP, et al. Range of joint motion and disability in patients with osteoarthritis of the knee or hip. Rheumatology (Oxford). 2000;39(9):955–61.
19. Akbari Shandiz M, et al. Changes in knee kinematics following total knee arthroplasty. Proc Inst Mech Eng H. 2016;230(4):265–78.
20. Song SJ, Park CH, Bae DK. What to know for selecting cruciate-retaining or posterior-stabilized total knee arthroplasty. Clin Orthop Surg. 2019;11(2):142–50.
21. Donadio J, et al. Control of paradoxical kinematics in posterior cruciate-retaining total knee arthroplasty by increasing posterior femoral offset. Knee Surg Sports Traumatol Arthrosc. 2015;23(6):1631–7.
22. Murakami K, et al. Kinematic analysis of stair climbing in rotating platform cruciate-retaining and posterior-stabilized mobile-bearing total knee arthroplasties. Arch Orthop Trauma Surg. 2017;137(5):701–11.
23. Komnik I, et al. Compromised knee internal rotation in total knee arthroplasty patients during stair climbing. PLoS One. 2018;13(10):e0205492.
24. Victor J, Banks S, Bellemans J. Kinematics of posterior cruciate ligament-retaining and -substituting total knee arthroplasty: a prospective randomised outcome study. J Bone Joint Surg Br. 2005;87(5):646–55.
25. Harato K, et al. Midterm comparison of posterior cruciate-retaining versus -substituting total knee arthroplasty using the genesis II prosthesis. A multicenter prospective randomized clinical trial. Knee. 2008;15(3):217–21.
26. Broberg JS, et al. Comparison of contact kinematics in posterior-stabilized and cruciate-retaining total knee arthroplasty at long-term follow-up. J Arthroplasty. 2020;35(1):272–7.
27. Verra WC, et al. Retention versus sacrifice of the posterior cruciate ligament in total knee arthroplasty for treating osteoarthritis. Cochrane Database Syst Rev. 2013;(10):CD004803.
28. Verra WC, et al. Similar outcome after retention or sacrifice of the posterior cruciate ligament in total knee arthroplasty. Acta Orthop. 2015;86(2):195–201.
29. Li N, et al. Posterior cruciate-retaining versus posterior stabilized total knee arthroplasty: a meta-analysis of randomized controlled trials. Knee Surg Sports Traumatol Arthrosc. 2014;22(3):556–64.
30. Peters CL, et al. Comparison of total knee arthroplasty with highly congruent anterior-stabilized bearings versus a cruciate-retaining design. Clin Orthop Relat Res. 2014;472(1):175–80.
31. Lützner J, et al. Similar stability and range of motion between cruciate-retaining and cruciate-substituting ultracongruent insert total knee arthroplasty. Knee Surg Sports Traumatol Arthrosc. 2015;23(6):1638–43.
32. Jang SW, et al. Comparison of anterior-stabilized and posterior-stabilized total knee arthroplasty in the same patients: a prospective randomized study. J Arthroplasty. 2019;34(8):1682–9.

33. Heyse TJ, et al. Kinematics of a bicruciate-retaining total knee arthroplasty. Knee Surg Sports Traumatol Arthrosc. 2017;25(6):1784–91.
34. Iriuchishima T, Ryu K. Bicruciate substituting total knee arthroplasty improves stair climbing ability when compared with cruciate-retain or posterior stabilizing total knee arthroplasty. Indian J Orthop. 2019;53(5):641–5.
35. Hansson U, et al. Mobile vs. fixed meniscal bearing in total knee replacement: a randomised radiostereometric study. Knee. 2005;12(6):414–8.
36. Haider H, Garvin K. Rotating platform versus fixed-bearing total knees: an in vitro study of wear. Clin Orthop Relat Res. 2008;466(11):2677–85.
37. Oh KJ, et al. Meta-analysis comparing outcomes of fixed-bearing and mobile-bearing prostheses in total knee arthroplasty. J Arthroplasty. 2009;24(6): 873–84.
38. Dennis DA, et al. Mobile-bearing total knee arthroplasty: do the polyethylene bearings rotate? Clin Orthop Relat Res. 2005;440:88–95.
39. Ball ST, et al. Fixed versus rotating platform total knee arthroplasty: a prospective, randomized, single-blind study. J Arthroplasty. 2011;26(4):531–6.
40. Fantozzi S, et al. Dynamic in-vivo tibio-femoral and bearing motions in mobile bearing knee arthroplasty. Knee Surg Sports Traumatol Arthrosc. 2004;12(2):144–51.
41. Hasegawa M, Sudo A, Uchida A. Staged bilateral mobile-bearing and fixed-bearing total knee arthroplasty in the same patients: a prospective comparison of a posterior-stabilized prosthesis. Knee Surg Sports Traumatol Arthrosc. 2009;17(3):237–43.
42. Kim YH, Yoon SH, Kim JS. The long-term results of simultaneous fixed-bearing and mobile-bearing total knee replacements performed in the same patient. J Bone Joint Surg Br. 2007;89(10):1317–23.
43. Rahman WA, Garbuz DS, Masri BA. Randomized controlled trial of radiographic and patient-assessed outcomes following fixed versus rotating platform total knee arthroplasty. J Arthroplasty. 2010;25(8):1201–8.
44. Woolson ST, Epstein NJ, Huddleston JI. Long-term comparison of mobile-bearing vs fixed-bearing total knee arthroplasty. J Arthroplasty. 2011;26(8):1219–23.
45. Moskal JT, Capps SG. Rotating-platform TKA no different from fixed-bearing TKA regarding survivorship or performance: a meta-analysis. Clin Orthop Relat Res. 2014;472(7):2185–93.
46. Post ZD, et al. Mobile-bearing total knee arthroplasty: better than a fixed-bearing? J Arthroplasty. 2010;25(6):998–1003.
47. Smith H, et al. Meta-analysis and systematic review of clinical outcomes comparing mobile bearing and fixed bearing total knee arthroplasty. J Arthroplasty. 2011;26(8):1205–13.
48. Murray DW, et al. A randomised controlled trial of the clinical effectiveness and cost-effectiveness of different knee prostheses: the knee arthroplasty trial (KAT). Health Technol Assess. 2014;18(19):1–235, vii–viii.
49. Morgan H, Battista V, Leopold SS. Constraint in primary total knee arthroplasty. J Am Acad Orthop Surg. 2005;13(8):515–24.
50. Sumino T, et al. Semi-constrained posterior stabilized total knee arthroplasty reproduces natural deep knee bending kinematics. BMC Musculoskelet Disord. 2020;21(1):107.
51. Sadhwani S, Picache D, Eberle R, Shah A. Achieving progressive constrained kinematics following primary complex total knee arthroplasty: the trapezoidal femoral component box. In: Orthopaedic proceedings. 2020. The British Editorial Society of Bone & Joint Surgery.
52. Avino RJ, et al. Varus-valgus constraint in primary total knee arthroplasty: a short-term solution but will it last? J Arthroplasty. 2020;35(3):741–746.e2.
53. Cottino U, et al. Long-term results after total knee arthroplasty with contemporary rotating-hinge prostheses. J Bone Joint Surg Am. 2017;99(4):324–30.

Alignment Options for Modern Total Knee Arthroplasty

Sivan S. Sivaloganathan, Loic Villet, and Charles Riviere

Introduction

Total knee arthroplasty (TKA) procedures have been performed widely since the 1970s; annually, more than 650,000 TKAs are carried out in the United States [1], and in excess of 80,000 in the United Kingdom and France [2]. TKAs are successful in relieving pain and improving knee function in people with advanced arthritis of the knee joint. Although TKA has become a more common procedure than total hip arthroplasty, patient satisfaction following TKA surgery remains inferior in comparison to its hip arthroplasty counterpart [3]. The exact reasons remain unclear; the knee is a complex joint and errors in both rotation and translation of the implant can lead to alteration in knee kinematics and can potentially compromise patient outcome.

There are a number of factors that determine whether a patient is satisfied with their TKA outcome. Techniques to improve overall functional outcomes using TKAs continue to evolve. One such aspect is the TKA alignment technique. Over the past few decades, various alignment techniques have been performed that fall into two broad groups—systematic and personalised.

Systematic alignment techniques include: Mechanical Alignment (MA), adjusted Mechanical Alignment (aMA) and Anatomical Alignment (AA); Personalised alignment techniques include: Kinematic Alignment (KA), restricted Kinematic Alignment (rKA), Functional (or smart) Alignment (FA) and Inverse Kinematic Alignment (IKA) [4].

This chapter will focus on alignment options for modern TKA.

Mechanical Alignment (MA) (Fig. 2.1)

Overview

Performance of early TKA designs was poor. It was Insall and Freeman who endeavoured to improve the longevity of early TKA designs by propagating the technique of Mechanical Alignment. MA TKA creates a straight limb by positioning both the femoral and tibial components perpendicular to the mechanical axis of each bone [4]; this results in a hip-knee-ankle (HKA) angle of the limb of 180° (this is considered neutral alignment). Suppositionally, this allows even load distribution between the medial and lateral compartments to minimise wear and the potential for component loosening. By standardising this procedure and making it more

S. S. Sivaloganathan
South West London Rotation, St George's University Hospital, London, UK

L. Villet · C. Riviere (✉)
Clinique du Sport, Merignac, France
e-mail: c.riviere@imperial.ac.uk

© The Author(s), under exclusive license to Springer Nature Switzerland AG 2023
A. J. Deshmukh et al. (eds.), *Surgical Management of Knee Arthritis*,
https://doi.org/10.1007/978-3-031-47929-8_2

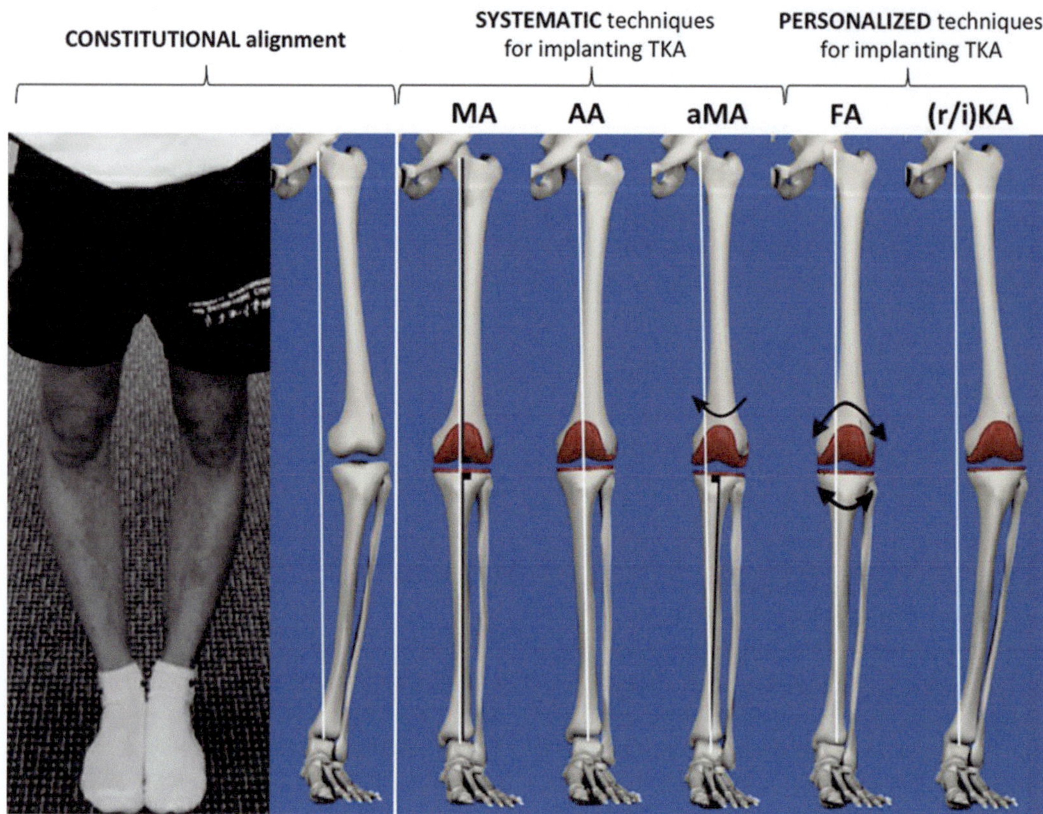

Fig. 2.1 Alignment techniques. Constitutional varus alignment when standing. Systematic techniques including mechanical alignment (MA), anatomical alignment (AA) and adjusted mechanical alignment (aMA). Personalised techniques including functional (smart) alignment (FA) and kinematic alignment (KA)/restricted KA/inverse KA. (Reproduced from *Charles Riviere* et al. *Kinematic alignment of medial UKA is safe: a systematic review. Knee Surgery, Sports Traumatology, Arthroscopy.* https://doi.org/10.1007/s00167-021-06462-6. Copyright © 2021. Elsevier Masson SAS. All rights reserved)

reproducible, the expectation was that correcting any lower limb deformity would effectively sustain better distribution of joint stress, which in the end would improve implant survival.

Technical

The distal femoral cut is performed perpendicular to a line drawn from the centre of the femoral head to the centre of the knee (the mechanical axis of the femur). Generally, for the distal femoral cut, most surgeons use an intramedullary rod in the distal femur set at a fixed valgus cut angle (usually 5° or 6°). The proximal tibial cut is perpendicular to a line drawn from the centre of the knee to the centre of the ankle (the mechanical axis of the tibia) and is made with the use of an extramedullary guide. These cuts achieve the extension gap. The sagittal alignment is determined by the patient's anatomy while femoral rotation can be based on either femoral anatomy (measured resection) or the flexion gap (gap-balancing) [5].

Opinion

MA is the most widely used technique for TKA. Though this technique results in very good outcomes [6], reservations remain amongst orthopaedic surgeons about the efficacy of this technique. Ultimately, their concerns lay in the functional performance of MA TKAs; 15–20% of patients are dissatisfied with the outcome of MA TKAs [7, 8]. In the vast majority of patients, the overall alignment to neutral results in changes to the joint line obliquity, and this includes raising the joint line. When the joint line changes, there is an expectant compensatory change in the axial rotation of the femoral component to minimise the inevitable imbalance of the collateral and retinacular ligaments. Current literature has quoted that up to 40% of MA TKAs can have a gap imbalance, and up to 50% of patients may have residual symptoms [8]. These residual symptoms may be due to a resultant change in an individual's constitutional anatomy and laxity of the knee. These known outcomes have contributed to the recognised limitations of the MA technique for TKA and the introduction of more physiological alignment techniques.

Adjusted Mechanical Alignment (aMA) (Fig. 2.1)

Overview

The adjusted Mechanical Alignment (aMA) technique is a modification of the MA technique that was developed for medial osteoarthritis (varus patients). The goal of this technique is to undercorrect the coronal alignment to a maximum of 3° of the varus [4, 9] aMA builds on Bellemans' concept of a constitutional varus limb; Bellemans argues that for a number of patients, neutral mechanical alignment is abnormal and to produce a neutral alignment in these patients would be undesirable [10]. This technique is another example of a 'systematic technique' as it aims to achieve a similar implant anatomy in all patients similar to that of the MA technique. All patients have a prosthetic lower limb with a slight varus (2–3°) [10, 11].

Technical

The aMA technique is a measured resection technique which achieves a balanced ligament tension through a femoral correction. The aMA technique keeps the tibial implant mechanically aligned, and therefore to achieve the overall alignment, the implant positioning adjustments are made on the femoral side [12]. The maximum deviation of the femoral alignment in the coronal plane from neutral is approximately 2–3°. In order to achieve this, the distal femoral cut is executed with a slight varus. This has two effects; firstly, it promotes the reduction of the asymmetry in the extension gaps, and secondly, it minimises the number of ligament release procedures required for overall soft tissue balancing [13].

Opinion

The clinical benefit of aMA has not been demonstrated in the literature with few comparative studies that have reported very good functional outcomes and/or long-term survivorship for aMA TKA for varus knees.

Anatomical Alignment (AA) (Fig. 2.1)

Overview

Introduced in the 1980s by Hungerford and Krackow, the Anatomical Alignment technique is an example of the systematic technique. With the AA technique, all patients have a straight lower limb but with an oblique joint line (3–6° of valgus) relative to the mechanical axis of the limb. The rationale for this technique is that it reduces the risk of lateral retinacular ligament stretching during knee flexion; this promotes a better distribution of load over the tibial component, in addition to more natural patella biomechanics [4].

Technical

The AA technique results in a straight lower limb with an overall component joint line alignment of 3° oblique. This is achieved by performing a 3° varus cut in the tibia (relative to the mechanical axis of the tibia) and a 3° valgus cut on the femur (relative to the mechanical axis of the femur). The overall net effect is a lower limb alignment of 180° [4, 14]. From a technical perspective, an additional advantage of this technique is that there is no longer a need to externally rotate the femoral component to balance the flexion gap.

Opinion

In principle, the AA technique alters the average anatomy of the knee less than the MA technique. It was the technical challenge in the 1970s to achieve precise bone cuts that led to the widespread abandonment of the AA technique by most surgeons [15, 16]. Today, this lack of surgical accuracy has been overcome by two means: firstly, by the use of precision tools for implant positioning (navigation system and robotic technology) and secondly, by the development of asymmetric implants with a tilted joint line (e.g. Journey TM by Smith & Nephew) [17]. This effectively means that the surgeon can perform identical orthogonal cuts similar to the MA technique, but achieve the same joint line orientation as AA which is called 'AA-like' using modern implants. Though good mid- to long-term results have been published with these techniques (AA-like), there is little difference in outcomes when compared to the MA technique [18].

Kinematic Alignment: Personalised Physiological Implantation (Fig. 2.1)

Overview

The kinematic alignment (KA) technique for TKA was developed by Howell and Hull as an alternative approach to neutral mechanical alignment [4]. Their work built on research performed by Hollister et al. which developed the idea of three-dimensional alignment for knee kinematics; this differed from MA and AA techniques which considered only two-dimensional alignment [14]. KA TKA is a 'physiological' implantation technique where the goal is to restore the native anatomy and ligament balance to that of the pre-arthritic knee [19]. To this end, KA TKA produces anatomic rather than systematic component positions, a more physiological joint line obliquity and better physiological knee kinematics.

Technical

The KA technique was originally performed using proprietary cutting blocks designed based on an MRI/CT scan of the patient's knee. The software was used to recreate the pre-diseased tibiofemoral relationship by compensating for cartilage wear, and a cutting block was designed to enable the surgeon to recreate this anatomy when implanting the components. The technique has since evolved to allow targets to be identified intra-operatively, allowing KA TKA to be performed using manual instrumentation (caliper technique) or a navigation system. The intention of KA is the restoration of the normal three-dimensional orientation of the three axes that determine normal knee kinematics [20]. By definition, the three kinematic axes are a cylindrical (or transverse) axis in the femur around which the tibia flexes and extends; a transverse axis in the femur about which the patella tracks; and a longitudinal axis in the tibia about which the tibia

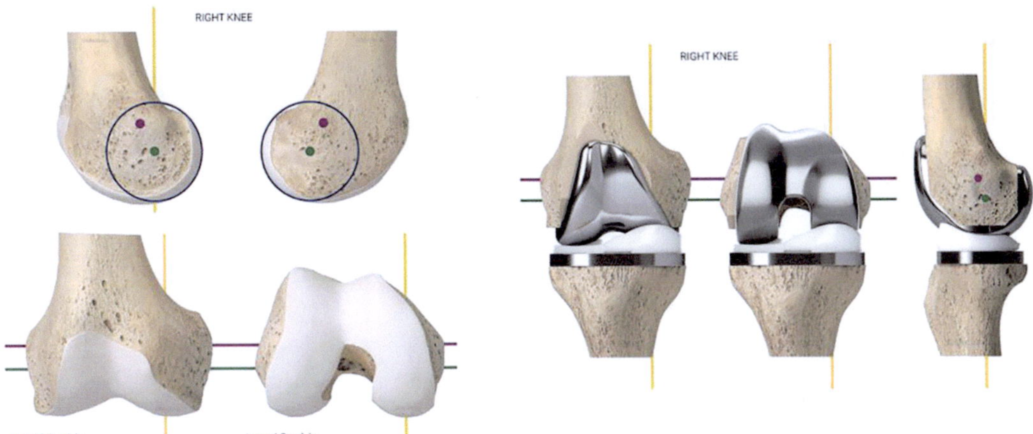

Fig. 2.2 The orange vertical lines demonstrate the longitudinal axis; the purple horizontal lines represent the transverse axis about which the patella flexes and extends; and the green horizontal lines represent the transverse axis about which the tibia flexes and extends (Reproduced from *Charles Riviere* et al. *Kinematic alignment of medial UKA is safe: a systematic review. Knee Surgery, Sports Traumatology, Arthroscopy.* https://doi.org/10.1007/s00167-021-06462-6. Copyright © 2021. Elsevier Masson SAS. All rights reserved)

internally and externally rotates on the femur [14] (Fig. 2.2). In principle, the parallel and orthogonal relationships between these three axes do not vary between knees [4].

Intra-operatively, kinematic alignment is performed with either manual instrumentation (calipered technique) (Fig. 2.3) or patient-specific guides [21] or computational navigation/robotics. The surgeon carries out bone resections after having compensated for cartilage wear. This is a measured resection technique, and the order for cutting bones (femur or tibia first) is left to the surgeon's preference.

For example, KA of the femoral component is achieved using this format: thickness of the two distal and two posterior bone resections + the thickness of the wear + the thickness of the kerf (from sawing the bone) = the thickness of the femoral component (Fig. 2.4). The tibial slope is matched to the patient's native medial plateau slope. The axial rotation of the femur is set according to the posterior condylar axis having compensated for wear. Axial rotation of the tibia is set parallel to the long axis of the ovoid shape of the lateral tibial plateau. In this manner, minimal, if any, soft tissue releases are required.

Opinion

The kinematic implantation of a TKA is physiological. The objective is to alter as little as possible and to recreate the normal anatomy, gap balance and kinematics of the pre-arthritic knee. Evidence in the literature suggests that KA reduces recovery time and improves functional outcomes as well as reducing the frequency of residual symptoms following a TKA [22]. The minor alterations in anatomy, laxity and the improvement in kinematics likely explain these good results [23]. Where significant deformity exists, a more cautionary restricted kinematic alignment (rKA) is recommended.

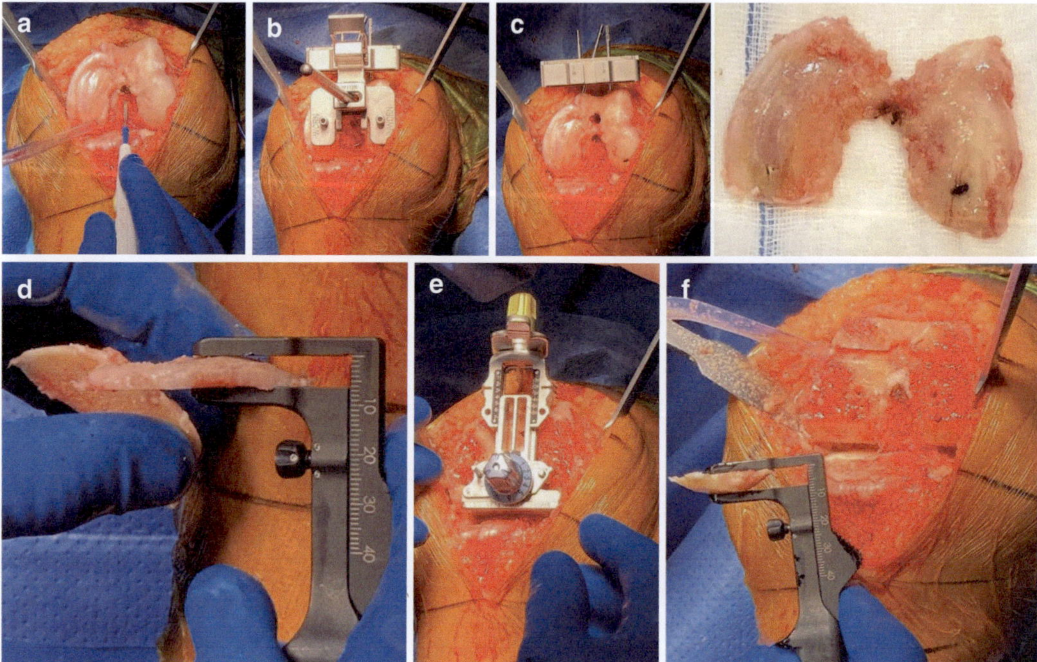

Fig. 2.3 (**a**) The medio-lateral positioning of the distal part of the sulcus is marked—This will serve to set the medio-lateral translational positioning of the femoral component. (**b**) An intramedullary rod is place in the distal femur in order to assist in setting the sagittal rotational positioning (flexion-extension) of the femoral component. The cutting guide is slid on to the intramedullary rod till contacting both medial and lateral distal condyles with the cartilage loss being compensated on the worn side by a 2-mm thick pad; this sets the frontal rotational positioning (varus-valgus) of the femoral component. (**c**) This composite image illustrates the cutting guide secured by three pins (left image) and the resulting distal femoral cut (right image). (**d**) The thickness of the medial distal condylar cut is approximately measured, using a caliper, at 6 mm. Considering a cartilage loss of 2 mm and a 1 mm thickness of the saw blade (kerf), the amount of bone and cartilage removed $(6 + 2 + 1)$ is equivalent to the thickness of the implant put instead (9 mm). (**e**) The posterior femoral cut is always made parallel to the posterior condylar line (zero degree rotation) using a posterior referencing technique. (**f**) The thickness of the medial posterior condylar cut is approximately measured, using a caliper, at 7 mm. Considering there is no cartilage loss and a 1 mm thickness of the saw blade (kerf), the amount of bone and cartilage removed $(7 + 1)$ is equivalent to the thickness of the implant put instead (8 mm). (**g**) The femoral trial component is positioned as to match the distal part of the prosthetic and native (electrocautery mark) groove. (**h**) This composite image illustrates methods to set the axial rotational positioning of the tibial component. A pin is inserted in the proximal tibia perpendicularly to the femoral component at knee extension (left image). The pin orientation often fairly coincides with the long axis of the oval shape of the lateral tibial plateau (right image). Those methods enable to set the tibial component parallel to the antero-posterior tibial axis, which is perpendicular to the cylindrical axis. (**i**) This composite image illustrates the technique to perform a KA tibial cut. A stylus sets the cut height on the healthy lateral plateau. An angel wing sets the posterior (parallel to the medial plateau posterior slope) and medial (exit point 8 mm below the worn medial articular surface—accounting for a 10-mm tibial implant) slopes. A pin (see Fig. 8) sets the axial rotation of the tibial cut. No attention is paid to where the extramedullary rod is positioned relative to the ankle; surgeon only pays attention to reading the joint and reproducing native knee anatomy. (**j**) This composite image illustrates visual aspects of the tibial cut before (upper image) and after (lower image) sawing. The thickness of the tibial cut is measured on both the medial and lateral plateaus by using a caliper. The healthy lateral plateau is measured at nearly 9 mm; considering there is no cartilage loss and a 1 mm thickness of the saw blade (kerf), the amount of bone and cartilage removed $(9 + 1)$ is equivalent to the thickness of the implant put instead (10 mm). (**k**) This composite image illustrates how final implants look intra-operatively (left image—extended prosthetic knee) and on the radiograph (right images)

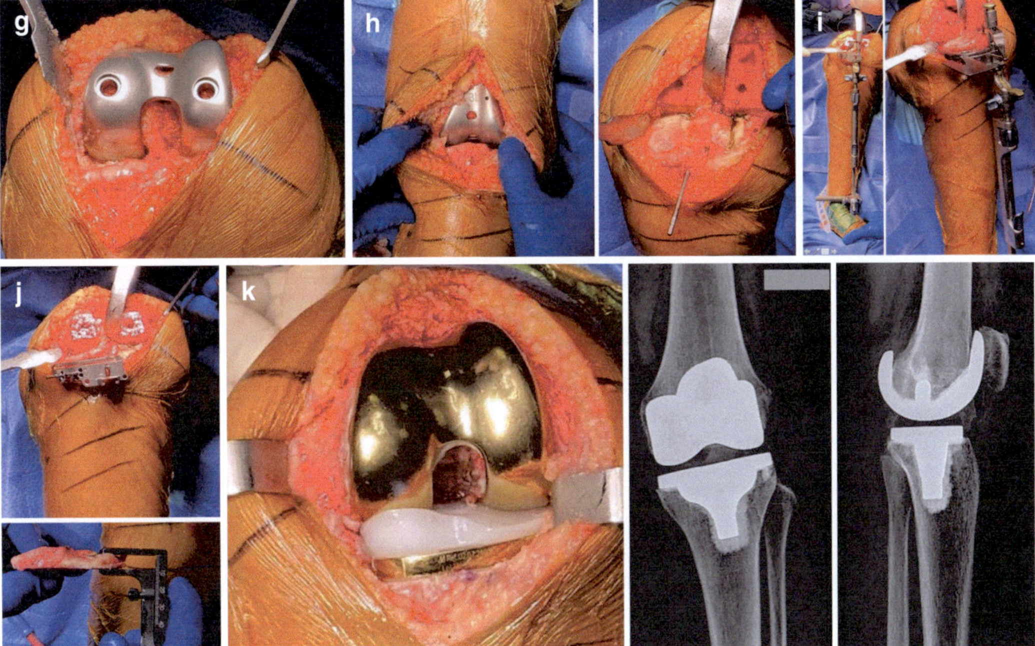

Fig. 2.1 (continued)

Fig. 2.4 Kinematic alignment technique: resected bone = implant thickness—saw blade KERF—cartilage wear (Reproduced from *Charles Riviere* et al. *Kinematic alignment of medial UKA is safe: a systematic review. Knee Surgery, Sports Traumatology, Arthroscopy*. https://doi.org/10.1007/s00167-021-06462-6. Copyright © 2021. Elsevier Masson SAS. All rights reserved). Calipered KA technique for TKA

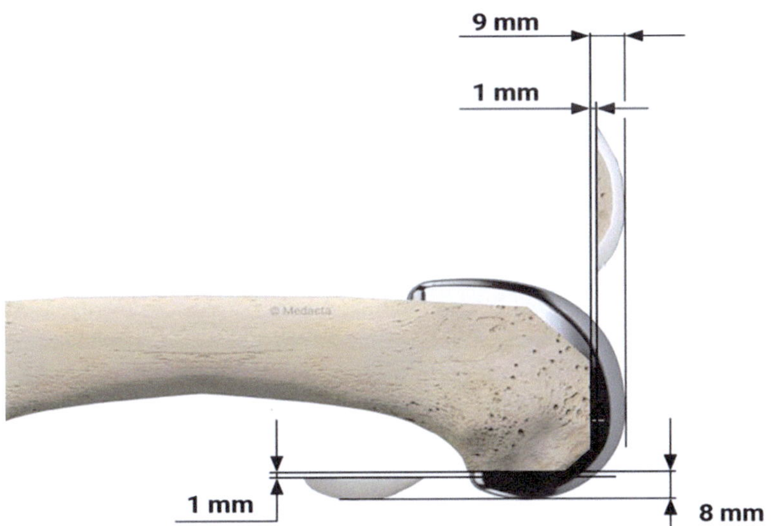

Restricted Kinematic Alignment (rKA) (Fig. 2.1)

Overview

The restricted kinematic alignment technique was developed as an alternative solution to the KA technique in scenarios where there is significant frontal limb deformity (coronal malalignment or joint line obliquity) [24]. Vendittoli proposed the rKA technique in which the tibial and distal femoral bone cuts must be within 5° from the bone's mechanical axis and the resulting hip–knee–ankle angle must not deviate more than 3° from a 180° alignment [25].

Technical

For the rKA technique, a software program/optical computer navigation is often used to assess overall limb alignment in addition to both femoral and tibial alignments. Patient-specific implantation (PSI) or robotic-assisted operative options are also acceptable. The values generated are used to assess the degree of existing malalignment and where there is severe deformity, the decision is taken to restrict the KA technique based on Vendittoli's rKA protocol.

The rKA protocol limits the femoral and tibial prosthesis coronal alignment to within 5° of neutral, with the overall combined lower limb orientation within 3° of neutral [26]. To resurface the posterior condyles, a posterior referencing guide is set to neutral rotation, thus resecting only the implant thickness of the posterior condyles and matching each patient's native femoral orientation. The tibial baseplate rotation can be set based on the long axis of the lateral tibial plateau or relative to the trial femoral component with the knee in extension [25]. Though the surgeon aims to recreate the patient's normal anatomy, resections are modified from the patient's anatomy if the measured angles fall outside the predefined safe range (constitutional frontal limb deformity (<3°) and a distal femoral or proximal tibial frontal joint line with less than 5° obliquity).

By applying the rKA protocol [26], the alignment is kinematically 'pure' in 51% of cases (true KA TKA); a slight adjustment (<1° on average) is needed to bring the patient's anatomy back into a safe zone in 32% of cases, and larger adjustments are needed in the remaining 17% of cases with more extreme malalignment. By applying these alignment thresholds, the resultant alignment is located in a range considered to be safe [4].

Opinion

The rKA protocol follows the main technical principle of the KA technique but also offers a satisfactory compromise for extreme limb constitutional deformities [24]. It allows the recreation of the normal patient anatomy for the majority of cases while avoiding the excessive corrections and ligamentous releases required with MA. The rKA technique also prevents any extremes of implant positioning that a standard KA technique may produce.

Functional (or Smart) Alignment (Fig. 2.1)

Overview

Functional (or smart) alignment is a technology-driven personalised implantation that has been performed since the introduction of advanced navigation and robotic surgery [5]. This alignment technique is performed through three-dimensional intraoperative simulation and real-time data on ligament tension. It allows the surgeon to modify the alignment until the component positioning and gap balance are deemed satisfactory [27]. Once the plan is validated by the surgeon, the robotic arm is used to precisely execute the bone cuts. Central to success is to use ligament tension throughout the range of motion of the knee to plan component positioning and the extent of bone cuts necessary.

Technical

The FA technique positions the femoral and tibial components to least compromise the soft tissue envelope of the knee. This restores the plane and obliquity of the joint to that which the soft tissues dictate. Once osteophytes are excised, the limb alignment is assessed intra-operatively. The software program calculates the potential flexion and extension gaps as any coronal malalignment is corrected through an applied varus or valgus force.

Unlike traditional alignment techniques, the FA technique achieves a gap balance by altering implant targets in three planes. For example, in practical terms, a smaller medial extension gap can be balanced by placing the tibial component in a more varus position or a tighter lateral flexion gap can be balanced by internally rotating the femoral component. All these offsets should be kept within safe zones (coronal alignment should be within 3° of varus or valgus) [5]. Joint line height is maintained by avoiding too much resection of the distal femur and a tight extension gap is prevented by under-resection.

Opinion

Published literature, though limited with respect to the follow-up period, suggests that FA techniques using robotic surgery improve the accuracy of implant positioning and reduce surgeon outliers in achieving the planned limb alignment compared to conventional MA TKA [28].

Inverse Kinematic Alignment (iKA) (Fig. 2.1)

Overview

This technique offers an alternative approach to personalised knee implantation. As described previously, the KA technique is a measured resection technique that aims to resurface the distal femur and maintain the native joint line obliquity. Inverse kinematic alignment aims to resurface the tibia first by maintaining the tibial joint line obliquity, with the flexion and extension gaps balanced by adjusting the femoral resections [29]. The main flaw of this technique is that patients with severe deformity would have their femoral anatomy altered during the iKA TKA, with the risk of creating a clinically deleterious kinematic compromise between femorotibial and femoro-patellar joints.

Technical

The tibial component is positioned first by planning a resection of equal amounts of bone on the medial and lateral on the tibia (factoring in bony wear). The aim is to restore the pre-arthritic medial proximal tibial angle (MTPA) within a safe zone of 84° (varus) to 92° (valgus). The tibial slope is set equal to the native medial tibial slope.

Once the tibial cut is performed, the femoral component is positioned to restore the medial joint line height both in extension and flexion. The flexion and extension gaps are balanced by adjusting the distal lateral and posterior lateral resection levels on the femur. The aim of the flexion gap is to attain residual laxity of 1–2 mm in the medial compartment and 1–3 mm in the lateral compartment. For the extension gap, a residual laxity of 1–2 mm in both compartments is desired whilst remaining within the hip-knee-angle safe zone of 174–183° [29].

Opinion

The literature is limited to support long-term outcomes for this technique. However, the advantage of this technique is that it avoids significant changes in the tibial alignment that have been associated with more detrimental effects [4].

Summary

Knee alignment techniques continue to evolve. Over the past few decades, both variations of systematic and personalised techniques have been developed to improve outcomes for TKA procedures. Further long-term studies are required to evaluate their true benefit.

Key Study Points

- Alignment options fall under two main groups—systematic vs. personalised alignment options.
- The limitations of systematic alignment options such as MA have led to advancements in alternatives such as KA.
- Further studies are required for mid- to long-term follow-up outcomes; however, early outcome results for physiological alignment options, such as KA, appear to be promising.

References

1. Carr AJ, Robertsson O, Graves S, Price AJ, Arden NK, Judge A, Beard DJ. Knee replacement. Lancet. 2012;379(9823):1331–40. https://doi.org/10.1016/S0140-6736(11)60752-6.
2. Rivière C, Villet L, Jeremic D, Vendittoli PA. What you need to know about kinematic alignment for total knee arthroplasty. Orthop Traumatol Surg Res. 2021;107(1S):102773. https://doi.org/10.1016/j.otsr.2020.102773.
3. Waterson HB, Clement ND, Eyres KS, Mandalia VI, Toms AD. The early outcome of kinematic versus mechanical alignment in total knee arthroplasty: a prospective randomised control trial. Bone Joint J. 2016;98-B(10):1360–8. https://doi.org/10.1302/0301-620X.98B10.36862.
4. Rivière C, Iranpour F, Auvinet E, Howell S, Vendittoli PA, Cobb J, Parratte S. Alignment options for total knee arthroplasty: a systematic review. Orthop Traumatol Surg Res. 2017;103(7):1047–56. https://doi.org/10.1016/j.otsr.2017.07.010.
5. Oussedik S, Abdel MP, Victor J, Pagnano MW, Haddad FS. Alignment in total knee arthroplasty: what's in a name? Bone Joint J. 2020;102-B(3):276–9. https://doi.org/10.1302/0301-620X.102B3.BJJ-2019-1729.
6. Patil S, McCauley JC, Pulido P, Colwell CW Jr. How do knee implants perform past the second decade? Nineteen- to 25-year follow-up of the press-fit condylar design TKA. Clin Orthop Relat Res. 2015;473(1):135–40. https://doi.org/10.1007/s11999-014-3792-6.
7. Collins M, Lavigne M, Girard J, Vendittoli PA. Joint perception after hip or knee replacement surgery. Orthop Traumatol Surg Res. 2012;98(3):275–80. https://doi.org/10.1016/j.otsr.2011.08.021.
8. Nam D, Nunley RM, Barrack RL. Patient dissatisfaction following total knee replacement: a growing concern? Bone Joint J. 2014;96-B(11 Suppl A):96–100. https://doi.org/10.1302/0301-620X.96B11.34152.
9. Deep K, Eachempati KK, Apsingi S. The dynamic nature of alignment and variations in normal knees. Bone Joint J. 2015;97-B(4):498–502. https://doi.org/10.1302/0301-620X.97B4.33740.
10. Bellemans J, Colyn W, Vandenneucker H, Victor J. The Chitranjan Ranawat award: is neutral mechanical alignment normal for all patients? The concept of constitutional varus. Clin Orthop Relat Res. 2012;470(1):45–53. https://doi.org/10.1007/s11999-011-1936-5.
11. Vanlommel L, Vanlommel J, Claes S, Bellemans J. Slight undercorrection following total knee arthroplasty results in superior clinical outcomes in varus knees. Knee Surg Sports Traumatol Arthrosc. 2013;21(10):2325–30. https://doi.org/10.1007/s00167-013-2481-4.
12. De Muylder J, Victor J, Cornu O, Kaminski L, Thienpont E. Total knee arthroplasty in patients with substantial deformities using primary knee components. Knee Surg Sports Traumatol Arthrosc. 2015;23(12):3653–9. https://doi.org/10.1007/s00167-014-3269-x.
13. Hommel H, Tsamassiotis S, Falk R, Fennema P. Adjustiertes mechanisches Alignment: Operative Technik—Tipps und Tricks [Adjusted mechanical alignment: operative technique—Tips and tricks]. Orthopade. 2020;49(7):562–569. German. https://doi.org/10.1007/s00132-020-03929-1.
14. Cherian JJ, Kapadia BH, Banerjee S, Jauregui JJ, Issa K, Mont MA. Mechanical, anatomical, and kinematic axis in TKA: concepts and practical applications. Curr Rev Musculoskelet Med. 2014;7(2):89–95. https://doi.org/10.1007/s12178-014-9218-y.
15. Srivastava A, Lee GY, Steklov N, Colwell CW Jr, Ezzet KA, D'Lima DD. Effect of tibial component varus on wear in total knee arthroplasty. Knee. 2012;19(5):560–3. https://doi.org/10.1016/j.knee.2011.11.003.
16. Manjunath KS, Gopalakrishna KG, Vineeth G. Evaluation of alignment in total knee arthroplasty: a prospective study. Eur J Orthop Surg Traumatol. 2015;25(5):895–903. https://doi.org/10.1007/s00590-015-1638-x.
17. Victor J, Mueller JK, Komistek RD, Sharma A, Nadaud MC, Bellemans J. In vivo kinematics after a cruciate-substituting TKA. Clin Orthop Relat Res. 2010;468(3):807–14. https://doi.org/10.1007/s11999-009-1072-7.

18. Yim JH, Song EK, Khan MS, Sun ZH, Seon JK. A comparison of classical and anatomical total knee alignment methods in robotic total knee arthroplasty: classical and anatomical knee alignment methods in TKA. J Arthroplasty. 2013;28(6):932–7. https://doi.org/10.1016/j.arth.2013.01.013.

19. Rivière C, Lazic S, Villet L, Wiart Y, Allwood SM, Cobb J. Kinematic alignment technique for total hip and knee arthroplasty: the personalized implant positioning surgery. EFORT Open Rev. 2018;3(3):98–105. Published 2018 Mar 29. https://doi.org/10.1302/2058-5241.3.170022.

20. Brar AS, Howell SM, Hull ML. What are the bias, imprecision, and limits of agreement for finding the flexion-extension plane of the knee with five tibial reference lines? Knee. 2016;23(3):406–11. https://doi.org/10.1016/j.knee.2016.01.005.

21. Howell SM, Papadopoulos S, Kuznik KT, Hull ML. Accurate alignment and high function after kinematically aligned TKA performed with generic instruments. Knee Surg Sports Traumatol Arthrosc. 2013;21(10):2271–80. https://doi.org/10.1007/s00167-013-2621-x.

22. Xu J, Cao JY, Luong JK, Negus JJ. Kinematic versus mechanical alignment for primary total knee replacement: a systematic review and meta-analysis. J Orthop. 2019;16(2):151–7. https://doi.org/10.1016/j.jor.2019.02.008.

23. McNair PJ, Boocock MG, Dominick ND, Kelly RJ, Farrington BJ, Young SW. A comparison of walking gait following mechanical and kinematic alignment in total knee joint replacement. J Arthroplasty. 2018;33(2):560–4. https://doi.org/10.1016/j.arth.2017.09.031.

24. Hutt JR, LeBlanc MA, Massé V, Lavigne M, Vendittoli PA. Kinematic TKA using navigation: surgical technique and initial results. Orthop Traumatol Surg Res. 2016;102(1):99–104. https://doi.org/10.1016/j.otsr.2015.11.010.

25. Blakeney WG, Vendittoli PA. Chapter 17. Restricted kinematic alignment: the ideal compromise? In: Rivière C, Vendittoli PA, editors. Personalized hip and knee joint replacement [internet]. Cham: Springer; 2020.

26. Laforest G, Kostretzis L, Kiss MO, Vendittoli PA. Restricted kinematic alignment leads to uncompromised osseointegration of cementless total knee arthroplasty. Knee Surg Sports Traumatol Arthrosc. 2022;30:705. https://doi.org/10.1007/s00167-020-06427-1.

27. Kayani B, Konan S, Pietrzak JRT, Huq SS, Tahmassebi J, Haddad FS. The learning curve associated with robotic-arm assisted unicompartmental knee arthroplasty: a prospective cohort study. Bone Joint J. 2018;100-B(8):1033–42. https://doi.org/10.1302/0301-620X.

28. Kayani B, Konan S, Ayuob A, Onochie E, Al-Jabri T, Haddad FS. Robotic technology in total knee arthroplasty: a systematic review. EFORT Open Rev. 2019;4(10):611–7. https://doi.org/10.1302/2058-5241.4.190022.

29. Winnock de Grave P, Luyckx T, Claeys K, Tampere T, Kellens J, Müller J, Gunst P. Higher satisfaction after total knee arthroplasty using restricted inverse kinematic alignment compared to adjusted mechanical alignment. Knee Surg Sports Traumatol Arthrosc. 2022;30:488. https://doi.org/10.1007/s00167-020-06165-4.

Individualizing Alignment in TKA with the Use of Image-Based Robotic Assistance

Tilman Calliess and Bernhard Christen

Introduction

Computer assistance was introduced in total knee arthroplasty (TKA) already in the late 1990s in order to improve surgical precision and to minimize errors. Current evidence on the conventional navigation tools affirms, that, in general, a higher precision in TKA component position and reduced outliers compared to manual instrumentation are achieved [1, 2]. However, it could not be shown that this automatically resulted in better patient outcomes [3, 4]. There is a growing discussion on whether this may be attributed to the unchanged surgical goal of a standardized mechanical alignment.

Now, robotic assistance is the latest evolutionary step in computer-assisted surgery. Compared to passive navigation systems, the robotic device actively helps the surgeon to conduct a computed plan for the TKA position. The resection plane is automatically adjusted by the robot and in certain systems also resection boundaries for the saw blade or burr are provided. This is meant to further increase precision and to actively protect the surrounding soft tissue. On the navigation side of these devices, now a virtual planning of the prosthesis position has been made possible, with the ability to customize the alignment to the individual patient's anatomy and the soft tissue envelope. Thus, these technologies are interesting not only to reduce surgical errors, but also to develop new methodologies and workflows to individualize alignment in TKA. This property is especially true for image-based systems, as the individual three-dimensional (3D) anatomy of the patient is visible beforehand and serves as a starting point for a customized planning. This also results in new surgical workflows. Intraoperatively, the focus is on validating the preplanning and conducting fine adjustments with respect to the individual soft tissue situation. The robot in the end supports the surgeon in the precise execution of the planning. Not only the resection plane is controlled but also important factors like relevant osteophytes are better visible in image-based systems, helping the surgeon to address these issues.

This chapter is meant to highlight the surgical technique of image-based robotic assistance to achieve individualized alignment in TKA and discusses basic principles and goals. The first section describes a step-by-step algorithm to analyze the knee and to preplan individualized alignment. This is primarily based on the principles of kinematic alignment (KA), but also a workflow for a restricted kinematic alignment (rKA) to correct for deformities is outlined.

In the second section, a distinct intraoperative workflow for KA using image-based robotics is outlined. It is based on a hybrid approach with a measured resection philosophy on the femur to

T. Calliess (✉) · B. Christen
Salem-Spital, Berne, Switzerland
e-mail: t.calliess@articon.ch; b.christen@articon.ch

A. J. Deshmukh et al. (eds.), *Surgical Management of Knee Arthritis*,
https://doi.org/10.1007/978-3-031-47929-8_3

restore the native joint surface and then a gap-balanced tibial resection to restore a rectangular extension space. In rKA, the need for additional soft tissue balancing is identified based on the implant planning and the analyzed gaps. For illustration, two clinical cases are discussed in terms of implant alignment and balancing algorithm for the mentioned two alignment philosophies.

Principles of Preoperative Planning for KA and rKA

Currently, there are different alignment concepts in terms of individualized TKA under debate, as outlined in this chapter. The best evidence is available for KA, so this is discussed as the standard planning algorithm. However, many surgeons have boundaries for KA, to stay within the yet established "safe zone" of 3° to the mechanical axis. Thus, also the concept of rKA is discussed with its underlying principles. This is applicable in case of necessary adaptions or compromises (e.g., due to the standard shape of the prosthesis does not ideally fit to the patient's knee morphotype), or intended corrections for pathologic situations (e.g., valgus osteoarthritis with a dysplastic lateral condyle).

To the author's experience, the best workflow to achieve a reproducible individualized alignment with image-based robotic-assisted surgery is to preplan the component position following the principle of KA or rKA, respectively. Based on the analysis of the knee morphotype, the philosophy to aim for is determined and possible pitfalls for the surgery are identified. Intraoperatively, this preplan is verified and fine-tuned with the cartilage and soft tissue information. Since there are only a few parameters left on which adjustments are made, surgery becomes more predictable and reproducible. Being a key factor for success, the planning should follow a standardized workflow, as described here.

True KA Planning Workflow

Femur

One basic principle of KA is to closely reconstruct the pre-arthritic surface of the knee joint with the prosthesis. Therewith, the natural joint line orientation and height, the overall limb alignment, and the physiological ligament tension are meant to be restored. Following these principles of KA, first, the distal and posterior resections on the femur are set symmetrically to match the thickness of the femoral condyles of the implant. As the model in image-based robotics is based on CT imaging and represents the bone level, the cartilage thickness needs to be taken into account to correctly restore the original joint line. Thus, the standard resection level on both the distal and posterior femur is **initially set at 6 mm** (bone resection), **resulting in** an average cartilage thickness of 2 mm [5] (6 mm + 2 mm = 8 mm = implant thickness) (Fig. 3.1). This results in an individual varus/valgus (v/v) orientation of the femur and an internal/external rotation of the component at 0° to the posterior condylar axis (PCA). The rotation to the transepicondylar axis (TEA) is of no interest. The orientation of the trochlea line does automatically match the prosthetic trochlea in this setting in a majority of cases (if not, this is an indication for adaptions, as described later for rKA).

After setting the distal and posterior resection, the femoral size is then determined. Focus is to best reconstruct the trochlea groove height and position without producing overhang. This is best visualized on axial cross sections in the planning model. From the author's experience, it is likely to select the largest component still fitting in the mediolateral (ml) dimensions of the knee.

Third and final planning step on the femur is to adjust the femoral component flexion. As the orientation, position, and size are already defined, it is used to create a smooth transition to the anterior femoral cortex with a low risk of notching. Care needs to be taken, not to influence the other

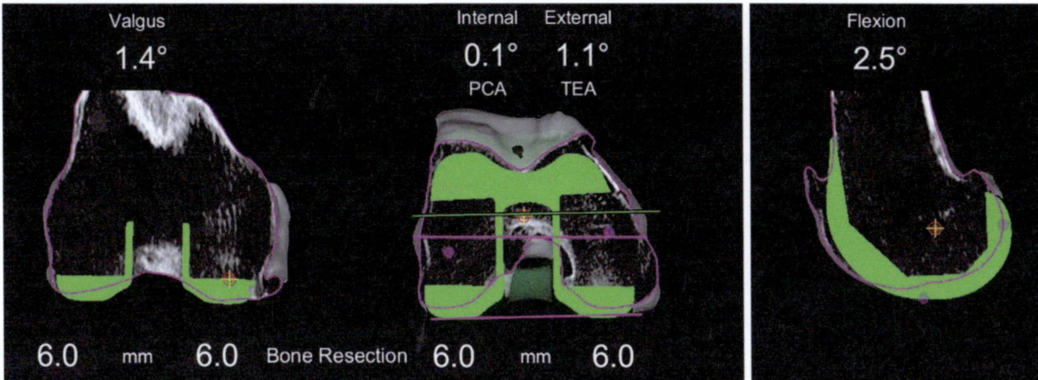

Fig. 3.1 Example of a preoperative planning of the femoral implant position following the KA principle. By default, distal and posterior resections are set to 6-mm bone resection. This sets the femoral component in 1.4° valgus and 1.1° external rotation to TEA in this example (transverse pink lines in the center image represent PCA and TEA). Size is adapted to best meet anterior offset and mediolateral dimensions. Flexion is adjusted for a smooth transition to the anterior cortex with the center of rotation approximately within the kinematic axis of the femur (red dot)

parameters when adjusting the flexion. Therefore, the center of rotation about which the component is flexed is positioned in the kinematic center of the prosthesis (Fig. 3.1).

Therewith, the femur is preplanned based on the KA principle. During surgery, only minor adaptions are made to this femoral plan, based on the cartilage thickness, potential defects, or the cartilaginous trochlea groove, as described in the *Bernese Surgical Workflow Robotic-Assisted KA TKA*. All adaptions that are necessary for balancing the knee are made on the tibia in the context of KA.

Tibia

The preplanning of a physiological tibia component orientation and position is a lot more difficult, as bone defects are much more likely on the tibia than on the femur and the native cartilage thickness has a greater variability [6]. Thus, the tibia plan is preliminary and conservative for slope, v/v angulation, and resection height, which leaves room for fine-tuning intraoperatively and recuts. The final tibia alignment is determined by the soft tissue balance in extension during surgery in order to create symmetric extension space (see *Bernese Surgical Workflow Robotic-Assisted KA TKA*).

Depending on the defect situation, we usually set the first parameter, which is the tibial component coronal plane close to what we think the original joint line obliquity is about with a maximum of 3° of varus to start with. Best visualization is on coronal CT-cross sections, aligning the tibia parallel to the (unworn) plateau (Fig. 3.2). Bringing the resection levels medial and lateral to a symmetric situation does not automatically mean the correct reconstruction of the joint line, as these values are very dependent on where the resection landmarks are set. Again, an intraoperative mapping of the tibia cartilage level can be used to verify and fine-tune the resection level and tibia orientation, as described in the *Bernese Surgical Workflow Robotic-Assisted KA TKA* section.

Second parameter on the tibia is the component rotation. In the proprietary planning protocol, tibia rotation is defined with reference to the posterior cruciate ligament insertion and the medial third of the tuberosity. However, this is error prone and does not follow the principles of KA [7]. Thus, in our protocol, the tibia rotation is set with reference to the transverse kinematic axis of the femur about which the tibia flexes and extends. Within the "Case Planning" screen in the systems software, the tibia rotation landmark can be set individually to the posterior condylar axis and centered to the trochlea groove. The A-P axis of tibial component is then oriented parallel to this landmark which sets the rotation of the implant parallel with respect to the A-P axis of the femoral component to 0°. Sizing and ml position are also addressed in this step, after defining the rotation.

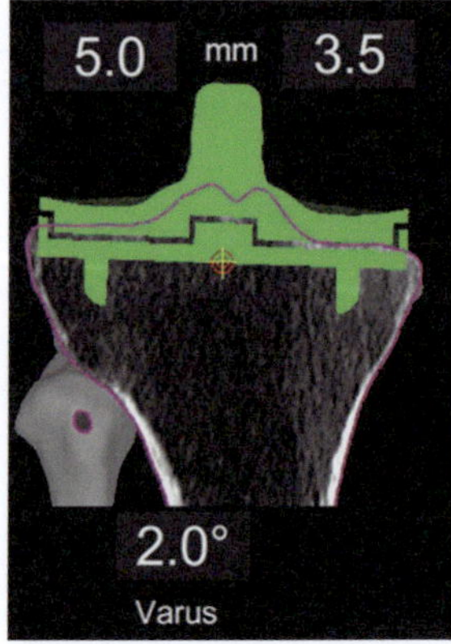
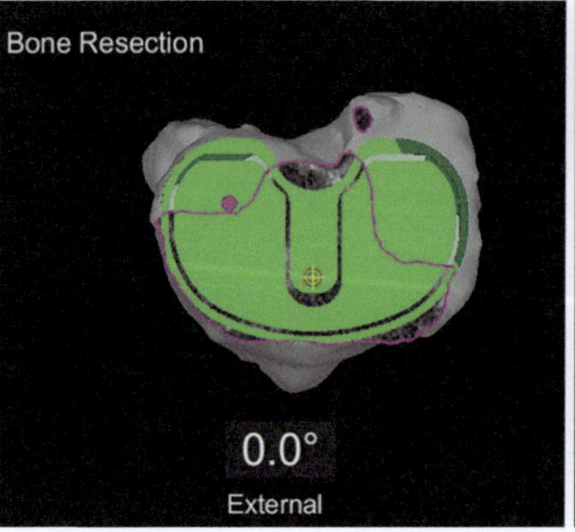
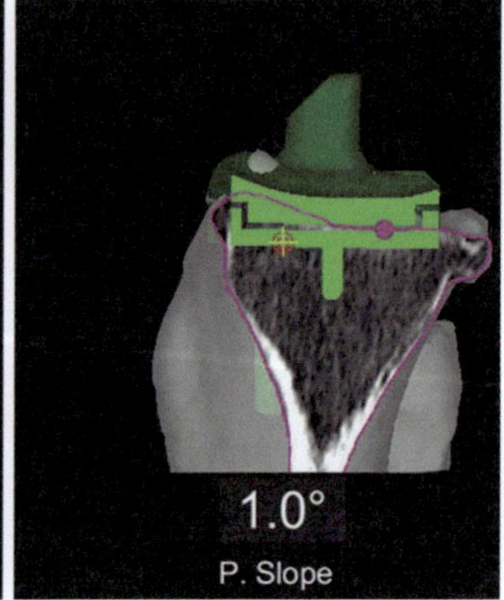

Fig. 3.2 Example of a preliminary plan of the tibia component orientation. The first parameter, which is the tibial coronal plane is aligned rather conservatively with respect to the visible joint line accounting for possible bone defects medially. The 2° varus and the resection level at 4–5 mm laterally is preliminary. Rotation is set at 0° in the axial plane, parallel to the described tibia rotation landmark. The tibia slope is orientated parallel to the posterior two-third of the medial plateau in the sagittal CT view of the medial plateau

Third parameter is the planning of the tibia slope. In KA, the idea is to reproduce the native tibia slope of the medial plateau. However, one must be careful with the common definition of the anatomical slope that usually refers to a tangent that is aligned to the most prominent anterior and posterior aspect of the tibia plateau. This measurement can be significantly affected by osteophytes with a tendency to overestimate the native slope. Thus, the slope should be adjusted conservatively and more to the posterior two-thirds of the medial tibia plateau without taking posterior osteophytes into account. According to Pinskerova and Freemann [8], this is the area where the femoral rollback on the medial plateau happens during flexion. In PS prosthesis, it might make sense even to reduce the slope to the native situation to account for the loss of the cruciate ligaments. If the slope cannot be estimated due to bone-defect situation, the recommendation is to start with a conservative alignment (0–3°) and to verify the slope based on the flexion space tightness during surgery.

Restricted KA Planning Workflow

Principle of Medial Column Reconstruction

As mentioned earlier, there are different situations conceivable in which adaptions to a pure KA make sense. However, one of the most critical questions is, where to make these adjustments.

There is growing evidence that the medial compartment stability plays an important role in knee kinematics and in the outcome of the patient [9]. In contrast to this, a lateral laxity or even a tensioning compared to the physiological situation seems to have a lesser impact. Based on this, our basic principle for adaptions made to the KA planning is, that all these adjustments are made on the lateral side, while the medial compartment is reconstructed anatomically. So, in any case, the posterior resection and the distal resection on the medial femur remain at 6 mm. This ensures the reconstruction of the isometric medial joint stability and limits the need for releases in the medial compartment. Also, the balancing is easier, as all release steps are to the lateral compartment only.

Asymmetric Varus Knee Morphotypes

In true KA, the femoral component is strictly aligned to the tibiofemoral joint line resulting in 0° rotation to the PCA. On average, the kinematic axis about which the patella flexes and extends is parallel to the primary kinematic axis in the femur [10, 11]. Thus, the trochlea axis is automatically reconstructed with the use of a symmetric prosthesis in most knees. However, there are some knee morphotypes where the condyles are asymmetric (different radii of the condyles) and/or the trochlea is not parallel to the tibiofemoral axis [12, 13]. This relationship between the PCA and the trochlea groove line is best visible on axial CT-cross sections in the preoperative planning. In the mentioned asymmetric knees, pure KA could result in a relative internal rotation of the groove and patella axis compared to the native situation. In those cases, a restricted KA is applicable with adjustment of the rotation alignment to neutrally align the prosthesis to the patella axis. It is important not to influence the medial condylar aspect, but only to reduce the posterior lateral resection. A clinical example is displayed in Fig. 3.3 with a resulting 6-mm posterior medial and 3.5-mm posterior lateral resection.

These adjustments typically have no influence on the tibia position or the distal femur alignment that follows the standard KA workflow.

Valgus OA with Dysplastic Lateral Condyle

Many osteoarthritic valgus knees present a pathological, distal, femoral joint-line angle of more than 3° valgus (<87° LDFA). This could be constitutional, but many of these knees also have bone defect situations that are more likely on the femoral side in valgus cases. With a planning that is made on the bony surface only, this might lead to too much valgus for the femoral component. In addition to that, valgus patients often also have relevant pathologies of the hip joint (e.g., abductor insufficiency, rotational instabilities) or the ankle (e.g., fixed hint-food valgus) which increase the dynamic valgus moment to the knee. If those knees are left in a relevant valgus, there is an increased risk for secondary medial or rotational instability and implant failure. Thus, those pathological valgus situations should be corrected to an overall neutral alignment.

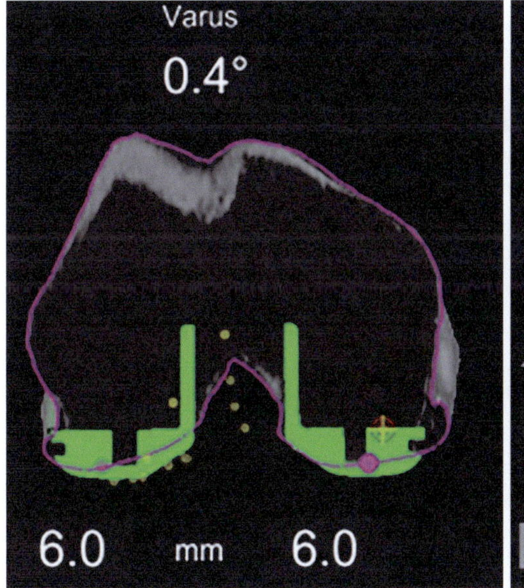

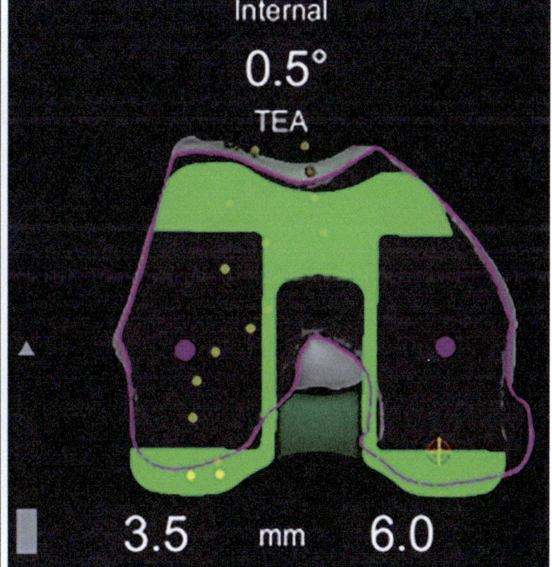

Fig. 3.3 Example of an rKA preoperative plan in a varus morphotype knee with asymmetric condyles. Distal femoral resections are planned symmetrically with 6-mm bone resection. To avoid relative internal rotation of the trochlea axis in the coronal plane, the posterior lateral resection is adjusted to 3.5 mm (external rotation of the component compared to the KA principle), while the medial resection level remains constant at 6 mm

Usually, the tibia joint line in said cases is much more horizontal at 0–2° varus, on average (88–90° MPTA). In combination with an LDFA below 88°, this would result in a valgus overall limb alignment that can be critical.

Now, to put these considerations for a correction into a schematic workflow we start again with the described KA workflow putting the distal femoral resection at 6-mm medial and lateral. If this results in more than 3° valgus, this is the trigger to go for rKA.

In our rKA planning workflow, we now proceed with the tibia planning instead of the femur. The tibia component is matched to the bone model with symmetric resection medial and lateral replicating the natural joint-line position (Fig. 3.4). This usually results in a neural or slight varus orientation in said cases. Valgus alignment of the tibia should be avoided and corrected to neutral (0°). If there is any varus in the tibia (2° varus like in our example, Fig. 3.4), this is the maximum valgus orientation we can put femoral component in (2° tibia varus +2° femoral valgus = neutral overall alignment). In the case of a 0° tibia alignment, the femur is also put to a 0° orientation. Planning the other way around, like adjusting the tibia varus to the natural valgus of the femur, it is very likely to produce medial over-resection on the tibia and has a high risk for resulting medial instability.

Now, the coronal position of the femur is aligned according to the tibia, keeping the 6-mm medial resection and reducing the lateral resection to achieve the desired angulation. With this, both neutral overall alignment and anatomic reconstruction of the medial column are achieved.

Next is again the rotation of the femoral component. The starting point can be the KA position with symmetric medial and lateral posterior resection levels. This very often results in an internal rotation with respect to the trochlea axis. The pivot point is then put to the medial condyle at a 6-mm resection level, so that this is not changed. Now, the component is externally rotated until the native trochlea line and the prosthetic trochlea match. This is typically close to the TEA. Very often, the distal and posterior resections are equal for both medial and lateral

compartments, which make sense when implanting a single radius prosthesis (medial compartment 6 mm, lateral compartment 3 mm, for example). Femoral flexion and tibia slope are adjusted according to the described KA principle. Also, the tibia rotation landmark can be orientated to the femur as described before; however, the dysplastic condyle needs to be adjusted the same way. A clinical example of rKA planning is displayed in Fig. 3.4.

Planning Boundaries for KA?

The other discussion when talking about KA are possible boundaries for its safe use. From the scientific standpoint, there are no unambiguous limits published or agreed on [14]. However, many surgeons stay within the accepted range of ±3° to the mechanical axis for the coronal alignment parameters. In this context, it has to be mentioned that, currently, the FDA approval for the described image-based robotic system is only granted for 2° deviation from neutral for each tibia and femur position and 3° for the resulting overall limb axis. For the femoral rotation, 0–3° external rotation with respect to the TEA is "allowed" and a tibia slope up to 3°. However, there are many cases in which KA results in an internal rotation to the TEA, but perfectly reconstructs the femoral anatomy. In those cases, we do not see the need for adjustments.

The ±3° boundary in the coronal plane, on the other hand, has its justification. Especially in neutral overall patients a joint line obliquity more than 3° should be avoided, as these patients typically do not have a great adduction of the limb during gait and thus do not bring the joint line horizontal to the floor when walking. Residual varus patients, on the other hand, seem to accept a higher degree of tibia vara without an increased risk for implant loosening or instability. With the natural adduction of the limb, the joint line is horizontal, and even the moments in the knee are reduced. Nonetheless, to our experience, the starting point for surgery should not be more than a 3° varus position to avoid medial instability in the first place. Adjustments can be made according to the described concept of medial column reconstruction.

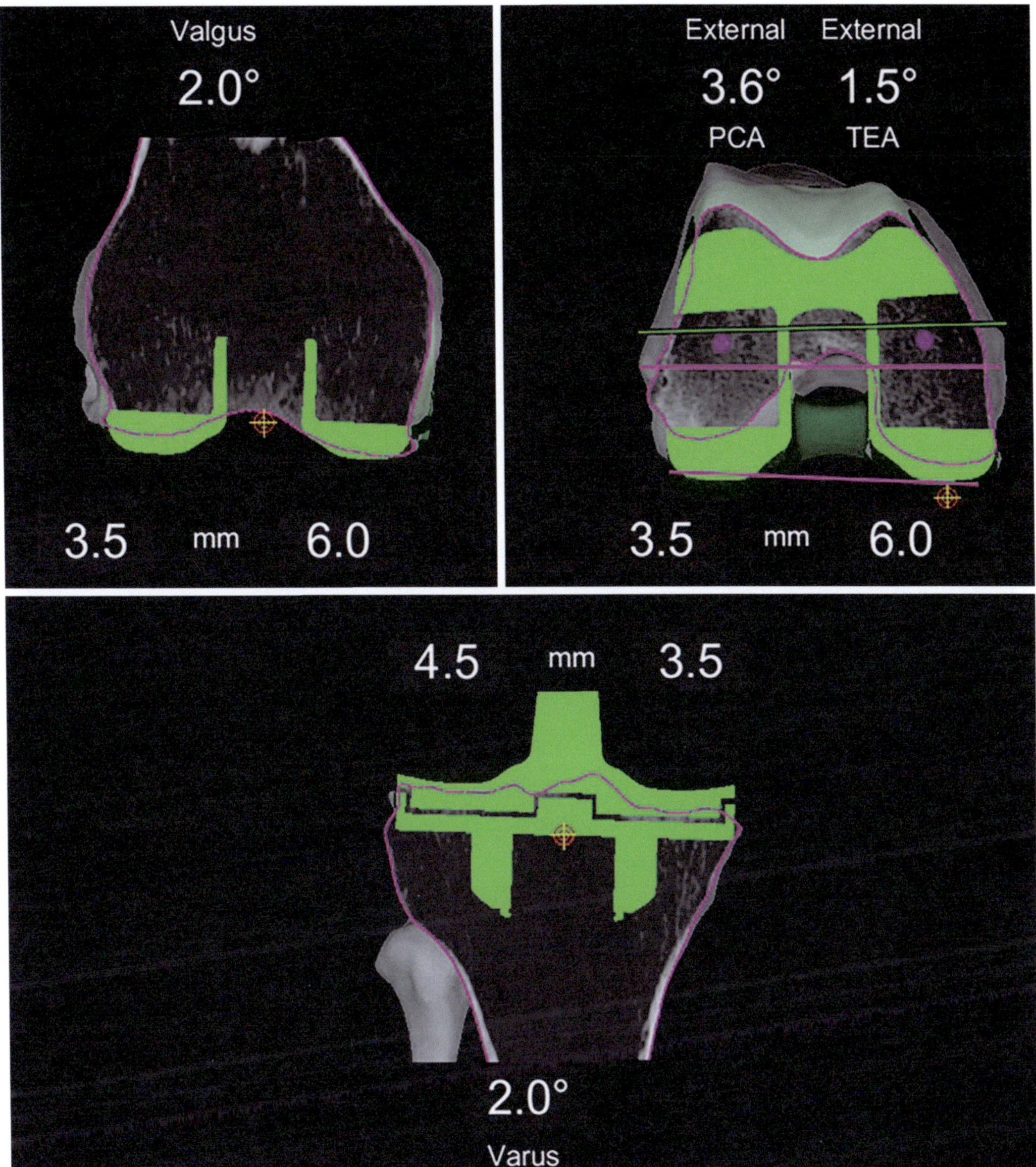

Fig. 3.4 Example of a preoperative planning of the implant position following the rKA principle. A 2°-varus orientation of the tibia component results in a nearly physiological reconstruction of the joint line. Thus, valgus orientation on the femur is limited to a 2° valgus maximum. To achieve this, distal and posterior medial resections remain at 6 mm, and lateral resections are adjusted to meet this 2° valgus and a neutral alignment to the trochlea axis. This results in a 1.5° external rotation with respect to the TEA in this example

Bernese Surgical Workflow Robotic-Assisted KA TKA

The customized component position might differ significantly from the mechanical standard planning provided by the robotic supplier. Thus, the authors recommend individualizing the planning before surgery, as it is complex to handle all parameters during surgery. Customization purely based on soft tissue information starting with the mechanical alignment plan has a higher risk of altering knee kinematics than the described workflow of a KA (or rKA) planning with fine-tuning based on soft tissue information.

As mentioned earlier, the main focus of the intraoperative workflow is (1) to verify the individualized preplan, (2) to reproducibly record the soft tissue situation, (3) to fine tune the implant position based on defined algorithms, and (4) to precisely execute the final plan. Most critical to the author's experience is the correct and as-objective-as-possible analysis of the joint spaces. Therefore, meticulous resection of all osteophytes is mandatory. To achieve this, it makes sense to start with a bone precut of some sort. This enables to approach all relevant osteophytes and to insert a balancer or spreader in order to bring the ligaments to tension. These considerations result in the following Bernese surgical workflow.

Setup, Incision, and Bone Registration

The robotic arm setup positioning and calibration protocol do not differ from the company's defined standards. The incision, exposure of the knee, position of the arrays in the tibia and femur, and the bone registration are also analogous to conventional robotic-assisted workflow. In contrast to imageless navigation, robotic system bone registration means that 40 random points on the surface of each bone are collected with a sharp probe that penetrates through the cartilage directly to

the subchondral bone or cortical surface. No specific landmarks have to be defined by the surgeon, but just the bone morphology. The computer matches the cloud of points to the segmented knee model, which is verified in a second step.

Intraoperative Verification of Preplan

First specific step in this workflow is the determination of the native cartilage thickness, where available, in order to verify the preselected resection levels. The cartilage surface is mapped as a second layer on the "Implant Planning" screen with the use of a blunt probe. Trochlea groove, distal and posterior femur, and the cartilage on the tibia plateau, close to the spine, are captured. Based on this information, the preplan is verified to better reproduce the actual joint surface with possible adjustment of the resection thickness (Fig. 3.5). Especially in large men, often the lateral resection results in less than the standard 6 mm.

Tibia Precut and Osteophyte Removal

For an individualized alignment that is adjusted to the soft tissue situation, one of the key steps is to correctly capture the flexion and extension space. Therefore, all osteophytes need to be removed before balancing. That usually cannot be achieved without conducting any bone cuts

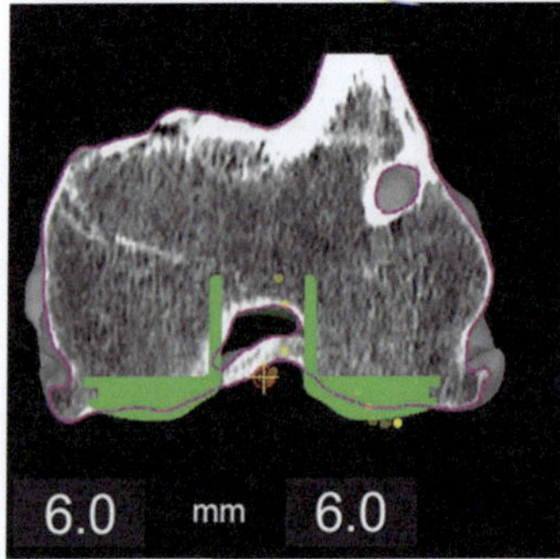
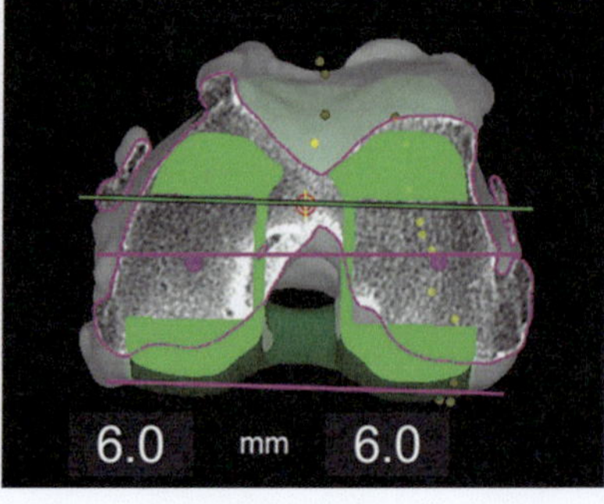
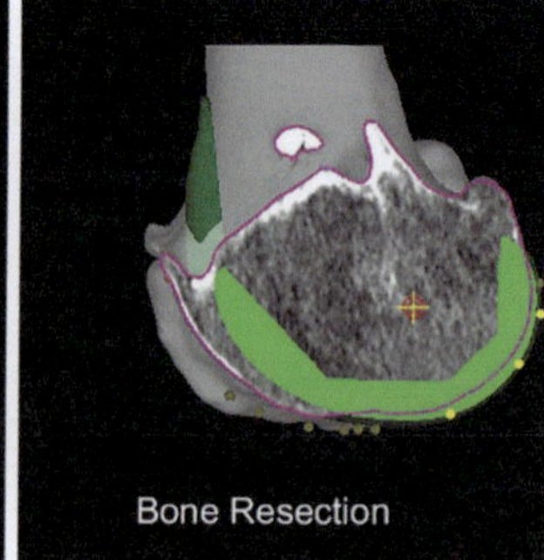

Fig. 3.5 Example of cartilage mapping on unworn lateral femur condyle and trochlea sulcus line (yellow dots added to the CT scan). The resection level is individually adjusted to reconstruct the original cartilaginous joint line with the prosthesis based on this information. Also, the femoral rotation is validated

beforehand. Especially in ACL-torn knees, osteophytes are likely to be in the posterior aspect of the knee influencing the extension space, which is critical for the KA component position. This is why it makes sense to start with a bone precut of some sort. In our routine, we start with the tibia for practical reasons. As outlined in the planning section, the orientation of this tibia cut is close to the estimated final alignment (v/v and slope) with a conservative resection of 4–5 mm. After that, it is likely to address the most relevant osteophytes both on the tibia and on the femur. Also, the flat surface of the tibia makes it easier to insert a balancer or a spacer block. In theory, the femoral cuts can also be conducted in the first place, as their positions are defined by the KA principle. However, with the tibia-first technique, the osteophytes and capsule appear a bit easier to access. In knees with severe extension deficit, we usually precut both the tibia and the distal and posterior femur. This is to create enough space to enable complete removal of osteophytes and capsule posteriorly, before analyzing the soft tissue. When aiming for a PS prosthesis, the PCL should also be resected before the gap evaluation.

Soft Tissue Analysis and Balancing Algorithm

Next is to include the soft tissue information to determine the definite component position. After the described tibia (and/or femur) precut and complete removal of the osteophytes and contractions, now, the extension and flexion spaces are analyzed using a balancer, two laminar spreaders, or a spacer block. The navigation captures the space between the two bones and predicts the space heights medial and lateral (in mm) with the current prosthesis alignment (Fig. 3.6a and b).

The primary target (for KA) is to produce a symmetric extension space. The flexion space is individual with the lateral gap generally being looser than the medial gap and both gaps typically a little looser in flexion than in extension. In the author's experience, the extension should be between 18- and 19-mm medial and lateral (for a

17-mm overall implant thickness) when analyzed with a spreader. The medial aspect in flexion should match the extension by ±1 mm. The lateral aspect in flexion ranges between 19 and 25 mm and is left that way.

To achieve the said parameters of a physiologically balanced knee, the position of the implants is adapted stepwise. In true KA, the key parameter to adjust is the v/v orientation of the tibia resection. Adapting the slope can be used to adjust the flexion space. A reduction of the slope often becomes necessary when using a PS prosthesis and the flexion gap opens up after resection of the posterior cruciate ligament. Care must be taken not to increase the slope to the natural situation, which has a higher risk of posterior tibial component overload that can cause early posterior subsidence or posterior insert wear [15]. According to the concept of KA, the distal and posterior femoral resections should not be increased to more than 6 mm on any occasion.

In restricted KA, not all situations or imbalances could or should be addressed with adjustments to the implant position. When a lateral tightness occurs in correcting a valgus OA to neutral, all implant adaptions would again result in a valgus orientation of the components or the overall limb alignment. Thus, soft tissue releases to the lateral structures are to be discussed. If only the extension space is involved, the release of the *IT band is* a vital option. For both extension and flexion tightness, it is most effective to address the lateral collateral ligament. If only flexion is too tight laterally, changing the femoral component rotation is a good option. Due to the protocol with anatomic resection on the medial compartment, no tightness can be present here— if the resection level is appropriate. In case of a too-loose medial gap, this should be better addressed with a higher implant constraint.

In this balancing context, attention must be drawn to a possible source of error. Depending on the technique to capture the flexion space, it is often outputted to be a little tighter than the extension space in the system. Most surgeons evaluate the flexion by resting the knee on the lower leg. This results in more pressure on the flexion space due to the body weight and explains

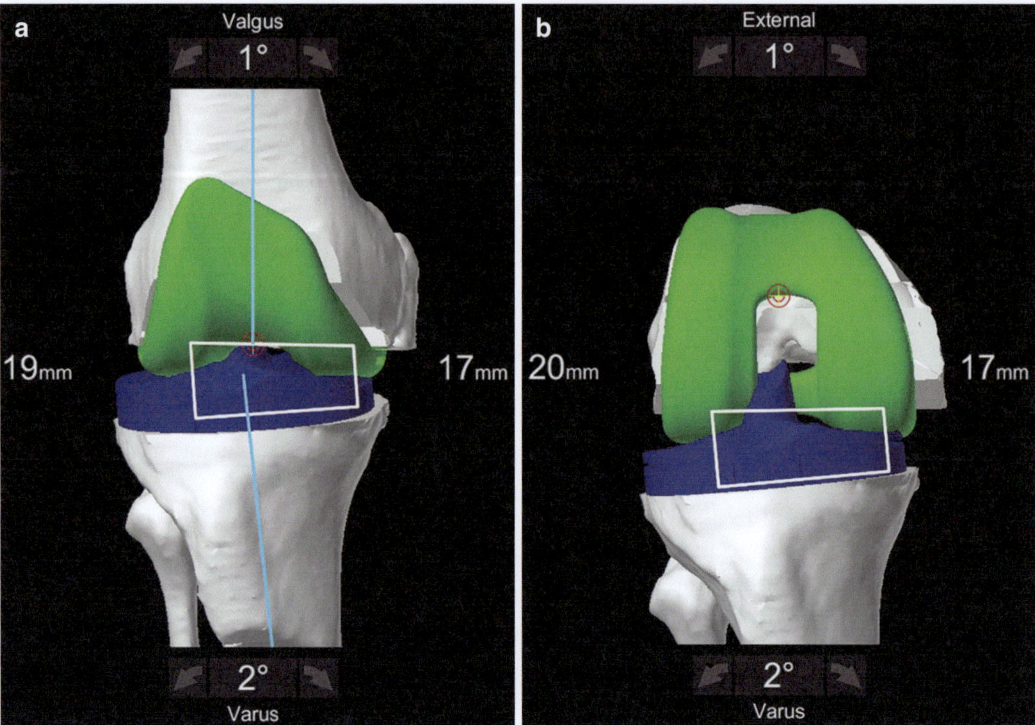

Fig. 3.6 Example of the computed extension (**a**) and flexion (**b**) spaces that would result with the current implant position in 1° femoral valgus, 1° femoral external rotation, and 2° tibia varus. The medial extension gap is at 17 mm, and the lateral extension gap is at 19 mm. In flex- ion, the gaps are at 17 mm medial and 20 mm lateral. For capturing the values, the gaps are tensioned with a spreader after a tibia precut and resection of the osteo- phytes in this example

the displayed tightness. Thus, in most cases, these values do not represent an accurate measure of the natural flexion space laxity. Accordingly, the balancing should primarily focus on the extension space. Increasing the slope or posterior femoral resections are usually not necessary in those situations. If in doubt, the flexion space should be reevaluated with the trial prosthesis in place. Only if the gap is too tight at that point (pop out of tibia inlay or femur trial), the tibia slope is adjusted and never the posterior femur.

In order to better illustrate the principles described, the intraoperative balancing situations of the earlier-mentioned KA (Figs. 3.1 and 3.2) and rKA (Fig. 3.4) cases are discussed in more detail in the following:

Balancing Example True KA

In this example, the femur component is planned strictly to the KA principle with 6-mm distal and posterior resection on the femur. This results in a 1.4° valgus orientation to the mechanical axis of the femur and 1.1° external rotation with respect to the TEA (0° to PCA) (Fig. 3.1). On the tibia, a precut in 2° varus, 1° slope, and 5-mm bone resection on the lateral plateau is planned (Fig. 3.2) and conducted after verification with cartilage points. Critical in this case is to address the posterior medial tibia osteophyte as this has a massive influence on the medial extension gap making it tighter. The tibia varus position can accordingly only be correctly determined if this is completely removed. If the osteophyte is not properly accessible, one should think about performing the femoral distal and posterior cuts, as these are not changed anymore in KA. After resection of all osteophytes, the flexion and extension spaces are captured (Fig. 3.6a and b). In this classic example, the lateral extension gap is already correct with 19 mm, whereas the medial extension gap is 2-mm too tight. The same applies to the flexion gap, which is of minor interest in KA.

So, the lateral tibia resection is already correct, whereas the medial resection is too low. In other words, the varus orientation of the tibia needs to be adjusted. Now, putting the tibia in a 3° varus orientation with a lateral pivot point results in a symmetric extension gap and a medial gap isometry in flexion (Fig. 3.7a and b). The physiological laxity of 20 mm on the lateral flexion gap is accepted. No changes are made on the femur, as this is reconstructed anatomically.

Balancing Example Restricted KA

The example in Fig. 3.4 is a typical valgus OA with a restricted KA preplanning. Planning this case purely on the bony anatomy would result in approximately 5° valgus of the femur component with massive internal rotation of the trochlea. With the physiological 2° varus on the tibia, the knee would result in an overall 3° valgus after surgery. Thus, the lateral femoral resection is reduced in order to create a neutral overall limb axis (2° femoral valgus, 2° tibia vara) and an anatomic reconstruction of the trochlea. This results in a 3.5 mm resection on the distal and posterior lateral condyle, whereas the medial remains at 6 mm.

Based on this preplan, tibia cut is conducted at 2° varus, 1° slope, and 4.5-mm resection level. After tiny osteophytes have been removed, the spaces are evaluated. As displayed in Fig. 3.8, this alignment results in a too-tight extension

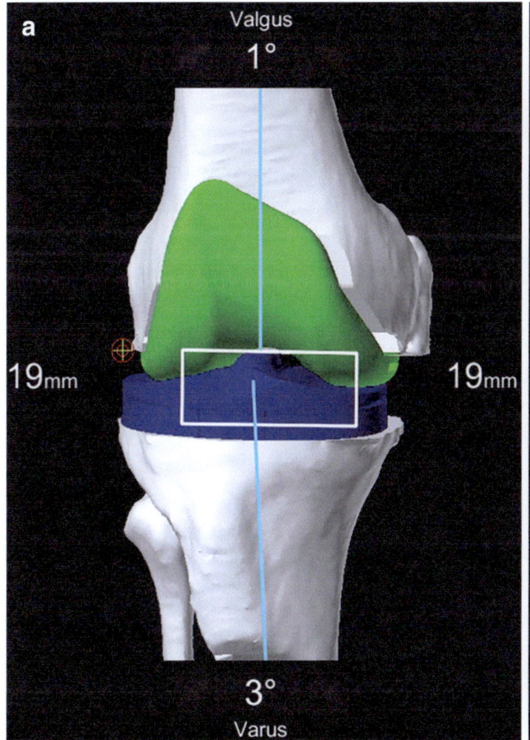

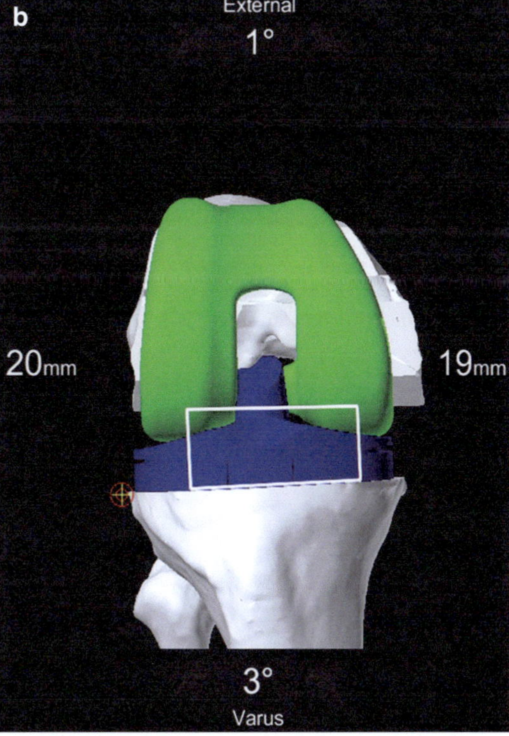

Fig. 3.7 Display of the resulting extension and flexion spaces after the tibia position is adjusted from 2° varus (see Fig. 3.6), to 3° varus. The pivot point for this adjustment is the lateral corner of the tibia (red dot). Now, a symmetric 19-mm extension space is achieved (**a**), and a gap isometry medial with 19 mm in flexion (**b**). Laterally, the physiological flexion laxity is reconstructed with 20 mm (**b**)

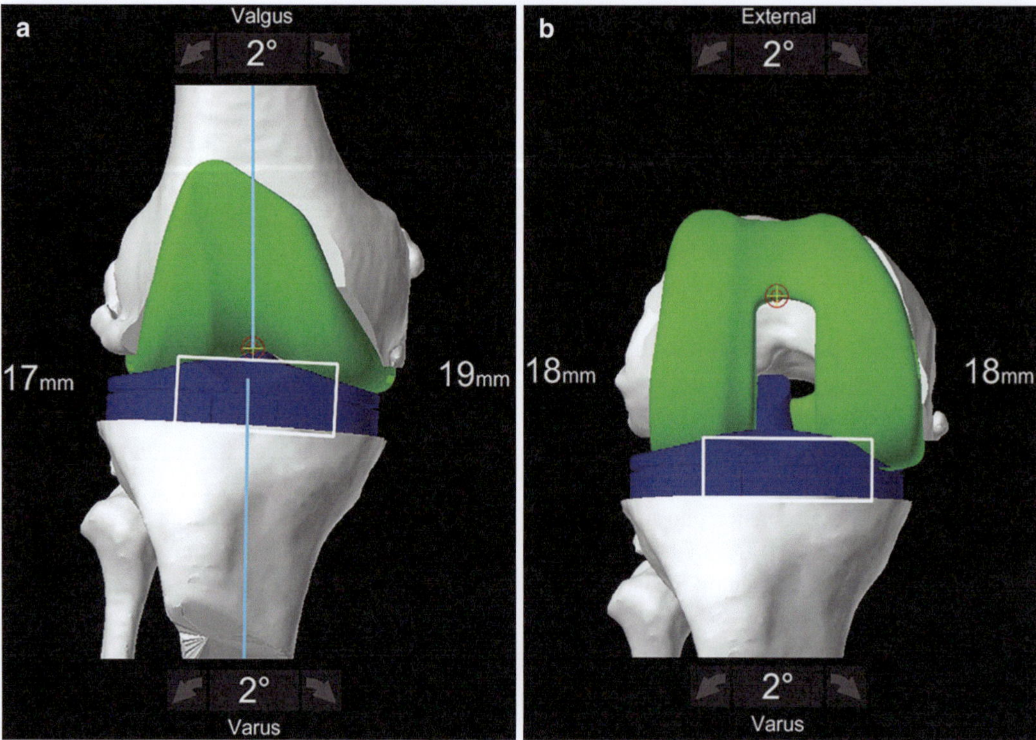

Fig. 3.8 Display of the computed extension (**a**) and flexion (**b**) spaces that would result in the rKA example with the implant position in 2° femoral valgus, 1.5° femoral external rotation (rounded to 2°), and 2° tibia varus. The medial extension gap is at 19 mm, and the lateral extension gap is at 17 mm. In flexion, the gaps are symmetric at 18 mm medial and lateral. For capturing the values, the gaps are tensioned with a spreader after a tibia precut and resection of the osteophytes in this example

space laterally in extension whereas medially the desired 19 mm is achieved. In contrast to this, the flexion gap is symmetrically balanced (displayed 1 mm tighter than it actually is, see earlier).

Now, to balance the extension space, the valgus position on the femur could be increased, but this is not recommended as this puts the knee into valgus. Thus, to balance the extension we would recommend soft tissue release on the lateral side in this case. This can even be controlled with recollecting the gaps. As the flexion space is well balanced, there is no need to adapt the femoral rotation or posterior resection. Only one could think about increasing the slope by 1 mm.

Final Bone Cuts, Verification Checks, and Trails

After having finalized the virtual KA planning with optimal extension balance, the bone cuts are conducted with the assistance of the robotic arm. All femoral cuts are made and the tibia recut, if necessary. Once all bone cuts have been made, the trial components are placed according to the planning. One trick is that the ml position of the components as well as the tibia rotation can also be controlled with the CT-based navigation. With the use of the blunt probe, the desired positioning of the trails can be visualized on the planning screen. This again is a benefit to standard techniques to realize a perfect rotational alignment of the tibia.

After insertion of the trial components, the balance can be re-checked and objectively evaluated with the navigation software of the robotic system. If an imbalance also occurs, a re-positioning of the tibia can be conducted as well as a recut, if necessary.

Summary

From the currently available technologies to assist total knee arthroplasty, the image-based robotic assistance appears to be a promising option to reproducibly individualize alignment. The workflow includes a preoperative, three-dimensional analysis of the knee and a preplanning of the alignment. This primarily follows the principles of kinematic alignment or identifies the need for adjustments like in a restricted KA approach. For a femoral component that is 8-mm thick distal and posterior, the femoral resections should be set to 6 mm both on the medial and the lateral condyle after compensating for 2 mm of cartilage. If corrections or adaptions are necessary, adjustments are made to the lateral aspect only so that the medial column is reconstructed anatomically. The tibia planning is preliminary in terms of varus/valgus orientation and resection height. Intraoperatively, it is adjusted to produce a stable and symmetric extension space. In the flexion space, the natural laxity of the lateral compartment is accepted.

The surgical workflow begins with additional mapping of the cartilage level onto the CT to fine tune the resection levels to the individual situation. For final implant position and balancing, a tibia precut is conducted, osteophytes are removed with navigation control, and gaps are evaluated. All adaptions to balance the knee are made on the tibia side or on the lateral femur only. In valgus cases aiming for a correction to a neutral overall limb alignment, sometimes lateral releases are applicable, but not to the medial structures. Overall, the surgical protocol follows a hybrid approach with a measured resection on the femur and a gap-balancing approach for the tibia orientation in order to create a stable and symmetrically balanced extension space. Different from established surgical techniques, the tibia is cut first in our robotic workflow, but, this is only preliminary to ensure correct analysis of the soft tissue with the computer assistance.

Key Study Points

- Image-based robotic assistance enables a 3D preoperative planning of individualized alignment in TKA.
- Based on the knee morphotype, a true kinematic alignment (KA) or restricted kinematic alignment (rKA) is selected.
- Basic principle in KA is to anatomically reconstruct the distal and posterior femoral surface with the prosthesis; the tibia is adjusted based on the soft tissue.
- In rKA, the medial column of the femur is reconstructed anatomically and adjustments are made on the lateral side and the tibia to achieve a certain overall alignment.
- Intraoperatively, the preoperative planning is verified based on cartilage level and soft tissue.
- A tibia precut is recommended to enable complete osteophyte removal and a reproducible analysis of the soft tissue envelope.
- This enables the definite alignment of the components to achieve a symmetrically balanced extension space and an isometric balance of the medial compartment in flexion. The physiological lateral flexion gap laxity is accepted.
- The robotic arm then helps the surgeon to precisely conduct this virtual, individualized TKA alignment.

References

1. Fu Y, Wang M, Liu Y, Fu Q. Alignment outcomes in navigated total knee arthroplasty: a meta-analysis. Knee Surg Sports Traumatol Arthrosc. 2012;20(6):1075–82.
2. Hetaimish BM, Khan MM, Simunovic N, Al-Harbi HH, Bhandari M, Zalzal PK. Meta-analysis of navigation vs conventional total knee arthroplasty. J Arthroplasty. 2012;27(6):1177–82.
3. Cheng T, Pan XY, Mao X, Zhang GY, Zhang XL. Little clinical advantage of computer-assisted navigation over conventional instrumentation in primary total knee arthroplasty at early follow-up. Knee. 2012;19(4):237–45.

4. Lee DY, Park YJ, Hwang SC, Park JS, Kang DG. No differences in mid- to long-term outcomes of computer-assisted navigation versus conventional total knee arthroplasty. Knee Surg Sports Traumatol Arthrosc. 2020;28(10):3183–92.

5. Nam D, Lin KM, Howell SM, Hull ML. Femoral bone and cartilage wear is predictable at 0 degrees and 90 degrees in the osteoarthritic knee treated with total knee arthroplasty. Knee Surg Sports Traumatol Arthrosc. 2014;22(12):2975–81.

6. Coleman JL, Widmyer MR, Leddy HA, Utturkar GM, Spritzer CE, Moorman CT 3rd, et al. Diurnal variations in articular cartilage thickness and strain in the human knee. J Biomech. 2013;46(3):541–7.

7. Brar AS, Howell SM, Hull ML. What are the bias, imprecision, and limits of agreement for finding the flexion-extension plane of the knee with five tibial reference lines? Knee. 2016;23(3):406–11.

8. Freeman MA, Pinskerova V. The movement of the normal tibio-femoral joint. J Biomech. 2005;38(2):197–208.

9. Risitano S, Indelli PF. Is "symmetric" gap balancing still the gold standard in primary total knee arthroplasty? Ann Transl Med. 2017;5(16):325.

10. Vercruysse C, Vandenneucker H, Bellemans J, Scheys L, Luyckx T. The shape and orientation of the trochlea run more parallel to the posterior condylar line than generally believed. Knee Surg Sports Traumatol Arthrosc. 2018;26(9):2685–91.

11. Eckhoff DG, Bach JM, Spitzer VM, Reinig KD, Bagur MM, Baldini TH, et al. Three-dimensional morphology and kinematics of the distal part of the femur viewed in virtual reality. Part II. J Bone Joint Surg Am. 2003;85-A(Suppl 4):97–104.

12. Maillot C, Leong A, Harman C, Morelli A, Mospan R, Cobb J, et al. Poor relationship between frontal tibio-femoral and trochlear anatomic parameters: implications for designing a trochlea for kinematic alignment. Knee. 2019;26(1):106–14.

13. Park A, Duncan ST, Nunley RM, Keeney JA, Barrack RL, Nam D. Relationship of the posterior femoral axis of the "kinematically aligned" total knee arthroplasty to the posterior condylar, transepicondylar, and anteroposterior femoral axes. Knee. 2014;21(6):1120–3.

14. Calliess T, Ettinger M. [Limits of kinematic alignment and recommendations for its safe application]. Orthopade. 2020;49(7):617–624.

15. Nedopil AJ, Howell SM, Hull ML. What mechanisms are associated with tibial component failure after kinematically-aligned total knee arthroplasty? Int Orthop. 2017;41(8):1561–9.

Mako Robotic Arm-Assisted Unicompartmental Knee Arthroplasty

4

Francesco Zambianchi, Valerio Daffara, and Fabio Catani

Introduction

Unicompartmental knee arthroplasty (UKA) has been shown to be a successful treatment in subjects presenting isolated unicompartmental knee osteoarthritis (OA) or osteonecrosis [1]. Optimizing patient selection is essential for a good outcome. In fact, the success of this procedure is strictly related to the quality of surgical indication. Shared indications for UKA include a preoperative diagnosis of symptomatic, primary, or post-traumatic unicompartmental knee OA or osteonecrosis and a passively correctable coronal plane deformity. Generally accepted exclusion criteria for medial and lateral UKA are coronal plane deformity >20°, a fixed flexion contracture >15° on the sagittal plane, lateral facet patellofemoral OA, functional incompetence of the anterior cruciate ligament (ACL), posterior cruciate ligament (PCL) or collateral ligaments, and presence of inflammatory arthropathies. While partial ACL incompetence may be acceptable in medial UKA in low-demand elderly patients and addressed by reducing the tibial component posterior slope, full ACL competence is a mandatory condition in lateral UKA. Thanks to the improved performance over total knee arthroplasty (TKA) in terms of blood loss, risk of infection, range of motion, perioperative complications, and faster rehabilitation [2], UKA has demonstrated to be an excellent surgical solution even in obese patients [3], in high-demand patients, and in those patients presenting with a number of medical comorbidities that could present a contraindication for TKA.

Over the last several years, the use of better implant designs and strict parameters for patient selection have led to improved outcomes and lower revision rates. However, the most common reasons for UKA revision are associated with inaccuracy in implant positioning, limb malalignment, and soft-tissue balancing [4–8].

UKA is considered a technically demanding procedure, whose success is partly related to the surgical technique. The advancement of technological innovations like robotics has led to considerable improvements in UKA in terms of reproducibility, accuracy, and lower implant revision rates [9, 10]. Robotic-arm assistance allows the surgeon to perform resurfacing arthroplasties, adapting implant placement to the patient's anatomy before bone preparation and avoiding limb overcorrection during implant positioning [11]. Thanks to the absence of conventional cutting jigs, robotic arm-assisted (RA) UKA can be easily performed even in patients with high BMI.

Preoperative and intraoperative planning are fundamental in this type of surgery to follow the concept of personalized knee arthroplasty as

F. Zambianchi (✉) · V. Daffara · F. Catani
Department of Orthopaedic Surgery, Azienda Ospedaliero-Universitaria di Modena, University of Modena and Reggio-Emilia, Modena, Italy
e-mail: fabio.catani@unimore.it

much as possible. These features are crucial, considering that on average only six operative cases are required to reduce operative times and become comfortable with the surgery, thereby reducing the learning curve of the surgeon. This allows even low case-volume UKA surgeons to achieve satisfactory results in terms of implant positioning [12] resulting in excellent short-term to mid-term RA-UKA survival rates [12–14].

Main Text: The Mako Robotic System

The Mako robotic system [Mako Surgical Corp. (Stryker), Fort Lauderdale, FL, USA] is a combination of software, hardware, and implants. The software starts with the upload of a CT scan of the patient's affected lower limb, which includes the hip, knee, and ankle. A three-dimensional reconstruction is made with dedicated software, in order to obtain the patient's virtual anatomy, which will be matched and validated with the real bony anatomy during the surgical procedure. This virtual anatomy is visible to the surgeon during surgery on a screen in the operating room. The hardware is composed of a robotic base which includes the engines moving the robotic arm, with its six degrees of freedom. At the end of the robotic arm there is a burr or saw blade, which is directly controlled by the surgeon. A haptic neurosensory feedback from different sensors drives the surgeon through the procedure and allows to respect anatomical structures during the surgical procedure, in order to remove only the predefined bone volumes. The Mako robotic system is a navigation-based system based on infrared optical arrays, with stable reflective sensors fixed to the patient's femur and tibia through bone pins and to an independent sensor array on the robotic arm. The Mako robotic system allows the following UKA procedures:

- Medial RA-UKA.
- Lateral RA-UKA.
- Patello-femoral RA-UKA.

Every Mako RA-UKA procedure is based on the sequence of five phases:

- System setting
- Preoperative planning and surgical setting
- System registration
- Intraoperative planning and soft-tissue balancing
- Haptically controlled bone preparation

Each of these phases is examined in the following paragraphs.

System Setting

Mako is an image-based system built on virtual three-dimensional implant positioning and evaluation of the lower limb alignment benchmarks. A 3D bone model of the patient's knee joint is obtained from the preoperative lower limb CT scan. At first, the surgeon has to check the correct position of the anatomical bone landmarks on CT images, since these allow computation of the anatomical coordinate system to assess flexion/extension, varus/valgus, and internal/external rotation angles relative to which the implant is positioned. The surgeon is able to plan the orientation, position, and size of the implants on the virtual bone model by scrolling the slices and rotating the models of the knee joint and the implants in the coronal, sagittal, and transverse planes. The ability to visualize the predicted implant configuration from different angles allows the surgeon to check for parallelism between femoral and tibial components before starting the surgical procedure. In addition, the position of the tibial and femoral implants can be fine-tuned based on the alignment parameters given by the robotic arm-assisted system, in combination with the surgeon's personal preferences and experience and evidence in the literature.

The CT-based knee model provides preoperative visualization of the subchondral bone bed, bone defects, osteophytes, regions of osteonecrosis, and hardware from previous surgical procedures (Fig. 4.1). Even though the 3D knee model does not show cartilage, a built-in cartilage map-

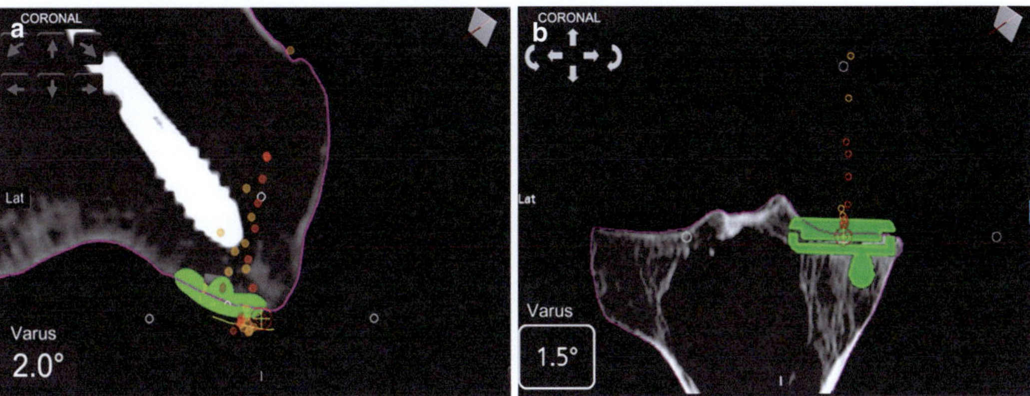

Fig. 4.1 CT-based knee models showing hardware from previous surgeries in the femur (**a**) and a wide bone defect in the tibia (**b**). The virtual femoral and tibial implant position is displayed

ping feature can account for this intraoperatively, allowing the surgeon to visualize cartilage location in relation to the bone.

The CT landmarks relative to which the anatomical coordinate system is built are the hip center, the lateral epicondyle and the medial sulcus of the distal femur, the medial and lateral malleoli, the tibial anterior-posterior (AP) axis, and the center of the tibial eminences. The orientation of the femoral and tibial components in the coronal, sagittal, and transverse planes is measured in relation to the axes derived from CT bone landmarks. Before starting the preoperative planning, the surgeon should check that the selected CT anatomical landmarks are correct. The CT-based approach allows preoperative implant selection and accurate registration to minimize error and improve intraoperative efficiency.

Preoperative Planning and Surgical Setting

A complete knee clinical assessment must be performed to evaluate ligamentous stability, joint laxity, deformity correctability, and range of motion. Preoperatively, patients should undergo weight-bearing full leg, AP, and lateral knee radiographs. The epiphyseal alignment of the distal femur and proximal tibia, as well as the posterior erosion of the tibial plateau in case of partial

incompetence of the ACL (in medial UKA), should be taken into account. Full leg, weight-bearing radiographs represent a reference for the affected limb alignment target if the contralateral leg is not affected by knee OA or concomitant arthropathies. The weight-bearing posterior-anterior flexed view (Rosenberg view) or varus stress radiographs at 20° of knee flexion are helpful to detect early antero-medial OA, as full-thickness cartilage loss could not appear on standing AP radiographs.

Due to the significant anatomic and kinematic differences between knee compartments, preoperative planning features for each of the Mako RA-UKA procedures will be discussed separately. Different surgical approaches can be performed for each type of RA-UKA. Moreover, robotic arm-assisted surgery enhances the use of mini-invasive approaches, since the lack of visualization is offset by haptic feedback and defined safe zones based on 3D knee reconstructions.

The patient is placed in supine position, with the option to use a dynamic leg positioner to hold the knee at 90° of flexion or in full extension. A tourniquet on the thigh is optional and depends on the surgeon's preferences. The operative leg is prepped, draped, and positioned in order to achieve full range of motion during the surgical procedure. The robotic system is positioned at the operative knee side, and the robotic arm must be aligned with the patient's knee.

- *Robotic arm-assisted Medial UKA*
- A crucial aspect of the medial UKA preoperative planning is the placement of the tibial component on the tibial cortical rim, which is the strongest part of the proximal tibia. Overhang of the tibial component also needs to be avoided, as it can cause soft-tissue pain [15]. Moreover, it is of fundamental importance that the tibial resection preserves the tibial spines and does not undercut the ACL fibers, and this can be verified in the coronal view of the 3D knee model. Tibial component coronal and sagittal alignment are set in order to reproduce the native tibia orientation, aiming a parallel orientation to the deepest point on the lateral tibial plateau in the coronal plane (Cartier angle) and sagittal plane (native posterior slope) [16]. It should be noted that

the polyethylene insert has a flat geometry, and thus the concave anatomy of the medial tibial plateau is not replicated. In case of partial incompetence of the ACL, which can be accepted in elderly, low-demand patients, the tibial posterior slope should be reduced. The amount of tibial resection should be planned with the goal of restoring the native joint line height (Fig. 4.2). Relative to femoral component placement, the implant sizing and positioning should shape-match the femoral condyle. In the coronal plane, the implant should be lateralized as close to the notch as possible [17]. In the sagittal plane, the femoral implant should be aligned with the sagittal profile of the femoral condyle, taking cartilage wear into account and adjusting femoral component flexion/extension to select the position

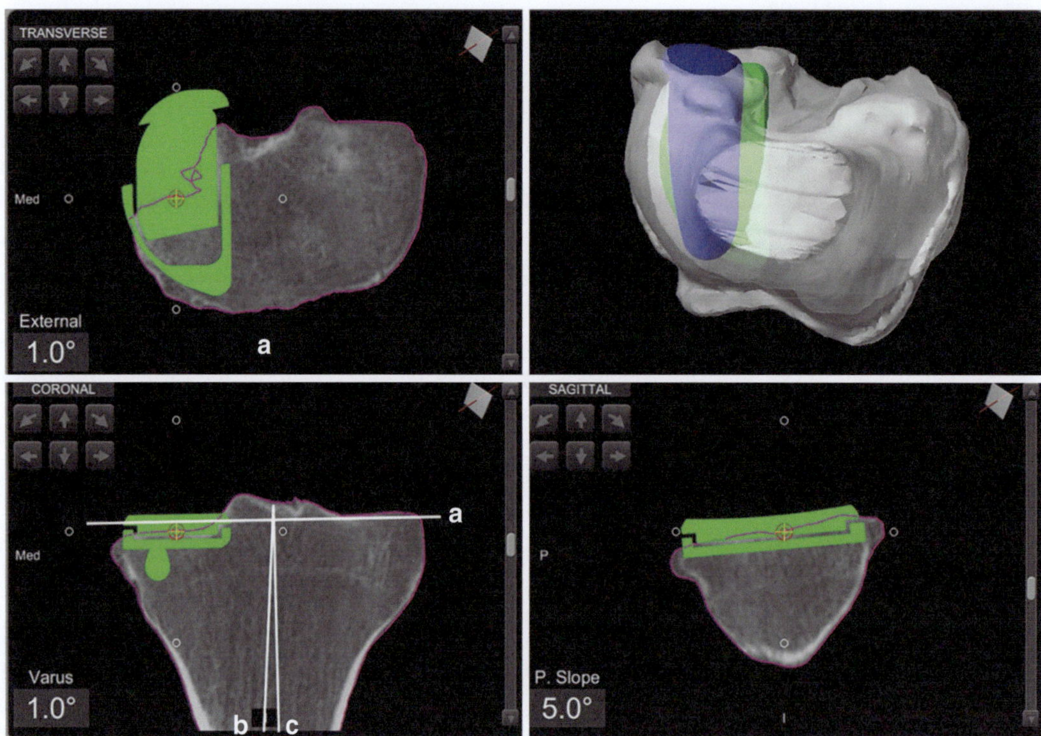

Fig. 4.2 Preoperative planning of the femoral and tibial components on the CT-based 3D model of the knee in medial UKA. The data relative to tibial component positioning is displayed. Tibial component coronal and sagittal alignment are set in order to reproduce the native tibia orientation. Implant size medio-lateral position is set to avoid undercut of the tibial spines. Parallelism between femoral and tibial components in the transverse plane is displayed in the top right of the figure. Tibial coronal alignment is set parallel to the tangent line to the deepest point of the lateral tibial plateau. The Cartier angle is the angle between the tibial mechanical axis (line B) and the perpendicular (line C) to the tangent line to the deepest point of the lateral tibial plateau (line A)

that best matches the native femoral "J-curve" [18] (Fig. 4.3). These solutions will allow the replication of the original joint line height and prevent anterior impingement of the femoral component against the patella. The surgeon can check intraoperatively the transition point from tibio-femoral to patello-femoral joint by putting the knee in full extension and marking the anterior contact point between femur and tibia. The femoral implant should not go beyond the tidemark, which represents the expected anterior termination of the component.

- These solutions will allow the replication of the original joint line height and prevent anterior impingement of the femoral component against the patella.
- A mini mid-vastus approach can be used for RA medial UKA [19–21]. The skin incision

should be performed from the superior-medial patellar pole to just below the joint line, slightly medial to the patellar tendon. After a medial parapatellar capsulotomy, the dissection is extended proximally to the vastus medialis, in order to follow its oblique fibers. The vastus medialis is split at approximately 2 cm and the patella is subluxated but not everted, to allow medial compartment exposure. The approach can be minimized as the surgeon can place the knee in various positions to allow the burr or saw to safely prepare the bone without direct visualization and prevent soft-tissue trauma. The patellar tendon and the medial collateral ligament are protected at all times during the procedure. If a patello-femoral procedure is associated, this approach can be extended as a standard medial parapatellar approach in order to evert the

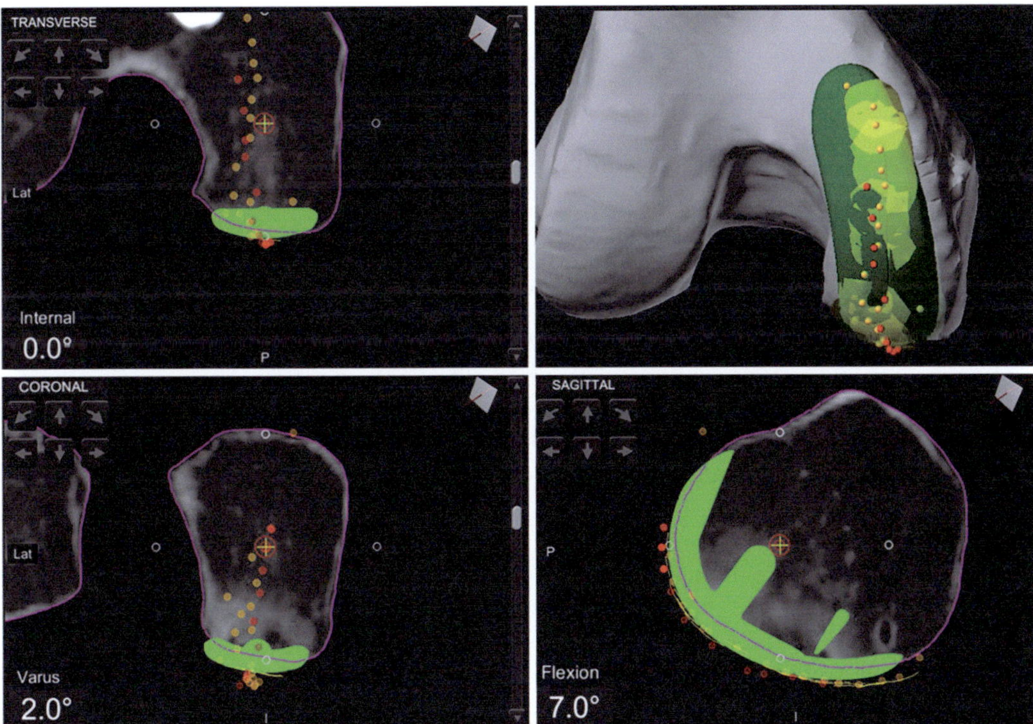

Fig. 4.3 Intraoperative planning of the femoral component on top of the CT-based 3D model of the knee in medial UKA. Preoperatively, the surgeon checks that the femoral component is aligned with the sagittal profile of the femoral condyle. Intraoperatively, the red dots depict implant tracking points on the femoral component model. With this information, the surgeon can centralize the tracking of the femoral component over the tibial component. The yellow dots and the yellow line express the profile of the mapped cartilage surface. The surgeon utilizes this feature to ensure that the implant volume compensates for worn cartilage

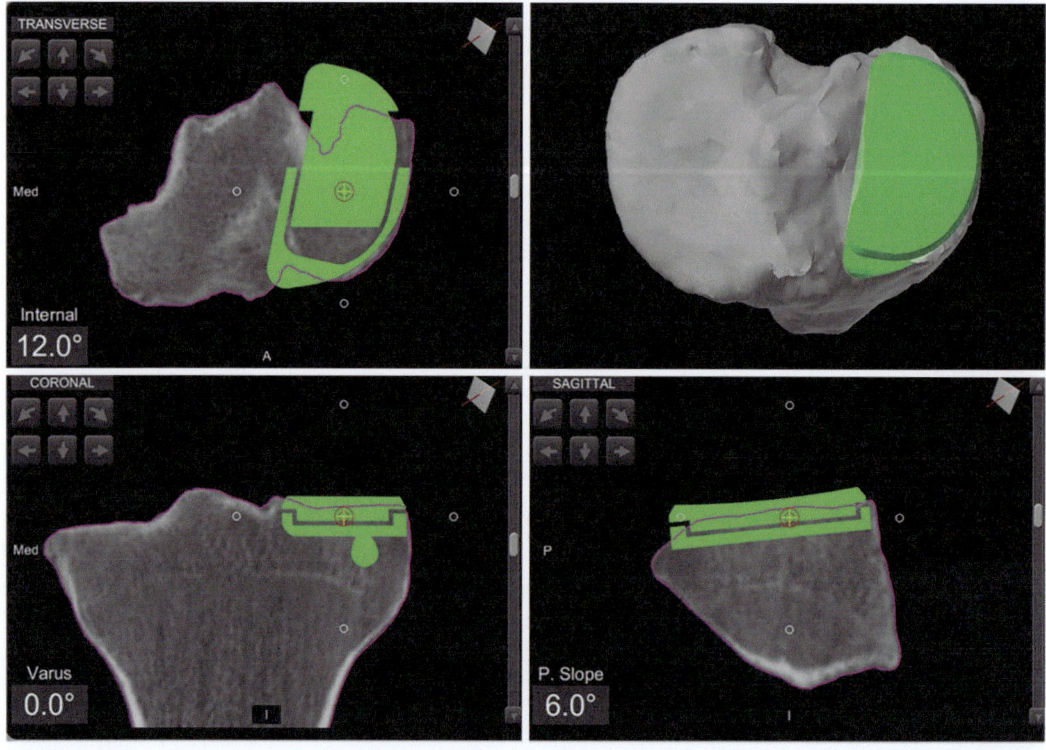

Fig. 4.4 Preoperative planning of the tibial component on the CT-based 3D model of the knee in lateral UKA. The tibial component is in internal rotation relative to the tibia AP axis to account for the "screw home" mechanism of the knee

patella. After bone exposure, the system registration phase is performed.

– *Robotic arm-assisted Lateral UKA*
– Similar to medial UKA, tibial component should maximize tibial bone coverage without overhang in the lateral compartment. Preoperatively, the surgeon should plan to align the tibial implant in order to respect tibial joint line orientation in the coronal and sagittal planes. The knee "screw-home" mechanism should be taken into account when performing preoperative implant planning. The "screw-home" mechanism is represented by the sharp femoral internal rotation relative to the tibia between 30° of flexion and full extension. This results in tightening of both the cruciate ligaments and knee locking in full extension. If this knee kinematic feature is not taken into account during implant planning, a risk of impingement between femoral implant and tibial spine eminence in full extension occurs [22]. Consequently, the femoral component should be planned to be positioned laterally as possible on the femoral condyle, with some degrees of external rotation, while the tibial component should be placed in internal rotation relative to the tibia AP axis (approximately 11–15°) and as close as possible to the tibial spine eminences (Fig. 4.4) [23]. In case of severe femoral condyle hypoplasia, the femoral component should not reproduce the femoral anatomy, but rather "augment" the dysplastic condyle distally and posteriorly. Preoperatively, the surgeon can check for the parallelism of the implants in full extension to confirm that the "screw-home" mechanism is respected.

– A standard lateral para-patellar longitudinal approach is used for RA lateral UKAs. The skin incision from the lateral pole of patella is extended distally over the lateral portion of tibial tubercle. A lateral parapatellar capsulotomy is extended from the lateral border of the quadriceps tendon, over the lateral margin of the patella, and ends 2 cm distal from the tibial tubercle. The patella is subluxated but not everted, in order to expose the lateral compartment. Most of the procedure is performed in mid-flexion, in order to relax the lateral pull of the patella and ensure good visualization of the lateral compartment. Intraoperatively, care must be taken not to damage the popliteus tendon, as the tendon drapes over the femoral condyle and is not tracked by the robotic system. After bone exposure, the system registration phase is performed.

– *Robotic arm-assisted Patello-Femoral UKA*
– Candidates for isolated patello-femoral UKA are subjects presenting with primary or post-traumatic symptomatic patello-femoral joint OA. Preoperative radiographs with skyline views and accurate clinical examination should rule out the presence of tibio-femoral joint arthritis before considering isolated UKA. Patello-femoral malalignment or dysplasia-induced OA is a common indication for patello-femoral UKA. Inflammatory arthropathies, tibio-femoral joint OA as well as coronal plane deformity >10°, increased Q angle, and fixed flexion contracture >15° are absolute contraindications for patello-femoral UKA. Patients should be attentively counseled on expectations and long-term outcomes.
– The primary goal of preoperative planning in RA-patello-femoral arthroplasty with the Mako system is accurate implant size selection and alignment relative to the bony anatomy. The largest trochlear component that does not overhang the medial and lateral cortical edges of the femur and gives anterior coverage should be selected. The trochlear component should be slightly externally rotated so that it is aligned perpendicular to the AP axis of the femur and parallel to the TEA. Excessive trochlear external rotation should be avoided as it will decrease lateral patellar jump height (decrease lateral patellar constraint), while internal rotation of the component should be accompanied by lateral

translation to offset the medialization due to internal rotation. A smooth transition between the anterior femoral cortex and the implant is advised, the distal tongue of the trochlear component should not interfere with the ACL and should be placed at the center of the femoral notch. To avoid impingement with the ACL the distal tip of the implant must be placed anteriorly to the Blumensaat's line (Fig. 4.5).
– A longitudinal skin incision extending from 2–3 cm proximal to the superior pole of patella to the superior pole of tibial tubercle is performed, followed by a medial parapatellar capsulotomy. While performing the arthrotomy, care should be taken to avoid damage to menisci, inter-meniscal ligament, and articular cartilage of the tibio-femoral compartments. With the knee in full extension, the patella can be everted using a Backhaus clamp. After bone exposure, the system registration phase is performed.

System Registration

After the exposure, the above-mentioned infrared arrays are secured to the femur and tibia shafts with bi-cortical, partially threaded pins. On the tibia, the pins are placed at approximately 5–8 cm distal to the incision on the medial side of the tibial crest. On the femur, the pins are placed starting approximately 5–7 cm superior to the superior pole of the patella. The femoral checkpoint is then located in a safe zone on the distal femur, and the tibial checkpoint is positioned in a safe zone on the tibial metaphysis, avoiding impingement with the planned implant. Once the robotic arm has been calibrated and the limb registered to obtain mechanical alignment, the surgeon validates the 3D knee reconstruction based on the preoperative CT scan, which has to be matched with the patient's anatomy, by using a sharp probe. In this phase, the surgeon has to acquire correct bone contact points, by piercing the cartilage residual surface, if present. A visual color code is used to facilitate the surgeon during this phase. Finally, the calibration procedure is validated by means of verification of bone points

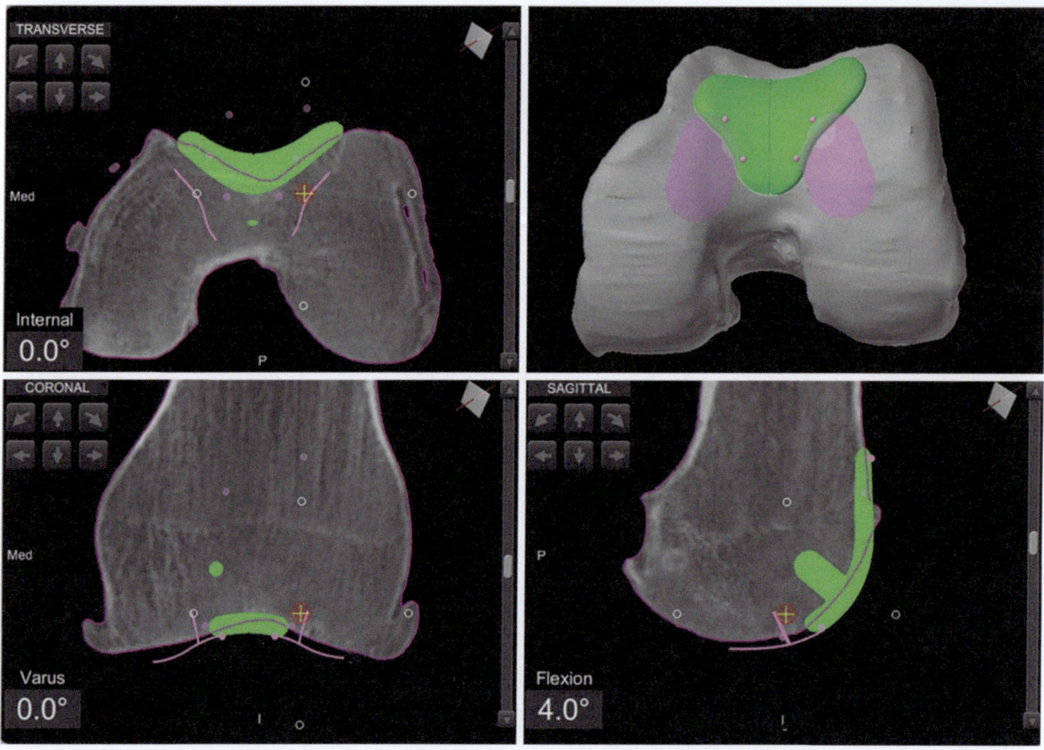

Fig. 4.5 Preoperative planning of the trochlear component on top of the CT-based 3D model of the femur in patello-femoral UKA. The trochlear component does not enter the femoral notch or overhang medial or laterally, nor the tip protrudes distally

planned by the system, and the CT scan results matched with patient anatomy.

Intraoperative Planning and Soft-Tissue Balancing

After the tibial and femoral osteophytes have been removed and ACL status has been inspected, limb deformity correctability can be assessed throughout the full arc of motion. While traditional techniques for UKA have relied on gap balancing in full extension and at 90° of flexion, Mako RA-UKA relies on the surgeon to choose data capture points throughout the whole range of motion.

While applying a valgus (for medial UKA) or varus (for lateral UKA) stress force to restore the pre-arthritic soft-tissue tension, the surgeon must put the knee throughout a full range of motion (Fig. 4.6). If unaffected from arthritic conditions, the contralateral limb can be taken as an align-ment target reference. During the varus/valgus stress maneuver the robotic software will gather gap-balancing data, tracking the contact points between the virtually planned femoral and tibial components and measuring the gaps between the planned implant models. A graph depicting detailed implant tracking gaps throughout the arc of motion is then displayed on the system's screen and visualized by the surgeon. Negative gap values indicate ligamentous tightness, while positive gap is suggestive of ligamentous laxity. Implant position can be customized and fine-tuned according to the surgeon's preferences. While changing the orientation and position of the femoral and tibial components, the graph automatically shows the adjusted gap-balancing information (Fig. 4.7). The gap-distance information provided by the robotic system is dependent on the manually applied valgus or varus load on the knee by the surgeon. Therefore, gap-distance information can vary between sur-

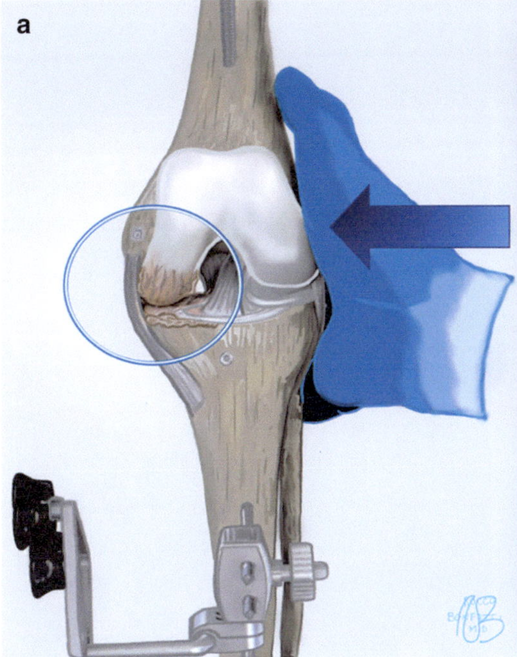

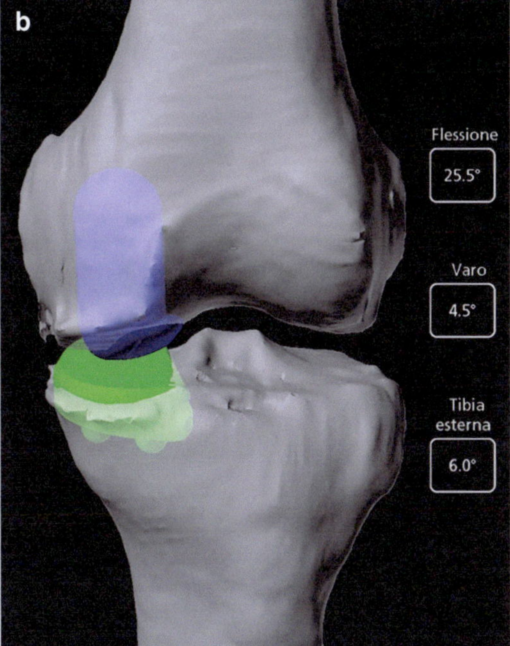

Fig. 4.6 Pose capture procedure in a medial RA-UKA. The surgeon puts the knee throughout a full range of motion, while applying a valgus stress force (**a**). During the maneuver, the surgeon focuses on the amount of correction applied and the knee flexion degree (**b**)

geons. However, the goal of dynamic gap balancing in UKA is in general to create a slightly lax gap throughout the arc of motion by adjusting the implant position without performing any ligament release. In medial UKA, on average the ligament balancing curve shows relative tightness in full extension, slight laxity between 20° and 40° of flexion, followed by relative tightness (femoro-tibial gap of approximately 0.5–1 mm) between 50° and 90° of flexion. Beyond 90° of flexion, relative laxity should be obtained [18] (Fig. 4.8). The implant tracking points are also depicted on the system screen. With this information, the surgeon can centralize the tracking of the femoral component over the tibia, in order to avoid edge loading throughout the entire arc of knee flexion (Fig. 4.3).

After implant fine-tuning is done, the blunt probe is used to check the planned implant position and sizing before bone preparation. The surgeon can then examine the coronal and sagittal alignment of the virtual tibial and femoral components and if the posterior femoral offset is restored. Cartilage mapping can be used to ensure that the implant volume compensates for worn cartilage on both articular surfaces (Fig. 4.3). After validation of the surgical plan, bone resections can be performed.

When performing a patello-femoral UKA, the tibia is not registered, pins are secured on the femoral shaft only, and the varus/valgus load maneuver is not performed. The goal of intraoperative patello-femoral UKA planning is to map cartilage surface and fine-tune the implant position and orientation for proper implant proudness, and smooth transition from the component to the mapped cartilage surfaces. Bone intercondylar osteophytes should be removed, and care should be taken to avoid interference between the tip of the trochlear component and the ACL. The patella is usually resurfaced using standard TKA principles, including medialization of the patellar button and a measured resection technique to avoid patello-femoral joint overstuffing. Osteotomy of the lateral patellar facet is advised to improve tracking and avoid lateral patellar impingement.

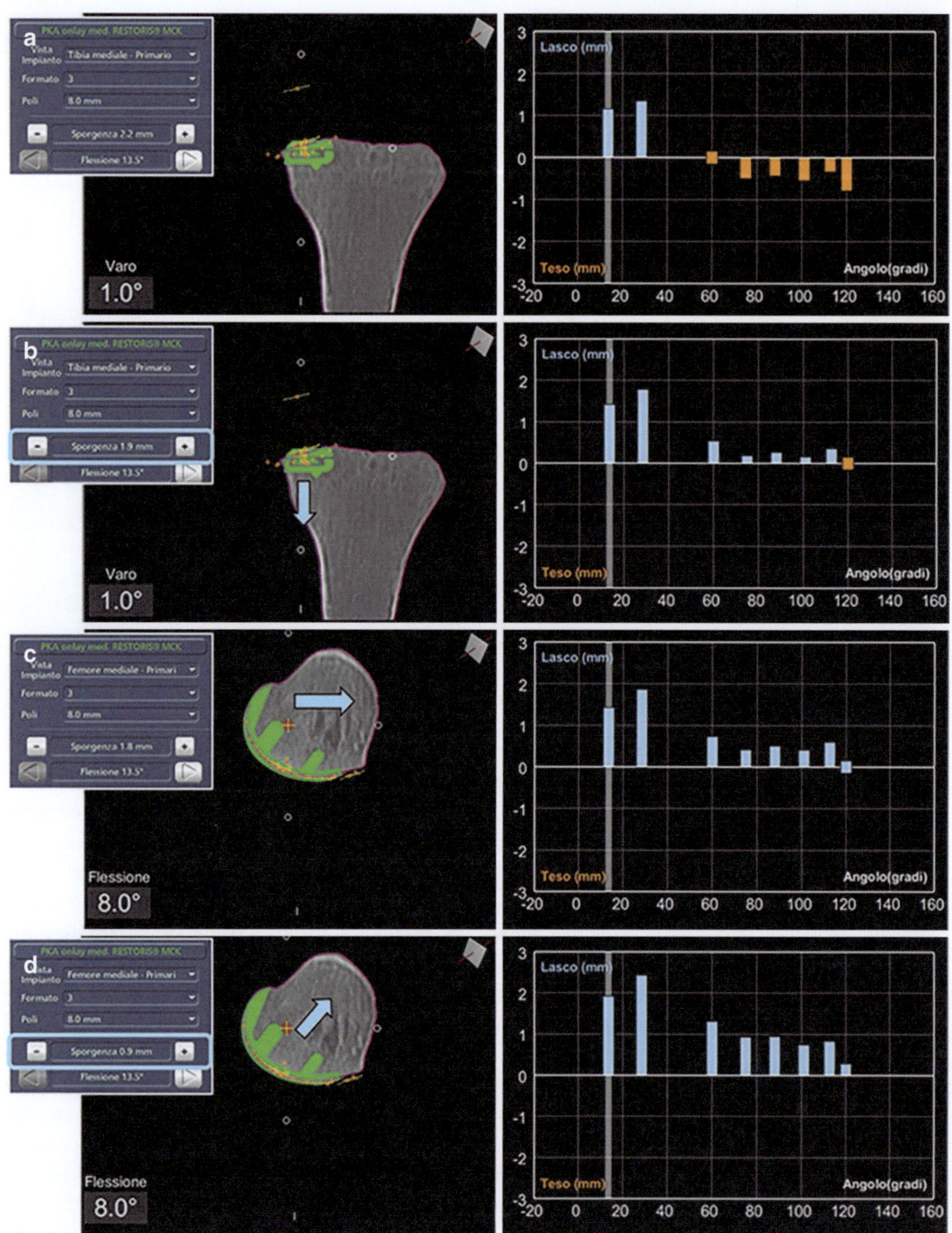

Fig. 4.7 Intraoperative graph depicting the gap between the planned implant positioning at different degrees of knee flexion. Implant positioning is fine-tuned to obtain the desired laxity pattern. If the knee is too tight throughout the full arc of flexion (**a**), the tibial component can be placed more inferior (decrease proudness) to loosen the soft tissue, causing the graph to increase over the entire arc of motion (blue bars) (**b**). When the knee has the desired gap in extension, but it is tight in flexion, the surgeon can shift the femoral component anteriorly, causing the graph to increase over the deeper flexion (blue bars) (**c**). If slight laxity is desired in mid-flexion, the surgeon can shift the femoral component toward the direction of the pegs (decrease proudness) to increase the gap between 60° and 90° of knee flexion (**d**)

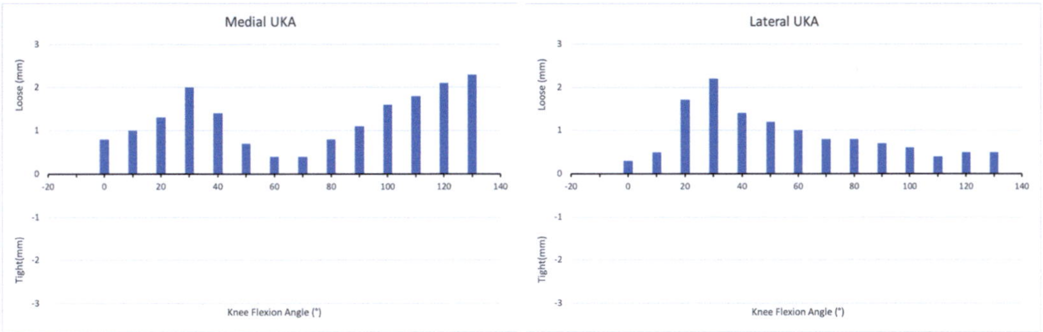

Fig. 4.8 Intraoperative ligament balancing of medial and lateral RA-UKA based on femoro-tibial gaps throughout knee range of motion [18, 23]

Haptically Controlled Bone Preparation

The planned volume of bone that needs to be removed to receive the implant is displayed on the system screen. The bone preparation procedure is performed with the burr/saw at the end of the robotic arm. The burr or saw is placed close to the joint, and the trigger at the end of the robotic arm is pressed, enabling the arm to perform surgeon-controlled self-alignment to align the resection tool with the stereotactic boundary. The haptic feature prevents the saw or burr from exceeding the predefined borders, which helps to ensure that only the planned bone is removed and prevents inadvertent soft-tissue injury (Fig. 4.9). The coronal tibial cut and posterior femoral condyle cut are usually performed first with the haptically controlled saw blade. Afterwards, distal femoral bone milling and tibial sagittal bone preparation are performed with the high-speed haptically controlled burr. The femoral keel and pegs for the femur and tibia are prepared with the motorized burr under haptic control. Lateral UKA does not allow the use of the haptically controlled saw blade due to the risk of patellar tendon damage, therefore only the use of the high-speed burr is allowed for bone preparation.

After bone cuts, trial prosthetic components are implanted, and the alignment and gaps can be checked. If thicker polyethylene trials are required, they can be inserted, and the limb reevaluated. If additional bone adjustment is required, the plan can be fine-tuned and the robotic arm reengaged. Once the trial components are accepted, the final components are implanted with cement and the polyethylene bearing is inserted and impacted. The bone pins and checkpoints are removed, and surgical sites are irrigated and closed in a standard fashion.

Evidence and Challenges Supporting the Use of Robotic Arm-Assisted UKA with Mako

Robotic assistance has brought substantial improvements in UKA practice in terms of clinical outcomes, implant survivorship, and technical challenges. As described by different studies, functional better outcomes in comparison with conventional UKA have been obtained in RA procedures. Kayani et al. have reported reduced postoperative pain and a reduced number of inpatient physiotherapy sessions, increased knee flexion, shorter time to straight leg raise, decreased mean time to hospital discharge, and improved short-time functional outcomes in highly active patients [24].

RA-UKA performed with Mako allows the surgeon to perform surgery with higher accuracy and reproducibility in implant positioning, respecting the patient's normal anatomy and limb alignment compared to conventional techniques [11]. This limits the risk of progression of osteoarthritic disease on the unsurfaced compartment, granting better functional outcomes and higher implant survivorship rates. In addition, the use of

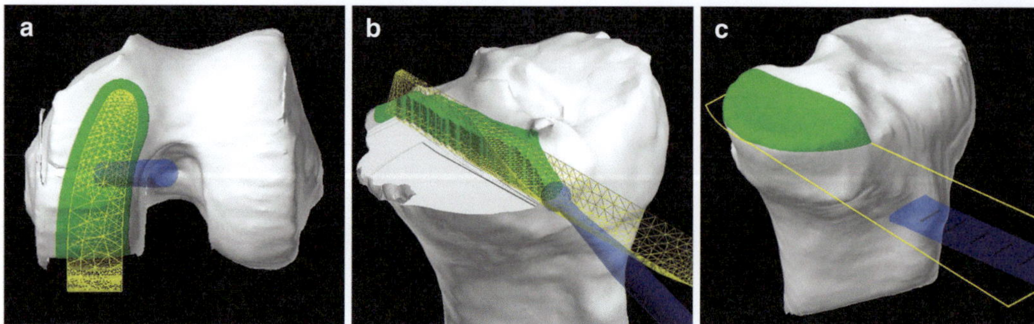

Fig. 4.9 Haptically controlled bone preparation. When the trigger at the end of the robotic arm is pressed, the resection tool is aligned to the stereotactic boundary. The distal femoral surface (**a**) and the sagittal profile of the tibia (**b**) are milled with the haptically controlled high-speed burr (blue), which removes only the predefined volume of bone (green). In medial UKA, the coronal tibial cut and the posterior femoral condyle cut can be optionally performed with the haptically controlled saw blade (**c**)

a CT-based system in combination with a haptically controlled tool for bone preparation has been demonstrated to grant enhanced precision in bone preparation, improved accuracy in implant positioning, and more conservative bone cuts [11, 25]. All these aspects help to preserve the bone stock and reduce bone edema, which has often been accounted for postoperative pain.

Several studies have reported encouraging results concerning RA-UKA short-time survival rates. Pearle et al. reported a 98.8% survival rate at a minimum of 2 years of follow-up, while a study by our group demonstrated a 99.0% survivorship for medial UKAs and 100% survivorship for lateral UKAs at an average of 3 years of follow-up [26, 27]. While long-term outcomes have not yet been reported, mid-term survivorship rates have been analyzed in other studies, with likewise promising results. A study by our group showed a 97.8% survivorship rate at an average of 5.9 years of follow-up for medial RA-UKA, while Kleeblad et al. reported a 97.5% survival rate at a minimum of 5 years of follow-up [14, 28]. Similar survivorship rates in different studies highlight the efficacy of robotic assistance in achieving high UKA survival independently from the volume of UKA performed per center. In fact, robotic arm-assisted surgery learning curve is shorter than conventional procedures, allowing even low- and mid-volume UKA centers to achieve satisfactory comfort in performing this type of surgery [25] and determining

RA-UKA to be a cost-effective procedure in centers with a case volume between 32 and 48 cases per year [29].

Summary

The Mako robotic system is a CT-based robotic surgical tool enabling performance of partial knee replacement with high reproducibility and accuracy. Short- to mid-term follow-up studies have demonstrated excellent clinical results and survival rates for RA-UKA.

- This system enables performance of three types of partial knee replacement: medial, lateral, and patello-femoral RA-UKA.
- Every RA-UKA procedure is based on the sequence of five phases: (1) system setting, (2) preoperative planning and surgical setting, (3) system registration, (4) intraoperative planning and soft-tissue balancing, and (5) haptically controlled bone preparation.

References

1. Burn E, Sanchez-Santos MT, Pandit HG, Hamilton TW, Liddle AD, Murray DW, et al. Ten-year patient-reported outcomes following total and minimally invasive unicompartmental knee arthroplasty: a propensity score-matched cohort analysis. Knee Surg Sports Traumatol Arthrosc. 2018;26(5):1455–64.

2. Palumbo BT, Scott RD. Diagnosis and indications for treatment of unicompartmental arthritis. Clin Sports Med. 2014;33(1):11–21. https://doi.org/10.1016/j.csm.2013.06.001.

3. Plate JF, Augart MA, Seyler TM, Bracey DN, Hoggard A, Akbar M, et al. Obesity has no effect on outcomes following unicompartmental knee arthroplasty. Knee Surg Sports Traumatol Arthrosc. 2017;25(3):645–51. https://doi.org/10.1007/s00167-015-3597-5.

4. van der List JP, McDonald LS, Pearle AD. Systematic review of medial versus lateral survivorship in unicompartmental knee arthroplasty. Knee. 2015;22(6):454–60. https://doi.org/10.1016/j.knee.2015.09.011.

5. van der List JP, Chawla H, Villa JC, Pearle AD. Different optimal alignment but equivalent functional outcomes in medial and lateral unicompartmental knee arthroplasty. Knee. 2016;23(6):987–95. https://doi.org/10.1016/j.knee.2016.08.008.

6. Chatellard R, Sauleau V, Colmar M, Robert H, Raynaud G, Brilhault J. Medial unicompartmental knee arthroplasty: does tibial component position influence clinical outcomes and arthroplasty survival? Orthop Traumatol Surg Res. 2013;99(4 Suppl):S219–25. https://doi.org/10.1016/j.otsr.2013.03.004.

7. Zambianchi F, Digennaro V, Giorgini A, Grandi G, Fiacchi F, Mugnai R, Catani F. Surgeon's experience influences UKA survivorship: a comparative study between all-poly and metal back designs. Knee Surg Sports Traumatol Arthrosc. 2015;23(7):2074–80. https://doi.org/10.1007/s00167-014-2958-9.

8. Barbadoro P, Ensini A, Leardini A, d'Amato M, Feliciangeli A, Timoncini A, et al. Tibial component alignment and risk of loosening in unicompartmental knee arthroplasty: a radiographic and radiostereometric study. Knee Surg Sports Traumatol Arthrosc. 2014;22(12):3157–62. https://doi.org/10.1007/s00167-014-3147-6.

9. Rauck RC, Blevins JL, Cross MB. Component placement accuracy in unicompartmental knee arthroplasty is improved with robotic assisted surgery: will it have an effect on outcomes? HSS J. 2018;14(2):211–3. https://doi.org/10.1007/s11420-017-9593-1.

10. Lonner JH, John TK, Conditt MA. Robotic arm-assisted UKA improves tibial component alignment: a pilot study. Clin Orthop Relat Res. 2010;468(1):141–6. https://doi.org/10.1007/s11999-009-0977-5.

11. Bell SW, Anthony I, Jones B, MacLean A, Rowe P, Blyth M. Improved accuracy of component positioning with robotic-assisted unicompartmental knee arthroplasty. J Bone Joint Surg Am. 2016;98(8):627–35. https://doi.org/10.2106/JBJS.15.00664.

12. Begum FA, Kayani B, Morgan SDJ, Ahmed SS, Singh S, Haddad FS. Robotic technology: current concepts, operative techniques and emerging uses in unicompartmental knee arthroplasty. EFORT Open Rev. 2020;5(5):312–8. https://doi.org/10.1302/2058-5241.5.190089.

13. Zambianchi F, Daffara V, Franceschi G, Banchelli F, Marcovigi A, Catani F. Robotic arm-assisted unicompartmental knee arthroplasty: high survivorship and good patient-related outcomes at a minimum five years of follow-up. Knee Surg Sports Traumatol Arthrosc. 2020;29:3316. https://doi.org/10.1007/s00167-020-06198-9.

14. Burger JA, Kleeblad LJ, Laas N, Pearle AD. Mid-term survivorship and patient-reported outcomes of robotic-arm assisted partial knee arthroplasty. Bone Joint J. 2020;102-B(1):108–16. https://doi.org/10.1302/0301-620X.102B1.BJJ-2019-0510.R1.

15. Chau R, Gulati A, Pandit H, Beard DJ, Price AJ, Dodd CAF, et al. Tibial component overhang following unicompartmental knee replacement-does it matter? Knee. 2009;16(5):310–3. https://doi.org/10.1016/j.knee.2008.12.017.

16. Takayama K, Matsumoto T, Muratsu H, Ishida K, Araki D, Matsushita T, et al. The influence of posterior tibial slope changes on joint gap and range of motion in unicompartmental knee arthroplasty. Knee. 2016;23(3):517–22. https://doi.org/10.1016/j.knee.2016.01.003.

17. Belvedere C, Leardini A, Giannini S, Ensini A, Bianchi L, Catani F. Does medio-lateral motion occur in the normal knee? An in-vitro study in passive motion. J Biomech. 2011;44(5):877–84. https://doi.org/10.1016/j.jbiomech.2010.12.004.

18. Zambianchi F, Franceschi G, Rivi E, Banchelli F, Marcovigi A, Nardacchione R, Ensini A, Catani F. Does component placement affect short-term clinical outcome in robotic-arm assisted unicompartmental knee arthroplasty? Bone Joint J. 2019;101-B(4):435–42. https://doi.org/10.1302/0301-620X.101B4.BJJ-2018-0753.R1.

19. Haas SB, Cook S, Beksac B. Minimally invasive total knee replacement through a mini midvastus approach: a comparative study. Clin Orthop Relat Res. 2004;428:68–73. https://doi.org/10.1097/01.blo.0000147649.82883.ca.

20. Laskin RS, Beksac B, Phongjunakorn A, Pittors K, Davis J, Shim JC, et al. Minimally invasive total knee replacement through a mini-midvastus incision: an outcome study. Clin Orthop Relat Res. 2004;428:74–81. https://doi.org/10.1097/01.blo.0000148582.86102.47.

21. Reid JB, Guttmann D, Ayala M, Lubowitz JH. Minimally invasive surgery-total knee arthroplasty. Arthroscopy. 2004;20(8):884–9. https://doi.org/10.1016/j.arthro.2004.07.021.

22. Ollivier M, Abdel MP, Parratte S, Argenson J-N. Lateral unicondylar knee arthroplasty (UKA): contemporary indications, surgical technique, and results. Int Orthop. 2014;38(2):449–55. https://doi.org/10.1007/s00264-013-2222-9.

23. Zambianchi F, Franceschi G, Banchelli F, Marcovigi A, Ensini A, Catani F. Robotic arm-assisted lateral unicompartmental knee arthroplasty: how are components aligned? J Knee Surg. 2021;35:1214. https://doi.org/10.1055/s-0040-1722346.

24. Kayani B, Konan S, Tahmassebi J, Rowan FE, Haddad FS. An assessment of early functional rehabilitation and hospital discharge in conventional

versus robotic-arm assisted unicompartmental knee arthroplasty: a prospective cohort study. Bone Joint J. 2019;101-B(1):24–33. https://doi.org/10.1302/0301-620X.101B1.BJJ-2018-0564.R2.

25. Kayani B, Konan S, Pietrzak JRT, Huq SS, Tahmassebi J, Haddad FS. The learning curve associated with robotic-arm assisted unicompartmental knee arthroplasty: a prospective cohort study. Bone Joint J. 2018;100-B(8):1033–42. https://doi.org/10.1302/0301-620X.100B8.BJJ-2018-0040.R1.

26. Pearle AD, van der List JP, Lee L, Coon TM, Borus TA, Roche MW. Survivorship and patient satisfaction of robotic-assisted medial unicompartmental knee arthroplasty at a minimum two-year follow-up. Knee. 2017;24(2):419–28. https://doi.org/10.1016/j.knee.2016.12.001.

27. Zambianchi F, Franceschi G, Rivi E, Banchelli F, Marcovigi A, Khabbazè C, Catani F. Clinical results and short-term survivorship of robotic-arm-assisted medial and lateral unicompartmental knee arthroplasty. Knee Surg Sports Traumatol Arthrosc. 2020;28(5):1551–9. https://doi.org/10.1007/s00167-019-05566-4.

28. Kleeblad LJ, Borus TA, Coon TM, Dounchis J, Nguyen JT, Pearle AD. Midterm survivorship and patient satisfaction of robotic-arm-assisted medial unicompartmental knee arthroplasty: a multicenter study. J Arthroplasty. 2018;33(6):1719–26. https://doi.org/10.1016/j.arth.2018.01.036.

29. Moschetti WE, Konopka JF, Rubash HE, Genuario JW. Can robot-assisted unicompartmental knee arthroplasty be cost-effective? A Markov decision analysis. J Arthroplasty. 2016;31(4):759–65. https://doi.org/10.1016/j.arth.2015.10.018.

Medial Pivot Implants and Patient-Specific Instrumentation

5

Peter P. Koch and Sandesh Rao

Introduction

In this chapter, we will review native knee anatomy and kinematics, especially as it pertains to tibiofemoral articulation and motion during flexion and extension. The kinematic function of the native knee is the foundation for which the medial pivot-based implant was created. The chapter will then focus on features of design and outcomes for medial pivot implants. We will also discuss the use of patient-specific instrumentation, specifically in the use of medial pivot implants.

The Anatomy and Kinematics of the Native Knee

The native knee joint is comprised of the bony articulation between the distal femur and the proximal tibia. The unique anatomical shape of both bones, in addition to contributions from ligament, muscle, and soft tissue attachments, results in a very complex joint with six degrees of freedom during motion. The radius of curvature and the center of rotation of the distal and posterior femoral condyles differ between the medial and lateral sides. Similarly, the medial and lateral tibial plateaus have anatomical differences. The differences lead to the unique and dynamic articulation of the distal femur and proximal tibia to form the knee joint and also what contributes to much of the differential freedom during movement.

The tibia articulates with the distal femoral condyles between 0 and 100°. The tibia articulates with the posterior femoral condyles from 100 to 150° [1]. The center of rotation of the distal femur sits anterior to the center of rotation of the posterior femur on both the lateral and medial sides. This contributes to femoral rollback during knee flexion, which allows for maximal deep knee flexion and avoidance of impingement on the posterior femoral cortex by the posterior tibial plateau. However, the center of rotation of the distal femur and posterior femur is far closer within the medial femoral condyle, compared to the lateral femoral condyle. On the tibia, the

P. P. Koch (✉)
Gelenkzentrum Winterthur, Winterthur, Switzerland
e-mail: peter.koch@gzw.ch

S. Rao
Washington Orthopaedics & Sports Medicine,
Washington, DC, USA

medial tibial plateau is a concave surface in the sagittal plane, while the lateral tibial plateau is a flat or even convex surface. These anatomical findings contribute to the medial femoral condyle effectively serving as a pivot point, as it has minimal anterior and posterior translation. The lateral femoral condyle freely translates and rotates on the lateral tibial plateau during flexion and extension. This results in internal rotation of the tibia with flexion and external rotation with extension. Medial pivot implants attempt to recreate the natural bony anatomy that allows for the effective natural rollback kinematics of the knee through the use of unique designs [2].

Considerations for a Change in Design of Total Knee Arthroplasty

The existing total knee arthroplasty designs, especially the cruciate-retaining designed TKA, resulted in paradoxical anterior translation of the femur during flexion of the knee [3]. The paradoxical anterior translation was thought to contribute to mid-flexion instability. In the posterior stabilized knees, where both the ACL and PCL were sacrificed, a post was incorporated within the polyethylene and a cam within the femoral component to allow for symmetric graduated femoral rollback which was thought to mimic the "four bar linkage" theory of knee kinematics, where the center of rotation of the knee was not fixed. However, asymmetric rollback where the lateral femoral condyle pivots around a relatively stationary medial femoral condyle was increasingly accepted as the kinematics of a normally functioning knee [4, 5] (Fig. 5.1). This understanding resulted in increased interest in designing implants that recreated or preserved the medial pivot beginning in the 1990s.

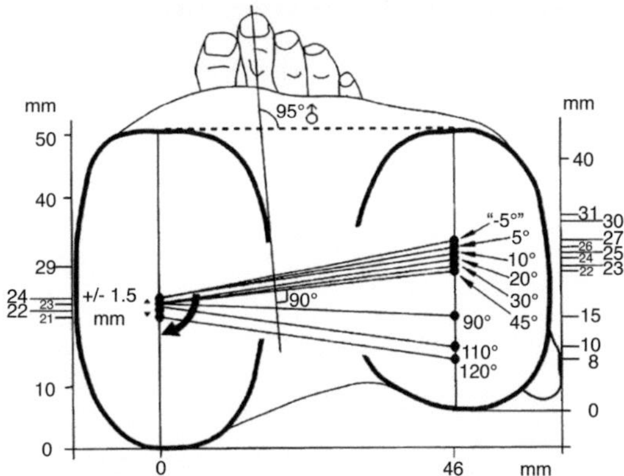

A diagram to show the articular surface of the tibia and the position of the centers of rotation of the medial and lateral condyles in various degrees of flexion (from -5° to 120°). Adapted from (Freeman MA 2005)

Fig. 5.1 Depiction showing the pivoting that occurs at the medial tibial plateau compared to the lateral tibia. (Reprinted with permission from Medacta)

The Design of Medial Pivoting Implants

Medial pivoting implants were designed with specific features to preserve the native knee kinematics described above. Specifically, the polyethylene tibial insert is designed with a concave, highly conforming medial tibial component that results in a "ball and socket" like articulation with the medial femoral condyle. Additionally, the anterior aspect of the polyethylene on the medial side is elevated, creating a raised ridge to allow for added stability in full extension while also preventing paradoxical anterior translation in mid-flexion. The lateral aspect of the polyethylene is relatively convex or less conforming, allowing for increased freedom of motion of the lateral femoral condyle. The medial femoral condyle of the femoral component is designed with a single radius of curvature for the distal and posterior femur mimicking the native femur, which has a center of rotation very close to each other for both the posterior and distal femur. Finally, because there is increased conformity between the femoral component and the polyethylene, the femoral component is placed in a few degrees of relative internal rotation to mimic the native femur and its articulation with the tibia. Engineering total knee arthroplasty in this manner theoretically allows for motion more consistent with native knee kinematics with a focus on a combination of both femoral rollback and medial pivoting (Fig. 5.2).

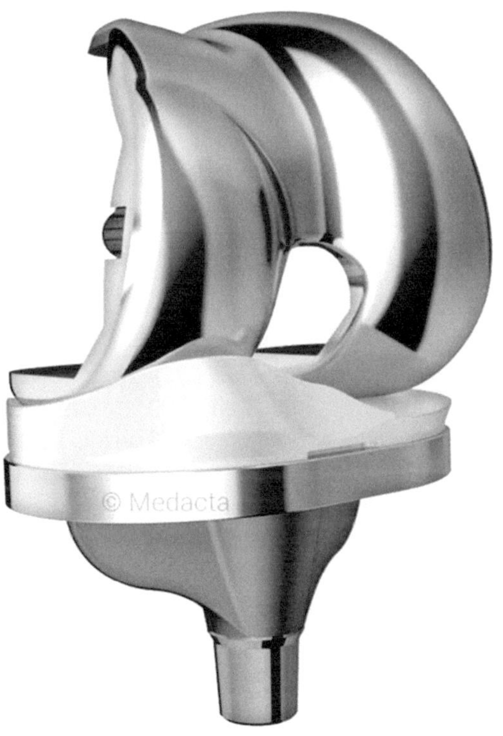

Fig. 5.2 Example of medial pivoting implants with a highly conforming medial aspect of the polyethylene. (Reprinted with permission from Medacta)

Given that the medial pivoting implant is designed to recreate native knee kinematics, a patient must have a knee that does not require any added level of constraint or stability beyond what would be accomplished in a standard posterior stabilized knee where both anterior and posterior cruciate ligaments would be sacrificed. If further level of constraint is needed, the medial pivoting implant is not recommended to be used.

Outcomes of Medial Pivoting Implants

The medial pivoting implants were created as a solution to help reliably recreate native knee kinematics, a fact that has been successfully proven through in vivo studies [6–8]. Specifically, as designed, there is evidence of limited anterior and posterior translation in the highly conformed medial aspect of the component with maximal translation and freedom of movement in the lateral aspect when compared to the traditional cruciate-retaining and posterior stabilized designs [6–8]. This allows for tibial internal rotation with maximal flexion. Additionally, given that native kinematics are effectively mimicked, the rate of condylar liftoff is decreased in medial pivoting implants compared to both PS and CR knees [7]. As a result of the improved congruence, the contact stresses are more evenly distributed and reduced, resulting in a decreased rate of polyethylene wear compared to CR-designed knees [9]. The improved medial congruence, which also represents increased constraint, however, did not result in increased failure or loosening compared to CR knee prostheses [9].

Successful kinematic mimicking does translate to improved clinical results, especially when compared to preoperative assessments. The use of medial pivoting implants has been shown to improve postsurgical extension and flexion when compared to presurgical native joint range of motion of the arthritic knee. The mean flexion is also on average 119–122° following prosthetic implantation, which is comparable to existing PS- and CR-implanted knees [8, 10, 11]. Additionally, there is a significant improvement in knee society scores, Western Ontario and McMaster University Osteoarthritis Index questionnaire score, and Oxford knee scores when compared to preoperative scores with survival rates greater than 95% at 17 years following implantation [10]. Patient-reported outcomes as defined by knee society scores, Western Ontario and McMaster University Osteoarthritis Index questionnaire score, and Oxford knee scores when compared to CR and PS prostheses may be equivocal as some studies do confirm significantly improved clinical score differences and even preference for the medial pivoting implant while others show no difference [12–15]. Furthermore, gait speed, gait cadence, push-off force, and stride length did not differ between medical pivoting implants and traditional CR or PS knees [13].

The Use of Patient-Specific Instrumentation

Patient-specific instrumentation involves the creation of specifically customized cutting blocks engineered to an individual patient's anatomy, and, as a result, is for one-time use only. They allow for measured resection and require little soft tissue balancing after the bone cuts are made and trial implants are tested. In order to manufacture PSI, patients require advanced three-dimensional imaging in the form of either an MRI or a CT scan of the knee. Although each proprietary implant system has a unique algorithm to create PSI including the preferred imaging modality, a CT scan, predictably, has more reliable bone modeling includ-

ing 3D architecture to allow reliable production of PSI compared to MRI [16]. After the creation of PSI, the resulting bone resections and subsequent placement of the prosthesis should reliably result in the appropriate position and orientation based on the preoperative plans [17]. This includes the mechanical alignment of the implants [18]. Although overall alignment when compared to conventional instrumentation is on average the same, the use of PSI does limit the outliers in terms of malpositioned instrumentation. Moreover, outliers defined as greater than 3 degrees of varus or valgus beyond physiologic parameters have been shown to have worse functional scores and higher wear rates as early as 2 years out from surgery [19].

Practically, comparing PSI to computer-navigated instrumentation, there are several benefits. The limitations of computer-guided systems include the time to set up the machine and the reference points, the need for additional incisions to place the reference points, and the associated increase in cost for both the initial investment on the machine and the added operative time. Moreover, the accuracy of the bone resection provided by PSI is as accurate as computer-navigated instrumentation [20]. Although PSI does have some added cost in the need for 3D imaging preoperatively, the generation of PSI results in less physical instruments needed within the operating room and quicker placement of PSI based on reliable landmarks (Fig. 5.3). This results in a reduction in the overall number of steps needed from start to finish of the case. So, although the outcomes are equivalent in traditional instrumentation versus PSI, an argument can be made for use when there is a concern for potential loss of traditional bone landmarks on which to determine angulation and rotation of bone resection is required in traditional instrumentation (Fig. 5.4). Furthermore, the reduction in overall instruments needed overall may result in a net decrease in cost in comparison to traditional reusable instrumentation when accounting for storage and processing needs [21].

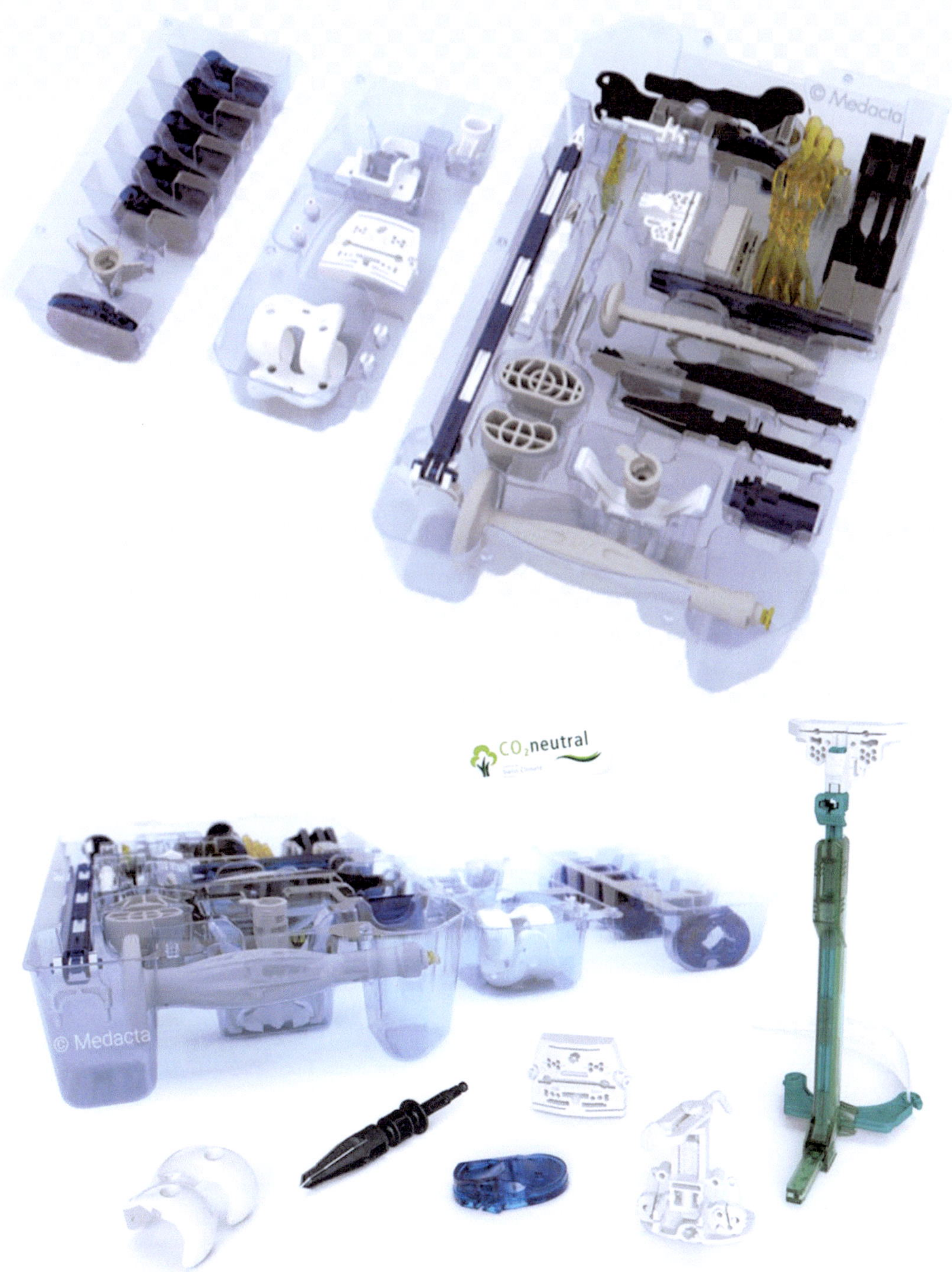

Fig. 5.3 An example of the PSI instruments that would be needed to perform a total knee arthroplasty with the use of the Medacta MyKnee excluding the traditional operating room instruments

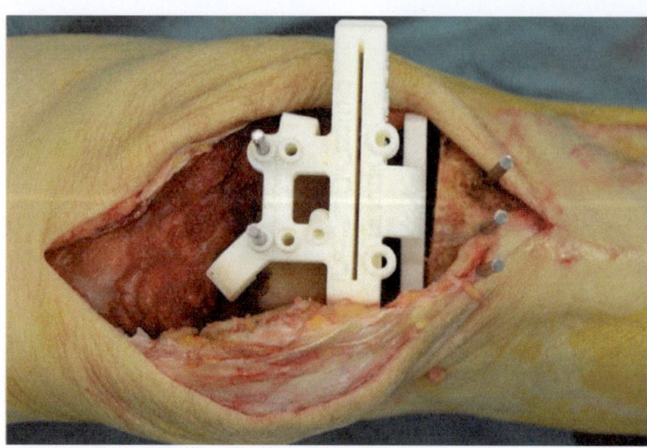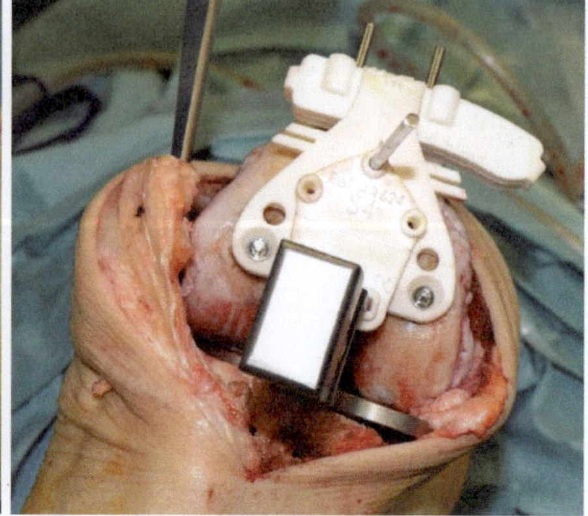

Fig. 5.4 Balancing the knee in extension and in flexion before cutting on the distal femur, allowing a proper judgment of gap tensioning with the help of PSI

Summary

The medial pivot implant designed to recreate native knee kinematics has been shown to accomplish this very goal both in vitro and in vivo when implanted within a patient. The clinical outcomes attributable to the use of medial pivot implantation, whether through implant design and/or patient-specific instrumentation, may be improved compared to traditional total knee arthroplasty prostheses, but further investigation is necessary. The use of PSI in both medial pivot implantation and traditional total knee arthroplasty allows for accurate recreation of the aimed alignment of the knee with a reduction in outliers. This in turn has the potential to reduce polyethylene wear rates, which is a leading cause of revision at 2 years postoperatively. Finally, operating room efficiency appears to be improved with the use of PSI.

References

1. Elias SG, Freeman MA, Gokcay EI. A correlative study of the geometry and anatomy of the distal femur. Clin Orthop Relat Res. 1990;(260):98–103.
2. Atzori F, Salama W, Sabatini L, Mousa S, Khalefa A. Medial pivot knee in primary total knee arthroplasty. Ann Transl Med. 2016;4(1):6. https://doi.org/10.3978/j.issn.2305-5839.2015.12.20.
3. Dennis DA, Komistek RD, Mahfouz MR, Haas BD, Stiehl JB. Multicenter determination of in vivo kinematics after total knee arthroplasty. Clin Orthop Relat Res. 2003;(416):37–57. https://doi.org/10.1097/01.blo.0000092986.12414.b5.
4. Freeman MA, Pinskerova V. The movement of the knee studied by magnetic resonance imaging. Clin Orthop Relat Res. 2003;(410):35–43. https://doi.org/10.1097/01.blo.0000063598.67412.0d.
5. Pinskerova V, Johal P, Nakagawa S, Sosna A, Williams A, Gedroyc W, Freeman MA. Does the femur roll-back with flexion? J Bone Joint Surg Br. 2004;86(6):925–31. https://doi.org/10.1302/0301-620x.86b6.14589.
6. Schütz P, Taylor WR, Postolka B, Fucentese SF, Koch PP, Freeman MAR, Pinskerova V, List R. Kinematic evaluation of the GMK sphere implant during gait activities: a dynamic videofluoroscopy study. J Orthop Res. 2019;37(11):2337–47. https://doi.org/10.1002/jor.24416. Epub 2019 Aug 7. Erratum in: J Orthop Res. 2020 Sep;38(9):2083.
7. Schmidt R, Komistek RD, Blaha JD, Penenberg BL, Maloney WJ. Fluoroscopic analyses of cruciate-retaining and medial pivot knee implants. Clin Orthop Relat Res. 2003;(410):139–147. https://doi.org/10.1097/01.blo.0000063565.90853.a4.
8. Shimmin A, Martinez-Martos S, Owens J, Iorgulescu AD, Banks S. Fluoroscopic motion study confirming the stability of a medial pivot design total knee arthroplasty. Knee. 2015;22(6):522–6. https://doi.org/10.1016/j.knee.2014.11.011. Epub 2014 Dec 7.
9. Mannan K, Scott G. The medial rotation total knee replacement: a clinical and radiological review at a mean follow-up of six years. J Bone Joint Surg Br. 2009;91(6):750–6. https://doi.org/10.1302/0301-620X.91B6.22124.
10. Macheras GA, Galanakos SP, Lepetsos P, Anastasopoulos PP, Papadakis SA. A long term clinical outcome of the medial pivot knee arthro-

plasty system. Knee. 2017;24(2):447–53. https://doi.org/10.1016/j.knee.2017.01.008. Epub 2017 Jan 29.

11. Karachalios T, Roidis N, Giotikas D, Bargiotas K, Varitimidis S, Malizos KN. A mid-term clinical outcome study of the advance medial pivot knee arthroplasty. Knee. 2009;16(6):484–8. https://doi.org/10.1016/j.knee.2009.03.002. Epub 2009 Apr 5.

12. Young T, Dowsey MM, Pandy M, Choong PF. A systematic review of clinical functional outcomes after medial stabilized versus non-medial stabilized total knee joint replacement. Front Surg. 2018;5:25. https://doi.org/10.3389/fsurg.2018.00025.

13. Benjamin B, Pietrzak JRT, Tahmassebi J, Haddad FS. A functional comparison of medial pivot and condylar knee designs based on patient outcomes and parameters of gait. Bone Joint J. 2018;100-B(1 Suppl A):76–82. https://doi.org/10.1302/0301-620X.100B1.BJJ-2017-0605.R1.

14. Batra S, Malhotra R, Kumar V, Srivastava DN, Backstein D, Pandit H. Superior patient satisfaction in medial pivot as compared to posterior stabilized total knee arthroplasty: a prospective randomized study. Knee Surg Sports Traumatol Arthrosc. 2021;29(11):3633–40. https://doi.org/10.1007/s00167-020-06343-4. Epub 2020 Nov 5.

15. Pritchett JW. Patients prefer a bicruciate-retaining or the medial pivot total knee prosthesis. J Arthroplasty. 2011;26(2):224–8. https://doi.org/10.1016/j.arth.2010.02.012. Epub 2010 Oct 6.

16. White D, Chelule KL, Seedhom BB. Accuracy of MRI vs CT imaging with particular reference to patient specific templates for total knee replacement surgery. Int J Med Robot. 2008;4(3):224–31. https://doi.org/10.1002/rcs.201.

17. Cenni F, Timoncini A, Ensini A, Tamarri S, Belvedere C, D'Angeli V, Giannini S, Leardini A. Three-dimensional implant position and orientation after total knee replacement performed with patient-specific instrumentation systems. J Orthop Res. 2014;32(2):331–7. https://doi.org/10.1002/jor.22513. Epub 2013 Oct 30.

18. Vaishya R, Vijay V, Birla VP, Agarwal AK. Computerized tomography based "patient specific blocks" improve postoperative mechanical alignment in primary total knee arthroplasty. World J Orthop. 2016;7(7):426–33. https://doi.org/10.5312/wjo.v7.i7.426.

19. Anderl W, Pauzenberger L, Kölblinger R, Kiesselbach G, Brandl G, Laky B, Kriegleder B, Heuberer P, Schwameis E. Patient-specific instrumentation improved mechanical alignment, while early clinical outcome was comparable to conventional instrumentation in TKA. Knee Surg Sports Traumatol Arthrosc. 2016;24(1):102–11. https://doi.org/10.1007/s00167-014-3345-2. Epub 2014 Oct 19. Erratum in: Knee Surg Sports Traumatol Arthrosc. 2016;24(12):4013.

20. Koch PP, Müller D, Pisan M, Fucentese SF. Radiographic accuracy in TKA with a CT-based patient-specific cutting block technique. Knee Surg Sports Traumatol Arthrosc. 2013;21(10):2200–5. https://doi.org/10.1007/s00167-013-2625-6. Epub 2013 Aug 13.

21. Attard A, Tawy GF, Simons M, Riches P, Rowe P, Biant LC. Health costs and efficiencies of patient-specific and single-use instrumentation in total knee arthroplasty: a randomised controlled trial. BMJ Open Qual. 2019;8(2):e000493. https://doi.org/10.1136/bmjoq-2018-000493.

Surgical Technique of Bicruciate-Retaining Total Knee Arthroplasty: Anatomic and Surgical Considerations of Bicruciate-Retaining TKA

Seth Stake, Pieter Berger, and Hilde Vandeneucker

Introduction

The "modern" era of total knee arthroplasty (TKA) started with the introduction of hinged knee prostheses in the 1950s. These led to the rotating-hinged knee prosthesis, which is now mostly used in revision, tumor, and cases with a high risk of instability [1]. Bicruciate retention has been considered since the advent of non-hinged TKA in the late 1960s.

The implants developed in the 1970s provided a foundation for the concepts and technologies used today. There were two philosophies to approach TKA: the functional approach and the anatomic approach. The functional approach preferred function and mechanics over anatomy. This approach simplified the mechanics of the knee by resecting the condyles and the cruciate ligaments. The anatomic approach aimed to mimic the native knee as closely as possible by preserving both cruciate ligaments and as much soft tissue as possible. Bicruciate-retaining

(BCR) implants adhere to the anatomic approach while most of the current TKAs follow the functional approach because of its simplicity and reliable results [2, 3].

A demographic shift toward a younger, active, and more demanding patient population made TKA a potentially valuable, albeit challenging surgical option. However, imperfect results were noted, including an unacceptable 20% patient satisfaction rate. The majority of these patients do not even come close to the daily activity levels of their healthy peers. Although multifactorial, the loss of proprioception and change in kinematics caused by sacrificing the anterior cruciate ligament (ACL) may play an important role in the suboptimal function and satisfaction of today's TKA patients. As such, resection of the ACL, described as intact in 60–80% of osteoarthritic knees, intuitively seems wrong (ref "ACL status in arthroplasty patients, why not to preserve?" [4]). A further potential advantage of ACL retention lies in improving implant longevity by lessening stress transmission to the implant and the bone-implant interface.

Nevertheless, interest in BCR design has been limited due to concerns regarding fixation strength, ligament balance issues, expected technical difficulties, and potential ACL failure in time. Moreover, studies have shown variable survival rates and discouraging clinical results, which explains why the BCR implant type so far has not been widely used.

S. Stake (✉)
Virtua Medical Group,
Moorestown, NJ, USA

P. Berger
University Hospitals Leuven, Leuven, Belgium
e-mail: pieter.berger@uzleuven.be

H. Vandeneucker
University Hospitals Leuven, Catholic University
Leuven, Leuven, Belgium
e-mail: Hilde.vandenneucker@uzleuven.be

However, promising results of some BCR designs led to the introduction of new designs, aiming to improve previously mentioned concerns.

History

The timeline of BCR implants and corresponding images are displayed in Fig. 6.1. In the mid-1960s, Frank H. Gunston developed a BCR implant and coined it the polycentric knee. This prosthesis utilized two semicircular runners on the femoral condyles which articulated with two corresponding separate tibial components.

In 1972, a group from the Mayo Clinic described the Geometric Total knee, with a single femoral component, consisting of two spherical femoral weight-bearing surfaces joined by a bridge, thereby eliminating the need to separately align each condylar replacement [9]. A prospective study performed by Cracchiolo et al. in 1979 demonstrated similar outcomes comparing subjects treated with polycentric and geometric prostheses.

The anatomic total knee, created by Townley in the later 1970s, included a bilobed horseshoe-shaped femoral implant allowing limited bone resection and retention of both cruciate ligaments [5]. In 1977 in Montreal, Cloutier introduced a modern condylar femoral component combined with a flat U-shaped tibial tray. This unlinked metal-on-plastic prosthesis allowed for unconstrained rotation, rolling, and sliding motion [10]. The prosthesis had a reported 91% good to excellent function.

Up to the 1990s, numerous BCR TKA iterations followed. However, following this period and up until recently, the use of these implants dropped due to technical difficulty, inconclusive benefits, and increased risk of complications.

Kinematics

The fundamental role of the cruciate ligaments in the kinematic behavior of the native knee has been extensively investigated. The ACL is responsible for the majority of the anterior translation restraint of the tibia. The posterior cruciate ligament (PCL) creates, in conjunction with the asymmetrical anatomical articular configuration of the medial and lateral tibial plateau, the external tibial rotation at terminal extension in the so-called screw-home mechanism. As the knee moves again to flexion, the posterior tibial glide

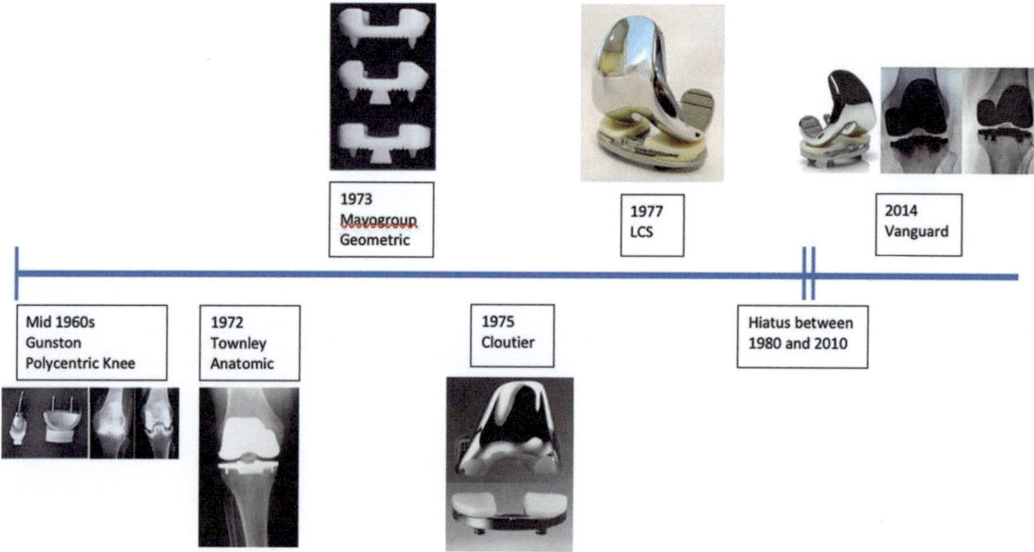

Fig. 6.1 Timeline of BCR TKA implant designs [5–8]

on the longer anteroposterior medial condyle dimension and the ACL are responsible for the tibial internal rotation. As such, the ACL plays an important role in the consistency of anteroposterior contact patterns between femur and tibia [11].

In a study using roentgen stereophotogrammetric analysis (RSA), Karrholm et al. measured a continuously abnormal, reduced internal rotation and tibial adduction in knees with chronic ACL deficiency, as compared to normal knees [12]. Berchuck et al. investigated gait patterns in subjects with ACL-deficient knees and found a significant avoidance of quadriceps contraction in injured patients, notably more abnormal during walking compared to jogging [13].

Therefore, it should not be surprising that many studies showed more normal and natural kinematics, resulting in more physiologic stability, when preserving both cruciate ligaments in TKA [14]. Halewood et al. used eight cadaver specimens to compare a BCR knee design to a cruciate-retaining (CR) TKA and the native knee. They demonstrated a significant difference in AP laxity between the CR TKA and the native knee while no significant differences were observed between BCR TKA and the native knee [15]. In this study, the BCR design had moved back by 65° of flexion, bringing the kinematics close to that in the normal knee, whereas the CR design showed a significant loss of femoral rollback in the absence of the ACL. They concluded that this mechanical improvement might then reduce the sense of instability of some TKA patients experience. Lo et al. investigated 14 cadaveric specimens following BCR TKA using robotic manipulation and a force sensor [16]. The investigators demonstrated that BCR-retaining TKA provided similar joint stability as the native knee, whereas PCL-retaining TKA's resulted in inferior joint stability in varus, valgus, external rotation, and anterior and posterior directions [16]. Moro-Oka et al. compared in vivo kinematics of BCR and PS TKA subjects with stair-stepping, treadmill gait, and fluoroscopic range of motion (ROM) studies. In all three of these activities, BCR TKA knees showed an increased ability to maintain physiologic femoral rollback activity

[6]. Stiehl et al. performed an in vivo weight-bearing fluoroscopic study comparing BCR and posterior cruciate-retaining implants and demonstrated a more anterior contact point in full extension, with gradual femoral rollback in flexion and limited anteroposterior translation in BCR knees [17]. In contrast, cruciate-retaining (CR) TKAs maintained a more posterior contact point in extension and demonstrated paradoxical progressive anterior femoral translation with flexion and exaggerated medial condyle translation on deep flexion [17]. The final conclusion was a more abnormal kinematic performance in the posterior cruciate-retaining designs. In a comparison of in vivo kinematic patterns of anterior cruciate-retaining TKA versus posterior stabilized TKA, Komistek et al. reported anteroposterior contact patterns, axial rotational patterns, and posterior femoral rollback magnitudes that more closely paralleled a healthy native knee in subjects with ACL-retaining implants [18]. In contrast with all these publications in favor of ACL retention, a recent kinematic gait analysis of patients with BCR TKA showed that sagittal plane motion, tibiofemoral articular contact pressures, and pivoting patterns were not fully replicated to natural values [19]. Overall, however, kinematic studies have consistently demonstrated more accurate replication of native knee kinematics in BCR TKA compared to designs that sacrifice one or both cruciate ligaments.

The ACL is also believed to have an added value of improved proprioception [20]. Relph et al. demonstrated decreased proprioception in patients with ACL injuries compared to their contralateral knee [20]. In ACL-sacrificing CR TKA, patients have been shown to have decreased proprioceptive abilities compared to healthy subjects [21]. Using sway analysis, Fuchs et al. compared subjects receiving a unicondylar prosthesis in both medial and lateral compartments with retention of both cruciates to the contralateral intact knee and to healthy controls. The study patients were asked to perform a single-leg stance on a force plate to test proprioception by calculating changes in the projected center of gravity [22]. Subsequent studies continued to show a superior static balance ability when preserving both cruciate ligaments, indicating better maintenance of physiologic proprioceptive ability [23, 24].

As the absence of ACL will cause an anterior translation of the tibia with a resulting slackening of the PCL, the geometry of the tibial inlay needs to compensate for this ACL insufficiency in ACL-sacrificing designs [25]. However, when preserving both cruciate ligaments, a design is needed that reproduces the natural articular geometry as anatomically as possible, respecting the curvature of the condyles, the differential tibial anatomy, the obliquity of the joint line, and the natural tibial slope differences, allowing the cruciate ligaments to carry out their normal function. A balance between articular geometry and the cruciate ligaments plays a crucial role in soft tissue tension and is mandatory to guide the unique normal motion during knee movement.

Design

A new BCR total knee should consider both specific design issues and the instrumentation technique. It should address historical design concerns. The femoral component does not need particular attention. It should have an open intercondylar notch accommodating the remaining tibial bone island containing the fixation of the natural cruciate ligaments. The CR type of a pre-existing design is mostly sufficient (Fig. 6.2). Care must be taken to avoid impingement of the femoral component on the central bone block [26]. The tibial component, however, provided most worries in the past. Due to the need for a central bone island, a central keel for stabilization is not possible. As this leads to limited contact area available for stability, tibial tray fixation has been of major concern [27]. Early prostheses in turn demonstrated a high incidence of loosening. In newer designs, a combination of a more anterior keel and pegs should ideally provide necessary stability. A "U"-shaped tibial tray, connecting the medial and lateral surfaces with a bridge across the anterior side, to fit around the bone island, ensures that the medial and lateral aspect of the trays lies in the same plane. Putting the keel under the anterior surface connection

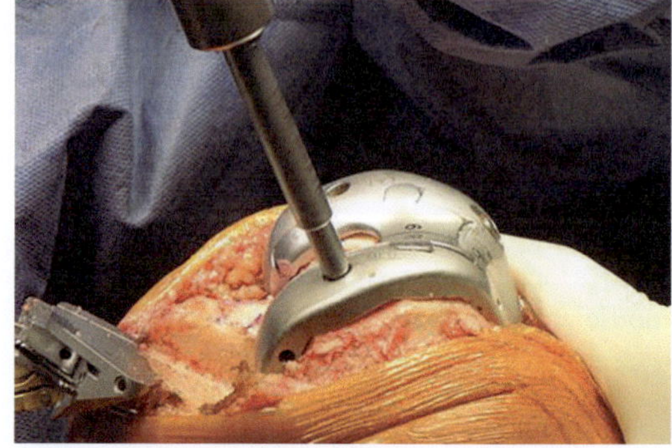

Fig. 6.2 Journey BCR TKA uses the standard femoral CR component (the property of Hilde Vandenneucker)

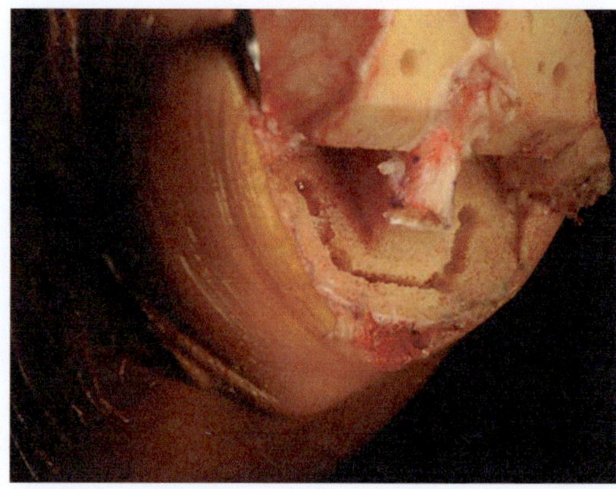

Fig. 6.3 Journey BCR TKA: preparation of anterior keel and fixation pegs (the property of Hilde Vandenneucker)

additionally reinforces the bridge, avoiding stress fractures (Fig. 6.3). The strength of the tibial baseplate should be high enough to withstand physiologic loading. On the other hand, thickness or width can jeopardize the ACL insertion and central bone island stock. Thus, an equilibrium must be found.

Optimized modified tibial instrumentation is necessary to allow for a controlled cut of the medial and lateral tibial surface and to guarantee the central bone island integrity and prevent it from undercutting, reducing the risk of postoperative fractures. Some features in the instrumentation of the newer designs incorporated additional protection for the island while making the bone cuts. The potential use of modern robot technology provides additional value in one of the new BCR designs.

The Vanguard XP (Zimmer-Biomet, Warsaw, IN) and the Journey BCR (Smith & Nephew, Memphis, TN) are the most frequently used implants on today's market. They both have the ability to easily switch from a bicruciate-retaining implant to a CR implant within a single system in case of technical problems, complications during the procedure, or in cases where proper ligament balancing cannot be achieved intraoperatively.

Indications and Surgical Technique

Most frequently, a standard exposure through a medial parapatellar approach is used, although a midvastus or subvastus approach can be considered as long as the patella can be easily everted to guarantee a good view. It is most important to avoid damage to the ACL fibers intraoperatively. Major ligamentous releases should be avoided during the approach as cases of severe deformity usually include a functional ACL and are not an indication for bicruciate-retaining implants.

When choosing classical instrumentation, femoral component preparation is initiated using a standard CR technique with the distal femoral cut. A conservative accurate distal femoral resection is mandatory to maintain the natural joint line. However, insufficient resection can result in increased strain on the ACL fibers, creating a higher risk of avulsion of the island with terminal extension, or negatively influence ACL function. Instrumentation may include a tool to appreciate the amount of distal bone resection prior to moving to the next step (Fig. 6.4).

The femur is then sized in the standard way. A 4-in-1 cutting block is rotated with reference to the transepicondylar axis, perpendicular to Whiteside's line in the same way a CR or PS design would be. The anterior, posterior, and chamfer cuts are made, taking care not to damage the ACL fibers. It is recommended to protect the fibers while cutting (Fig. 6.5). Osteophytes in the notch should be removed in order to avoid ACL impingement.

Tibia preparation needs most of the attention. First, the tibial eminence resection is planned. The sizing template is aligned in the optimal

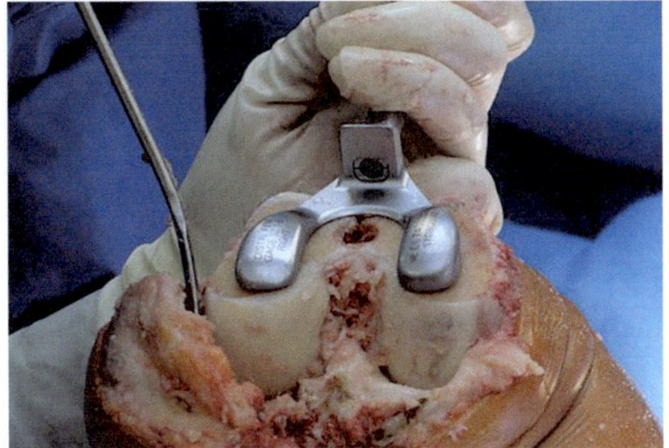

Fig. 6.4 Journey BCR TKA: distal femoral gauge to appreciate the amount of femoral distal bone resection and mark in extension the provisional level of tibial bone resection (the property of Hilde Vandenneucker)

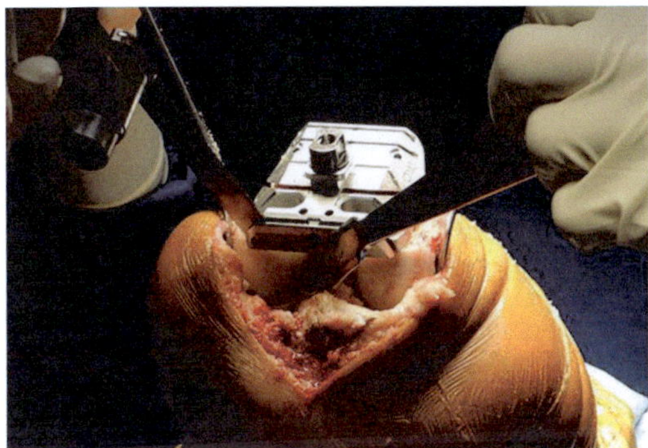

Fig. 6.5 Protection of ACL fibers when performing the femoral anterior, posterior, and chamfer cuts using the 4-in-1 guide (the property of Hilde Vandenneucker)

position for midline medial and lateral coverage, while avoiding significant underhang or overhang, adjusting rotation as necessary. The ACL fibers should be fully captured and protected. Tibia rotation should not be set linked to the placement of the femur, orientation of the ACL fibers, or the tibia tubercle. Optimal tibial coverage is of major importance (Fig. 6.6). An extramedullary tibial guide is placed in alignment with the mechanical axis. First, the valgus/varus position of the guide is checked, followed by setting the slope angle to restore the patient's natural tibial slope. In a third step, the depth of resection is determined at 8 mm from the medial or 11 mm from the lateral high point of the unaffected side of the tibial plateau in a design that restores the oblique natural joint line and therefore uses

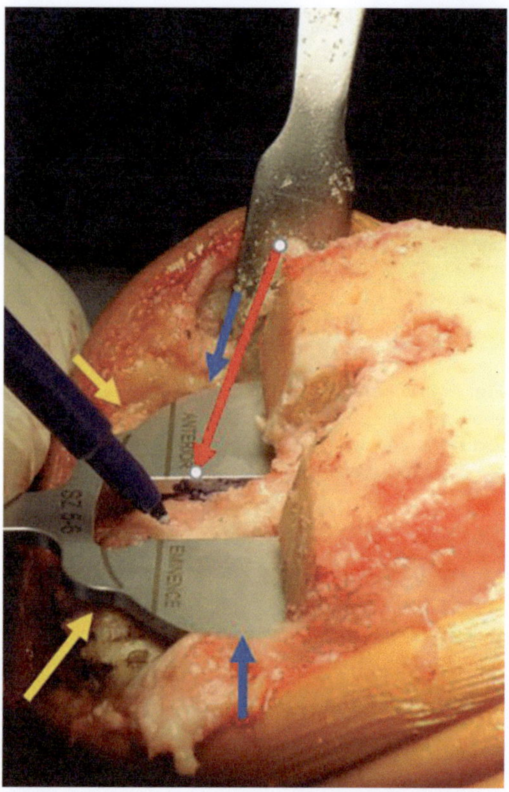

Fig. 6.6 Aligning the sizing template in the optimal position for midline medial/lateral coverage, avoiding overhang or insufficient covering with full capturing of the ACL fibers (the property of Hilde Vandenneucker)

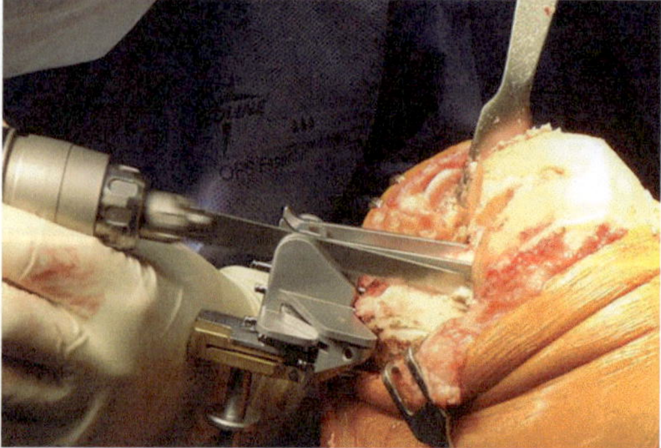

Fig. 6.7 A vertical cutting guide for a protected cut of the central bone island including the cruciate ligaments insertion (the property of Hilde Vandenneucker)

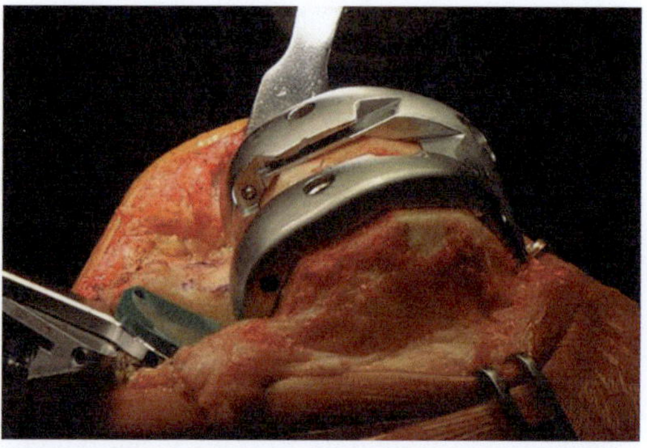

Fig. 6.8 Journey BCR TKA: balancing the medial site (the property of Hilde Vandenneucker)

asymmetrical thickness in the tibial plateau restoration. A vertical resection guide is then aligned to capture the bony island that includes the tibial spines and cruciate ligaments. This eminence stylus is designed to guide a reciprocal saw blade and protect the bone island and cruciate during the vertical cut. Diving and deflection of the saw blade has to be avoided and care should be taken not to damage the posterior tibial cortex (Fig. 6.7). Once the vertical cuts are performed, the horizontal medial resection is carried out and the medial bone of the plateau is removed. Osteophytes, meniscal tissue, and synovial proliferation are removed from the back of the medial side. A first balance check in flexion and extension is then performed using a medial polyethylene spacer block, which is available in different thicknesses and degree of slope. A decision

is made about the necessary additional bone resection and/or adaptation of slope (Fig. 6.8). If mandatory, corrections are performed. In the following step, the lateral horizontal cut is made, taking care to protect the patellar tendon. The lateral plateau is removed and the posterior side of the knee is cleaned of meniscal remnants and osteophytes (Fig. 6.9). A final full trial including both medial and lateral polyethylene inserts is done. A decision about PE implant thickness is made in a perfect balance between excessive laxity and tightness. The design is typically placed with slightly more laxity than a standard PS design. Medial and lateral inserts differ by 3 mm in height to reproduce joint line obliquity and are available in neutral and upslope. The last option may be necessary if the slope in the initial tibial bone cut has been considered too big for optimal

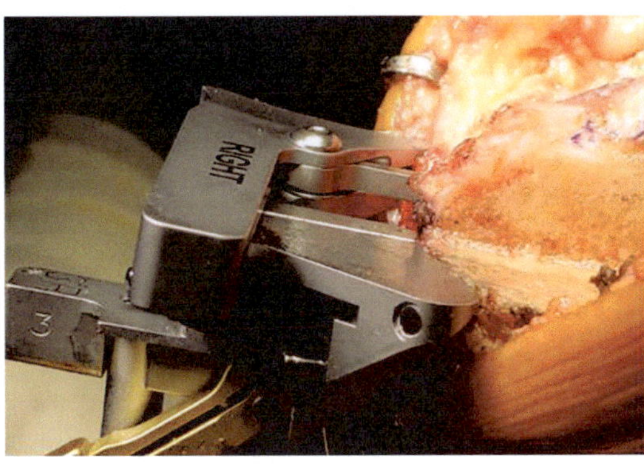
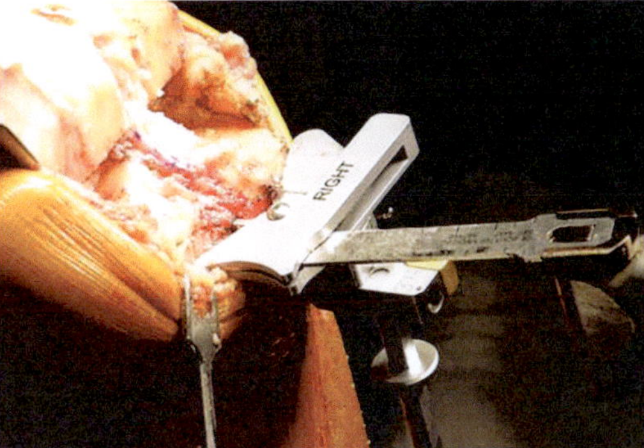

Fig. 6.9   Journey BCR TKA: lateral horizontal cut (the property of Hilde Vandenneucker)

flexion–extension balance (Fig. 6.10). Note that during trialing, the first extension check needs to be done with caution to protect the island from avulsion in case of unexpected high ACL fiber tension. Overextension should be avoided anyway.

The femoral component is then further prepared and patellar resurfacing is performed. Resurfacing of the patella is desirable as the preference for a bicruciate-retaining implant over a unicondylar knee implant is often triggered by concomitant patellofemoral disease. In the final tibia preparation, the anterior eminence resection is done using the available tools of the system. The anterior bridge should avoid the anterior overhang of the tray without creating damage to the tibial ACL insertion. The tibial fixation pegs and anterior keel are then precisely prepared. It is advised to check the strength and quality of the bone island before moving to the final implant placement. In this stage, conversion to a CR or PS implant can still be considered in cases of doubt, requiring only a few extra steps (Figs. 6.10 and 6.11).

The trial implants are removed, extra drill holes are made in sclerotic bone, and the surfaces are irrigated with pulse lavage and dried for cementation. Cement is placed in a thin layer on the tibial tray and additionally on the tibial bone. The tray is placed and impacted starting from the posterior side to push the excess of cement ante-

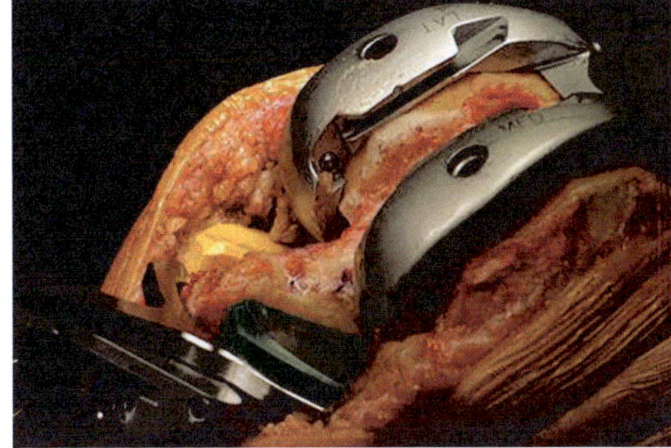

Fig. 6.10   Journey BCR TKA: final implant trial using medial and lateral PE inserts (the property of Hilde Vandenneucker)

riorly. The excess of cement is carefully removed with specific attention to the posterior side. Femoral and patellar components are then cemented in place, and trial PE inserts are positioned until the cement is completely hard, after which the final bearings are placed (Figs. 6.12 and 6.13).

The intraoperative challenges can be diminished using modern instrumentation. Exposure of the tibia is more difficult due to the intact ACL. Damage to the fibers should be avoided during femoral component preparation. The location of the vertical tibial eminence cutting guide determines the rotation and medial /lateral position of the tibial tray and therefore needs careful attention. During tibial preparation, the central

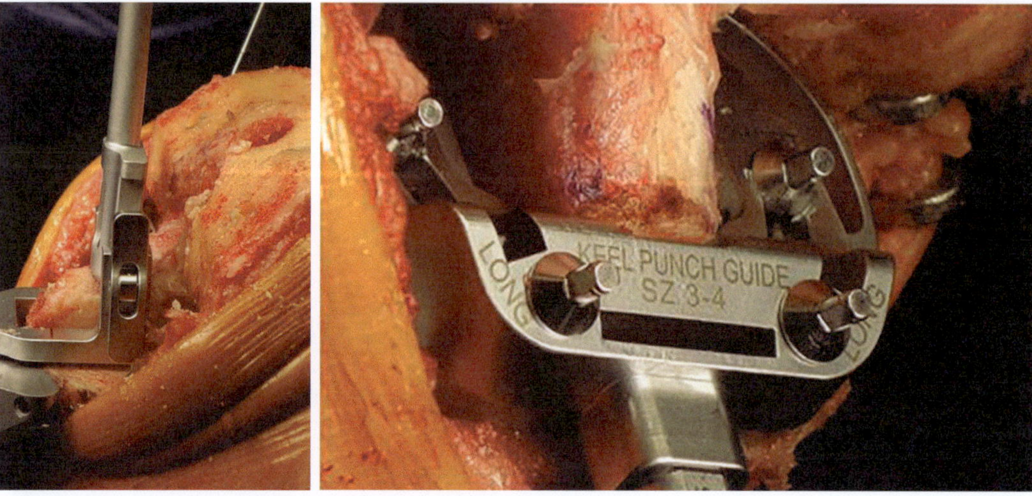

Fig. 6.11 Journey BCR TKA: final tray preparation: resection of anterior eminence and preparing fixation pegs and anterior keel (the property of Hilde Vandenneucker)

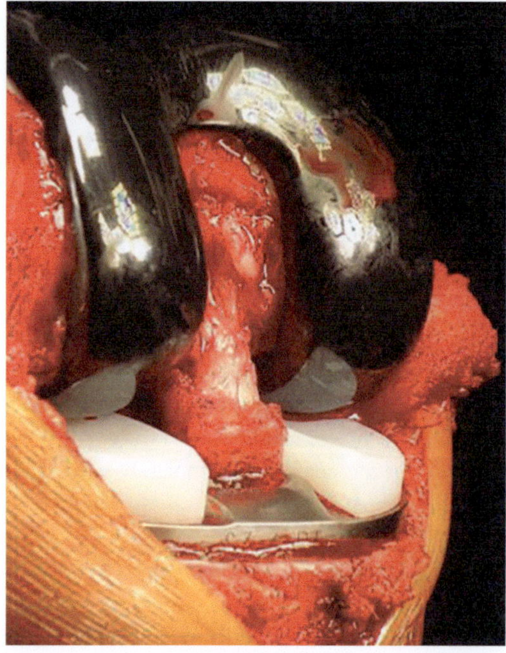

Fig. 6.12 Final clinical image of the Journey BCR TKA implant with medial and lateral polyethylene inserts (the property of Hilde Vandenneucker)

eminence bone island should be protected from undercutting. Island fracture or avulsion is a specific risk. While performing the lateral horizontal cut care should be taken to protect the patellar tendon. The most important design challenge lies at the tibial side. Independent medial and lateral PE implants and a U-shaped implant with a limited anterior bridge between medial and lateral plateau are needed. The rather small bridge is a point of concern due to the risk of fatigue fracture. Unavoidably, the tibial implant bone contact interface is smaller than in the standard implants, putting a challenge on fixation with pegs and an adapted keel.

Robotic-assisted surgery came with additional advantages, allowing to minutely plan the surgery before actually performing cuts. It avoids some of the perioperative risk factors and creates the possibility to adapt femoral and tibial position for an optimal ligament balance throughout the full range of motion.

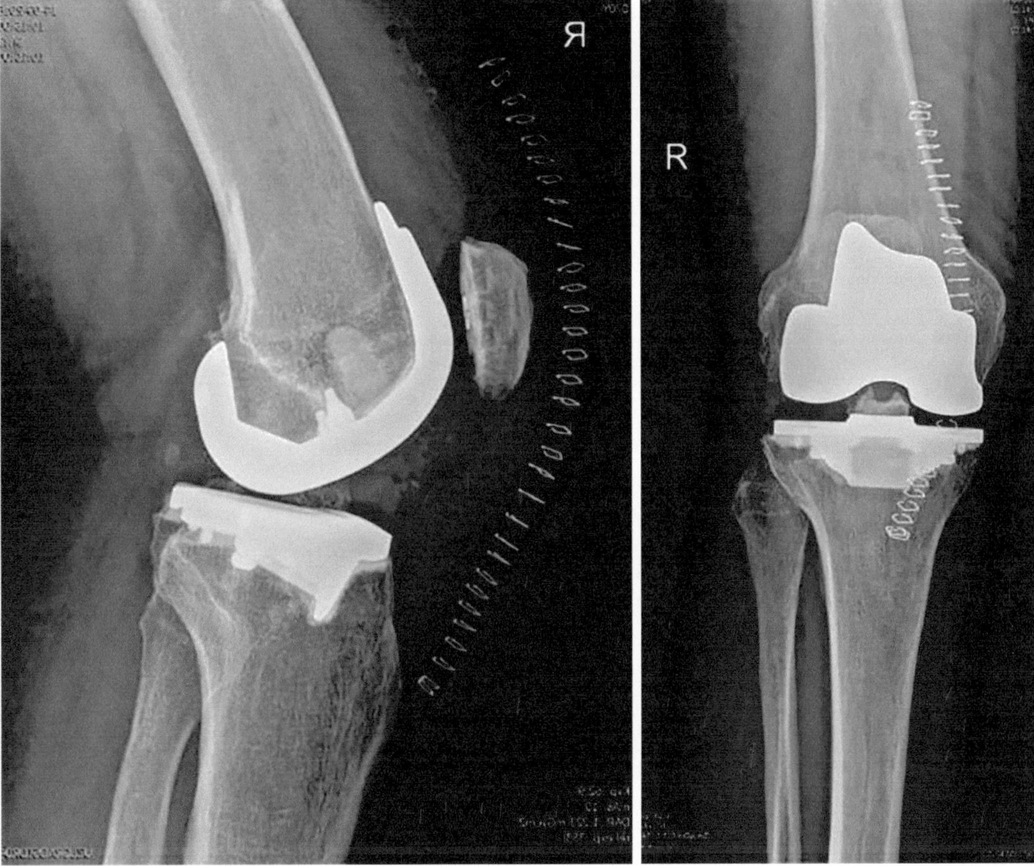

Fig. 6.13 Journey BCR TKA: fully cemented BCR implant with final PE medial and lateral inserts (the property of Hilde Vandenneucker)

Outcomes

Reports of poor clinical outcomes with initial designs, such as the geometric knee, published suboptimal short-term results, and concerns regarding modern designs, such as the Vanguard XR, have caused surgeons to be reluctant to use BCR implants. However, drastically improved designs and instrumentation have resulted in more promising outcomes comparable to those of CR TKA. In addition, a few older designs have demonstrated good long-term survival [27, 28].

Longevity

With a mean follow-up of 3.5 years, Cracchiolo et al. reported the failure rates in first-generation BCR TKA patients and mentioned 11% and 16% for polycentric and geometric knees, respectively. Lewallen et al. reported a survivorship of 66% at 10 years in polycentric implants [29].

While early long-term follow-up studies using first-generation components had poor longevity, survivorship improved with the use of more modern implants. In 1990, Buechel and Pappas published the first long-term outcome study specifically focusing on survivorship in BCR TKA using more modern implants [30]. A total of 46 patients who received low contact-stress, mobile-bearing BCR TKA were compared after 12 years to 57 PCL retaining subjects and 108 cruciate-sacrificing subjects. BCR TKA survivorship was 90.9% compared to 97.9% for the posterior cruciate-retaining design and 97.5% for the cruciate-sacrificing design. In 1999, Cloutier published a report on 10 years of follow-up of 163 BCR TKA knees, reporting a 95% survivorship at 10 years [31]. He concluded that his design offered a reasonable long-term option, even when the cruciate ligaments were partially degenerated. These same Hermes 2C design BCR implants were evaluated in 2013 by Sabouret et al. with a mean follow-up of 22.4 years [5]. The authors of this study preserved the ACL even if it had a partially degenerative appearance, as long as the anterior drawer and Lachman tests were normal [5]. Survivorship was 82% with the majority of revisions due to polyethylene wear.

Boese et al. published a literature review of 13 studies. Eight of them analyzed outcomes of the Vanguard XP implant and cited revision rates of 1–13.5% within 5 years postoperatively [28].

Complications

The polycentric TKA was found to have high complication rates of 34% [7]. Short-term studies demonstrated a high rate of loosening (1.8–10%) as well as a high rate of infection (2–7%) [7, 32–36]. Fractures and dislocations were also noted in these implants, often caused by malalignment, insufficient cementing, and poor fit. Long-term follow-up studies of polycentric TKA reported loosening rates of 4.2–7% [29, 36, 37]. In order to improve loosening rates, the wide-track polycentric knee was introduced, which was meant to increase the surface area. However, the incidence of lateral subluxation increased in these components [5].

The geometric prosthesis showed similar high rates of loosening and infections. Developers of this design noted a learning curve, with decreased complication rates as experience increased. The non-constrained natural LCS TKA (Depuy, West Chester, PA), Search TKA (Aesculap, Tuttlingen, Germany), Hermes 2C (Ceraver, Roissy-En-France, France), and Vanguard XP were developed with the aim to lower the rate of aseptic loosening and other early revision causes found in the early designs. The non-constrained natural TKA, developed by Cloutier based on the Townley anatomic TKA, showed good long-term

clinical results with reduced incidence of loosening (0.9–1.8%) [10, 30]. This implant has been largely abandoned as the metal-backed design carries a risk of metallosis. While loosening was found to be rare in the Hermes 2C implant (0.6% at 9–11 years), polyethylene failure was a reason for revision in 12.3% of knees at 22 years postoperatively [5, 30]. Despite continued design advancement, the Vanguard XP TKA reported lower than expected survivorship with aseptic loosening as the leading cause (5% at 3 years).

Patient Reported

BCR TKA has been shown to consistently improve the knee society score (KSS) compared to low preoperative scores [28]. The Townley Anatomic TKA, introduced in 1972, cited good to excellent outcomes in 89% of knees with an average KSS of 91 [8]. Cloutier found similarly encouraging results, even including patients with degenerative ACL changes, with 104 out of 107 patients reporting excellent results with an average KSS of 91 at 9–11 years postoperatively [31]. Studies on the Vanguard XP TKA have also demonstrated excellent outcomes, with a 94% satisfaction rate cited by Alnachoukati et al. [8].

However, postoperative ROM studies showed variable results. While some studies showed improved range of motion (ROM) postoperatively, others have demonstrated decreased ROM compared to preoperative values [28]. Boese et al. performed a meta-analysis of BCR TKA studies, finding mean terminal flexion below 110° in 4 studies and below 120° in 11 studies, with only 4 studies above 120° [28]. In second-generation studies, despite patient-reported outcomes being reported with higher frequencies, no significant differences were noted in terms of either KSS or ROM [28].

Direct functional comparisons between implant types have been made in patients with bilateral TKA. Pritchett examined patients who underwent staged-bilateral TKA using different prostheses on each side [38, 39]. In 1996 and 2011, 70% and 89.1% of subjects stated a preference for the BCR implant to the medial pivot, posterior stabilizing, or mobile-bearing contralateral implant. On the contrary, Jenny and Jenny performed a comparison of ACL-retaining components to ACL-sacrificing TKA at 2–3-year follow-up with less positive results [40]. The authors of this study found no difference in terms of KSS, postoperative ROM, or radiographic outcomes, concluding that there was no advantage of BCR TKA vs ACL-sacrificing implants [40].

Mixed literature regarding the benefit of ACL preservation in TKA has sparked controversy surrounding the utility of BCR TKA.

strate a high proportion of excellent functional scores following BCR TKA implantation.
- With difficult intraoperative visualization, a questionable track record of loosening rates, and mixed results in terms of proposed benefits (kinematics, proprioception, improved knee scores postoperatively), the utility of BCR TKA remained controversial. Significant improvement in design and instrumentation, together with the potential advantages of robot-assisted surgery, could make this design a valuable option in the portfolio of the knee arthroplasty surgeon.

Summary

Since the original BCR TKA was developed by Gunston in the late 1960s, numerous iterations of ACL-sparing implants have been introduced. Due to technical difficulties, inconclusive benefits, and the increased risk of complications such as aseptic loosening, the utility of these implants remained controversial. With improved designs and refined operative techniques, BCR TKA has the potential to re-emerge as a viable option in patients seeking a more kinematically designed implant for the treatment of end-stage knee osteoarthritis.

Key Study Points
- Gunston developed the first BCR TKA in the 1960s.
- The original modern ACL-sparing implant, the anatomic total knee, was developed by Townley in the 1970s.
- Cadaveric studies have revealed kinematics similar to native knees in BCR TKA specimens compared to posterior stabilized knees.
- Early implant designs showed high rates of aseptic loosening due to low implantation surface area in ACL-sparing components. Newer designs have displayed greater survivorship with decreased rates of loosening.
- Histopathologic studies on patients undergoing ACL-sparing TKA demonstrate significant degenerative change in the majority of subjects. However, even in patients with ACL degeneration, the majority of studies demon-

References

1. Aubriot JH, Deburge A, Genet JP. GUEPAR hinge knee prosthesis. Orthop Traumatol Surg Res. 2014;100:27.
2. Makridis K, Karachalios T. A brief history of total knee arthroplasty. In: Total knee arthroplasty: long term outcomes. 2015.
3. Schindler O. Insall & Scott surgery of the knee. J Bone Joint Surg Br. 2006;88-B:1678.
4. Johnson AJ, Howell SM, Costa CR, Mont MA. The ACL in the arthritic knee: how often is it present and can preoperative tests predict its presence? Knee Clin Orthop Relat Res. 2013;471(1):181–8.
5. Sabouret P, Lavoie F, Cloutier JM. Total knee replacement with retention of both cruciate ligaments: a 22-year follow-up study. Bone Joint J. 2013;95-B:917.
6. Moro-Oka TA, Muenchinger M, Canciani JP, Banks SA. Comparing in vivo kinematics of anterior cruciate-retaining and posterior cruciate-retaining total knee arthroplasty. Knee Surg Sport Traumatol Arthrosc. 2007;15(1):93–9.
7. Gunston FH. Polycentric knee arthroplasty. Prosthetic simulation of normal knee movement. J Bone Joint Surg Br. 1971;53-B:272.
8. Alnachoukati OK, Emerson RH, Diaz E, Ruchaud E, Ennin KA. Modern day bicruciate-retaining total knee arthroplasty: a short-term review of 146 knees. J Arthroplasty. 2018;33:2485.
9. Cracchiolo A, Benson M, Finerman GAM. A prospective comparative clinical analysis of the first-generation knee replacements: polycentric vs. geometric knee arthroplasty. Clin Orthop Relat Res. 1979;(145):37–46.
10. Cloutier JM. Results of total knee arthroplasty with a non-constrained prosthesis. J Bone Joint Surg Am. 1983;65:906.
11. Kim HY, Kim KJ, Yang DS, Jeung SW, Choi HG, Choy WS. Screw-home movement of the tibiofemoral

joint during normal gait: three-dimensional analysis. CiOS Clin Orthop Surg. 2015;7(3):303–9.

12. Kärrholm J, Selvik G, Elmqvist LG, Hansson LI. Active knee motion after cruciate ligament rupture: stereoradiography. Acta Orthop. 1988;59:158.

13. Berchuck M, Andriacchi TP, Bach BR, Reider B. Gait adaptations by patients who have a deficient anterior cruciate ligament. J Bone Joint Surg Am. 1990;72:871.

14. Andriacchi TP, Galante JO, Fermier RW. The influence of total knee-replacement design on walking and stair-climbing. J Bone Joint Surg Am. 1982;64:1328.

15. Halewood C, Traynor A, Bellemans J, Victor J, Amis AA. Anteroposterior laxity after bicruciate-retaining total knee arthroplasty is closer to the native knee than ACL-resecting TKA: a biomechanical cadaver study. J Arthroplasty. 2015;30(12):2315–9.

16. Lo JH, Müller O, Dilger T, Wülker N, Wünschel M. Translational and rotational knee joint stability in anterior and posterior cruciate-retaining knee arthroplasty. Knee. 2011;18(6):491–5.

17. Stiehl JB, Komistek RD, Cloutier JM, Dennis DA. The cruciate ligaments in total knee arthroplasty: a kinematic analysis of 2 total knee arthroplasties. J. Arthroplasty. 2000;15(5):545–50.

18. Komistek RD, Allain J, Anderson DT, Dennis DA, Goutallier D. In vivo kinematics for subjects with and without an anterior cruciate ligament. Clin Orthop Relat Res. 2002;404:315–25.

19. Tsai TY, et al. Bi-cruciate retaining total knee arthroplasty does not restore native tibiofemoral articular contact kinematics during gait. J Orthop Res. 2019;37:1929.

20. Relph N, Herrington L, Tyson S. The effects of ACL injury on knee proprioception: a meta-analysis. Physiotherapy. 2014;100(3):187–95.

21. Fuchs S, Thorwesten L, Niewerth S. Proprioceptive function in knees with and without total knee arthroplasty. Am J Phys Med Rehabil. 1999;78:39.

22. Fuchs S, Tibesku CO, Genkinger M, Laass H, Rosenbaum D. Proprioception with bicondylar sledge prostheses retaining cruciate ligaments. Clin Orthop Relat Res. 2003;(406):148–54.

23. Baumann F. Bicruciate-retaining total knee arthroplasty compared to cruciate-sacrificing TKA: what are the advantages and disadvantages? Expert Rev Med Devices. 2018;15:615.

24. Osmani FA, Thakkar SC, Collins K, Schwarzkopf R. The utility of bicruciate-retaining total knee arthroplasty. Arthroplast Today. 2017;3:61.

25. Fantozzi S, Leardini A, Banks SA, Marcacci M, Giannini S, Catani F. Dynamic in-vivo tibio-femoral and bearing motions in mobile bearing knee arthroplasty. Knee Surg Sport Traumatol Arthrosc. 2004;12(2):144–51.

26. Bellemans J. Bicruciate-substituting and bicruciate-replacing arthroplasty of the knee: technique and results. In: The knee: a comprehensive review. 2010.

27. Cherian JJ, Kapadia BH, Banerjee S, Jauregui JJ, Harwin SF, Mont MA. Bicruciate-retaining total knee arthroplasty: a review. J Knee Surg. 2014;27(3):199–205.

28. Boese CK, Ebohon S, Ries C, De Faoite D. Bi-cruciate retaining total knee arthroplasty: a systematic literature review of clinical outcomes. Arch Orthop Trauma Surg. 2020;141:293.

29. Buechel FF, Pappas MJ. Long-term survivorship analysis of cruciate-sparing versus cruciate-sacrificing knee prostheses using meniscal bearings. Clin Orthop Relat Res. 1990;(260):162–169.

30. Cloutier JM, Sabouret P, Deghrar A. Total knee arthroplasty with retention of both cruciate ligaments: a nine to eleven-year follow-up study. J Bone Joint Surg Am. 1999;81:697.

31. Bryan RS, Peterson LFA, Combs JJ. Polycentric knee arthroplasty. A review of 84 patients with more than one year follow up. Clin Orthop Relat Res. 1973;(94):136–9.

32. Bloom JD, Bryan RS. Wide-track polycentric total knee arthroplasty: one year follow-up study. Clin Orthop Relat Res. 1977;(128):210–13.

33. Ilstrup DM, Combs JJ, Bryan RS. A statistical evaluation of polycentric total knee arthroplasties. Clin Orthop Relat Res. 1976;(120):18–26.

34. Gunston FH, MacKenzie RI. Complications of polycentric knee arthroplasty. Clin Orthop Relat Res. 1976:(120):11–7.

35. Manske PR, Debender JOHNJ. Polycentric total knee arthroplasty. South Med J. 1977;70:1088.

36. Thomas BJ, Cracchiolo A, Lee YF, Chow GH, Navarro R, Dorey F. Total knee arthroplasty in rheumatoid arthritis. A comparison of the polycentric and total condylar prostheses. Clin Orthop Relat Res. 1991;(265):129–36.

37. Townley CO. The anatomic total knee resurfacing arthroplasty. Clin Orthop Relat Res. 1985;(192):82–96.

38. Pritchett JW. Patients prefer a bicruciate-retaining or the medial pivot total knee prosthesis. J Arthroplasty. 2011;26(2):224–8.

39. Pritchett JW. Patient preferences in knee prostheses. J Bone Joint Surg Br. 2004;86-B:979.

40. Jenny JY, Jenny G. Preservation of anterior cruciate ligament in total knee arthroplasty. Arch Orthop Trauma Surg. 1998;118:145.

Current Concepts in Predictive Modeling and Artificial Intelligence

Cécile Batailler, Timothy Lording, Daniele De Massari, Sietske Witvoet-Braam, Stefano Bini, and Sébastien Lustig

Introduction

Total knee arthroplasty (TKA) is an efficient surgical treatment for advanced osteoarthritis of the knee. The number of total knee replacements performed annually in the United States is expected to grow by 673% to 3.48 million procedures by 2030 [1]. However, despite the recent advances in knee arthroplasty, patient dissatisfaction, and suboptimal patient-reported outcomes are reported to be as high as 20% [2, 3]. With the rise of robotic surgery, a time may come when the procedure itself will no longer be considered a feature that significantly determines outcomes. A feature is considered as a variable or a factor. In such a scenario, understanding how other groups of variables such as patient-specific attributes, functional measures, socioeconomic indicators, or perioperative recovery location influence clinical outcomes will become increasingly important. Conceivably, using relevant data points incorporated into an algorithm, the insights derived for any given patient could impact surgical indications, procedure type, venue of surgery, and even recovery site.

The use of clinical criteria to predict the outcomes of surgery and, by extension, the indication for surgery, such as the use of Patient-Reported Outcome Measure (PROM) or radiographic findings, may not be as applicable in patients with multiple risk factors. Furthermore, these kinds of clinical parameters alone do not completely explain the results after TKA. Some publications have identified nonclinical features influencing patient satisfaction after TKA such as the patient's mental health, socioeconomic status, and demographic characteristics [4–9]. However, the relative importance and interplay between preoperative clinical parameters and demographic variables as predictors of postoperative satisfaction or functional outcomes are still not completely understood.

Predictive modeling is a discipline where algorithms are deployed to generate estimates for a specific target output. Predictive models learn (are "trained") to identify the relationships between a set of features, also called predictors (e.g., a patient's age, BMI, level of fitness, etc.), and the selected target (e.g., occurrence of a

C. Batailler (✉) · S. Lustig
Orthopedic Surgery Department, Lyon North University Hospital, Croix-Rousse Hospital, Hospices Civils de Lyon, Lyon, France

Université Lyon, Université Claude Bernard Lyon 1, IFSTTAR, LBMC UMR_T9406, Villeurbanne, France

T. Lording
Melbourne Orthopaedic Group, Windsor, Australia

D. De Massari · S. Witvoet-Braam
Stryker, Amsterdam, the Netherlands
e-mail: daniele.demassari@stryker.com; sietske.witvoet@stryker.com

S. Bini
University of California, San Francisco, CA, USA

© The Author(s), under exclusive license to Springer Nature Switzerland AG 2023
A. J. Deshmukh et al. (eds.), *Surgical Management of Knee Arthritis*,
https://doi.org/10.1007/978-3-031-47929-8_7

myocardial infarction). Statistical models (e.g., regression models) and machine learning techniques (e.g., random forest models or neural networks) are used to learn the complex target-predictors relationship hidden in the data [10]. Deep learning models (e.g., neural networks with several hidden layers) have seen wide success in image recognition and classification where the input is represented by unstructured data (e.g., pixel values) [11]. Predictive models are usually deployed in contexts where the measurement of the output is difficult, time demanding, and expensive or when an early estimate of the target can trigger a proactive intervention to modify the course of action and, for instance, avoid adverse events (e.g., re-admission to the hospital). The increasing availability of large digital healthcare data sets (i.e., large number of features and samples) has facilitated the application of predictive models in different healthcare settings such as lung cancer screening, cognitive impairment detection [12], prediction of heart failure patient re-admission [13], or medical image segmentation [14]. A similar trend is expected to occur in the orthopedic field where new technologies, such as surgical robots and wearable devices, are transforming the traditional data landscape by introducing new features that will provide a more comprehensive description of the patient journey. While this wealth of information can be overwhelming and difficult to be interpreted by a human, it generates the context where machine-learning models thrive and achieve the best performances [15, 16].

To address this unmet concern, several studies have published predictive models for TKA outcomes that have taken into account a number of features such as functional scores and preoperative pain [17], comorbidities [18], demographic characteristics, psychological features [19–21], and socioeconomic status [19]. The goal was to use these probabilistic models to estimate and predict the likelihood of improvements in function and satisfaction after TKA with the goal of supporting patient and surgeon decision-making [15]. Ever more complex algorithmic approaches have been developed, however none of these have so far been able to replicate standard surgeon

intuition [22] or become a practical tool for clinical use [23].

Currently, to our knowledge, no study summarizes which features have been identified as the most predictive of clinical outcomes or which algorithms have been most successfully used in predictive analytics following TKA. The purpose of this chapter is therefore to systematically review the relevant literature on predictive factors and predictive models for outcome after TKA. This chapter will describe the preoperative predictive features, which have been identified as having the strongest correlation with outcomes and patient satisfaction after TKA. Second, it will review the machine-learning models that have been identified as the most predictive of TKA results.

Methods

Article Identification and Selection Process

In April 2020, a query was performed to identify all available literature that described or used predictive models for outcomes after TKA. The search was performed through PubMed, EMBASE, and MEDLINE databases from 1996 to 2020 inclusive using the 2009 Preferred Reporting Items for Systematic Reviews and Meta-Analyses protocol (PRISMA).

Inclusion criteria for the search strategy included all English language studies reporting information regarding the use of predictive models or the identification of preoperative predictive factors for outcomes after TKA. The following terms were used: "total knee arthroplasty" or "total knee replacement"; "predictive factor" or "predictive model" or "predictive modeling" or "predictive feature"; and "outcomes," "satisfaction," "pain," or "PROM." Exclusion criteria consisted of (1) editorial articles, (2) systematic reviews or meta-analyses, (3) articles on revision TKA, and (4) articles evaluating joints other than the knee. The abstracts from all identified articles were independently reviewed by two investigators. Articles were excluded on the basis of the title and abstract if they did not assess predictive factors for TKA outcomes. Full-text articles were obtained for review to allow further assessment of inclusion and exclusion criteria when necessary.

Additionally, all references from the included studies were reviewed and reconciled to verify that no relevant articles were missing from this systematic review that met inclusion criteria.

Quality Assessment

The ROBINS-I tool (Risk Of Bias In Non-Randomized Studies of Interventions) [24] was used to evaluate the quality of the included studies and their relative risk of bias. This included bias due to confounding, selection of participants, classification of interventions, deviations from intended interventions, missing data, measurement of outcomes, and selection of reported results. The categories for risk of bias judgments are "Low risk," "Moderate risk," "Serious risk," and "Critical risk." The worst judgment bias assigned within any one domain gives the judgment score of the complete study. The level of evidence was also noted for each included study. To increase the reliability of this classification, the same observer evaluated all articles with the ROBINS-I tool two times separated by an interval of 4 weeks. If the assessment of the study quality was not the same during these two evaluations, a second observer evaluated the concerned article with the ROBINS-I tool.

Results

Included Articles and Study Characteristics

The PRISMA flow diagram for study selection is shown in Fig. 7.1. A total of 64 potential full-text articles were identified by the search strategy. Of the 64 articles, 13 were excluded as not relevant and 8 were excluded due to their scoring a "critical risk of bias" score, leaving 43 studies for inclusion. Twenty-one included studies had a

level of evidence of II, 21 had a level of evidence of III and 1 study had a level of evidence of IV. Of these, 5 studies presented a "low risk of bias" score according to the ROBINS-I [24], 28 studies presented a "moderate risk of bias," and 10 studies presented a "serious risk of bias" (Table 7.1). The reported follow-up periods ranged from 30 days to 5 years. The majority of the studies assessed postoperative outcomes in the first year after TKA and 22 studies had more than 500 patients in their cohorts. Ten studies proposed a predictive model for outcomes after TKA.

Predictive Factors

Several parameters were consistently identified in different studies as impacting outcomes after TKA. The "outcomes" after TKA corresponded to the reported functional results of patients after a TKA with varying follow-up. These parameters included satisfaction, pain during different activities, range of motion, and capacity to perform daily activities. These outcomes were mainly assessed using functional knee scores. The parameters we identified have been classified into three groups according to the strength and frequency of their association with any outcome: (1) a strong and consistent association; (2) a strong but inconsistent association; and (3) a weak and inconsistent association.

The predictive factors classified in group I (strong association) were significantly correlated with outcomes after TKA ($p < 0.05$) in all studies with low or moderate risk, which assessed these factors. The predictive factors classified in group II (strong but inconsistent association) were significantly correlated with TKA outcomes ($p < 0.05$) in low- or moderate- risk studies, but not in all. For this group, relevant studies found a significant correlation, but other relevant studies did not find the same strong association. The predictive factors classified in group III (weak association) were not significantly correlated with TKA outcomes in the low- or moderate-risk studies. The correlation between predictive factors and TKA outcomes for each study is reported in Tables 7.2 and 7.3.

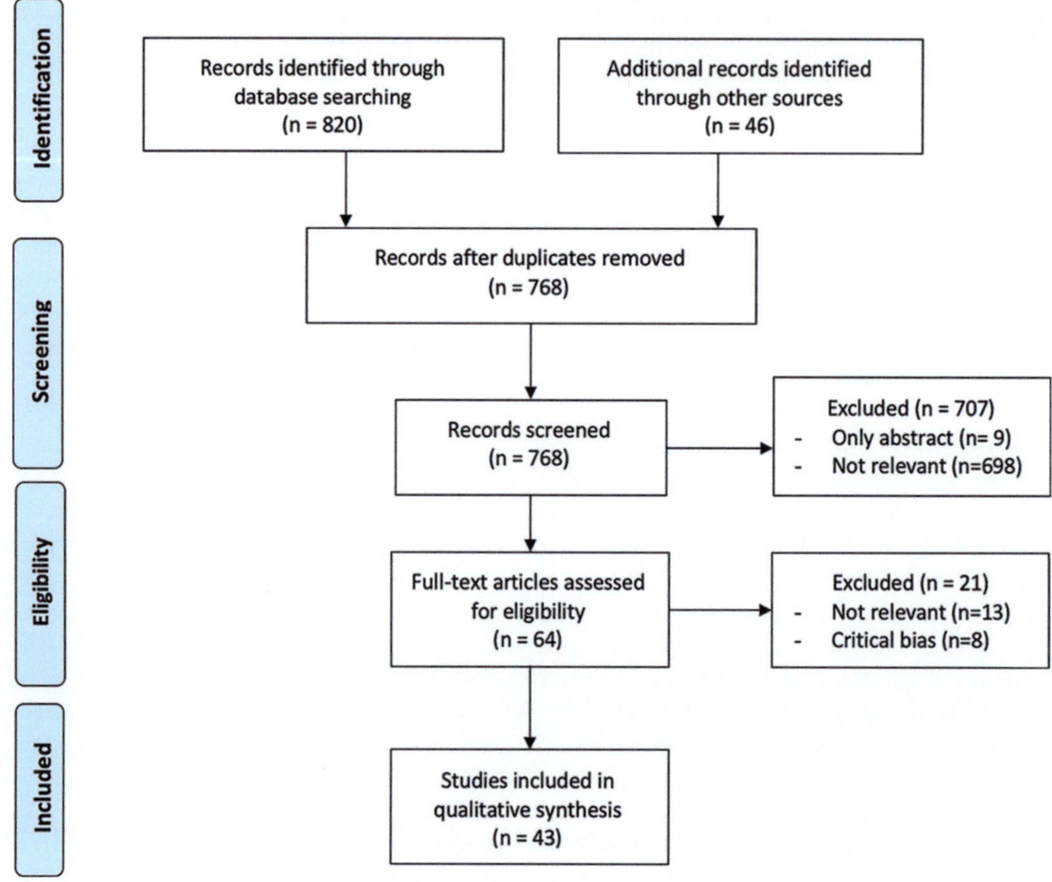

Fig. 7.1 Flow chart from initial literature search through to data extraction from the final list of included studies

Predictive Features with a Strong and Clear Association with Outcomes

Several features presented a clear association with postoperative outcomes after TKA in all studies and were identified as crucial to developing an effective predictive model.

- Preoperative pain

  Patients with higher levels of pain prior to TKA surgery had lower postoperative functional scores. However, improvements in pain scores, functional knee scores, and patient satisfaction were greater in this group. Huijbregts et al. found that a one-point increase in preoperative NRS pain (Numerical Rating Scale) resulted in a 1.73-point decrease in 1-year OKS [25]. And while preoperative pain also strongly correlated with early postoperative pain and opioid consumption during hospitalization, several other studies confirmed the association with improved postoperative satisfaction [26–29].

- Preoperative PROM score

  Preoperative PROM scores, particularly knee-specific measures, were strongly correlated with outcomes after TKA [18]. Tolk et al. found that the preoperative KOOS-PS question that included the sit-to-stand test (Knee injury and Osteoarthritis Outcome Score—Physical Function Short Form) was the strongest predictor for residual complaints associated with the sit-to-stand function for female patients (OR:1.61, 95% CI: 1.374–1.882) [30]. Similar results were described with other knee PROM scores [27, 28]. Clement et al. demonstrated that poorer

Table 7.1 Summary of quality assessment of the studies included in our analysis, according to the ROBINS-I tool (Risk Of Bias In Non-Randomized Studies of Interventions).[24] The categories for risk of bias judgments are "Low risk," "Moderate risk," "Serious risk," and "Critical risk." The worst judgment bias assigned within any one domain gives the judgement score of the complete study

Study	Confounding	Selection of patients	Classification of interventions	Deviations from intended interventions	Missing data	Measurement of outcomes	Selection of reported results	Study risk
Brander (2003)	Moderate	Low	Low	Low	Low	Moderate	Moderate	Moderate
Lingard (2004)	Moderate	Low	Moderate	Low	Moderate	Moderate	Moderate	Moderate
Bourne (2007)	Moderate	Moderate	Low	Low	Low	Moderate	Low	Moderate
Escobar (2007)	Moderate	Low	Low	Low	Low	Moderate	Low	Moderate
Davis (2008)	Moderate	Low	Low	Low	Moderate	Moderate	Moderate	Moderate
Franklin (2008)	Low	Low	Low	Low	Low	Low	Low	Low
Nilsdotter (2008)	Serious	Moderate	Moderate	Low	Moderate	Serious	Moderate	Serious
Rajgopal (2008)	Moderate	Low	Low	Low	Moderate	Low	Moderate	Moderate
Dowsey (2010)	Moderate	Low	Low	Low	Low	Moderate	Low	Moderate
Bourne (2010)	Moderate	Moderate	Moderate	Low	Low	Serious	Moderate	Serious
Blackbum (2012)	Moderate	Moderate	Moderate	Low	Moderate	Moderate	Low	Moderate
Judge (2012)	Moderate	Low	Moderate	Low	Serious	Serious	Moderate	Serious
Baker (2012)	Moderate	Low	Low	Low	Moderate	Moderate	Low	Moderate
Schnurr (2013)	Moderate	Moderate	Low	Low	Moderate	Moderate	Moderate	Moderate
Barlow (2014)	Serious	Moderate	Moderate	Low	Serious	Serious	Moderate	Serious
Lungu (2014)	Moderate	Moderate	Low	Low	Serious	Serious	Moderate	Serious
Sueyoshi (2015)	Moderate	Low	Moderate	Low	Moderate	Moderate	Low	Moderate
Huijbregts (2015)	Moderate	Low	Low	Low	Moderate	Low	Moderate	Moderate
Maratt (2015)	Moderate	Moderate	Moderate	Low	Moderate	Moderate	Moderate	Moderate
Feldmann (2015)	Serious	Moderate	Low	Low	Moderate	Serious	Low	Serious
Maempel (2016)	Low	Low	Low	Low	Low	Low	Low	Low
Van Onsem (2016)	Moderate	Moderate	Low	Low	Moderate	Moderate	Low	Moderate
Giurea (2016)	Moderate	Low	Moderate	Low	Moderate	Moderate	Moderate	Moderate
Hinarejos (2016)	Moderate	Low	Moderate	Low	Low	Moderate	Moderate	Moderate
Kremers (2017)	Low	Moderate	Low	Moderate	Serious	Moderate	Serious	Serious
Jain (2017)	Serious	Serious	Moderate	Low	Moderate	Serious	Moderate	Serious
Sanchez Santos (2018)	Low	Low	Low	Low	Low	Low	Low	Low
Clement (2018)	Moderate	Low	Low	Low	Moderate	Moderate	Low	Moderate

(continued)

Table 7.1 (continued)

Study	Confounding	Selection of patients	Classification of interventions	Deviations from intended interventions	Missing data	Measurement of outcomes	Selection of reported results	Study risk
Van Onsem (2018)	Serious	Moderate	Moderate	Low	Serious	Serious	Moderate	Serious
Clement (2018)	Moderate	Low	Moderate	Low	Moderate	Moderate	Moderate	Moderate
Abrecht (2019)	Moderate	Moderate	Moderate	Low	Low	Moderate	Low	Moderate
Calkins (2019)	Low	Serious	Moderate	Low	Low	Serious	Low	Serious
Twiggs (2019)	Low	Low	Low	Low	Low	Low	Low	Low
Tolk (2019)	Moderate	Low	Moderate	Low	Moderate	Moderate	Moderate	Moderate
Zabawa (2019)	Moderate	Moderate	Moderate	Low	Low	Moderate	Low	Moderate
Kunze (2019)	Low	Low	Moderate	Low	Low	Moderate	Low	Moderate
Clement (2019)	Moderate	Low	Low	Low	Moderate	Moderate	Moderate	Moderate
Ramkumar (2019)	Low	Low	Low	Low	Low	Low	Low	Low
Pua (2019)	Moderate	Low	Moderate	Low	Low	Moderate	Moderate	Moderate
Xu (2019)	Moderate	Moderate	Low	Low	Moderate	Moderate	Low	Moderate
Vissers (2020)	Moderate	Low	Moderate	Low	Low	Moderate	Moderate	Moderate
Kunze (2020)	Moderate	Moderate	Low	Low	Moderate	Low	Low	Moderate
Belford (2020)	Moderate	Moderate	Moderate	Low	Moderate	Moderate	Moderate	Moderate

Table 7.2 Different predictive factors and the strength of their correlation with TKA outcomes, for each included study

	Parameters	Brander (2003)	Lingard (2004)	Bourne (2007)	Escobar (2007)	Davis (2008)	Franklin (2008)	Nilsdotter (2008)	Rajgopal (2008)	Dowsey (2010)	Bourne (2010)
Quality assessment		Mod.	Mod.	Mod.	Mod.	Mod.	Low	Serious	Mod.	Mod.	Serious
Preoperative predictive factors	Pre-op VAS Pain	SA									
	Pre-op pain medication										
	Neurological disease / Backpain				SA						
	Pre-op KOOS score										
	Pre-op KSS score										
	Pre-op WOMAC	SA	SA						SA		IA
	Pre-op SF-12 PCS/SF-36		SA		IA		SA				
	Pre-op SF-12 MCS		SA				SA		SA		
	Pre op OKS Score										
	Pre-op EQ5D VAS										
	Pre-op ROM										
	Joint comorbidity/ Previous knee surgery										
	Severity osteoarthritis (Kellgren)										
	Pre-op knee alignment										
	Quadriceps strength						SA				
	Depression/ Anxiety	SA									
	Ability to cope										
	Allergy (>1 self-reported)										
	Medical co-morbidities / ASA score		IA								
	BMI	NA	IA	IA			SA	IA	IA	IA	NA
	Gender	NA	IA	NA	IA		NA	IA	NA		NA
	Age	NA	SA	SA	IA		SA	IA	NA		SA
	Geography (UK vs US/AUS)		SA								
	Income					IA					
	Decreased social support										
	Education / Socioeconomic status (SES)				IA	NA					
	Smoking / Drinking										
	Employment status										NA
	Expectation							NA			SA
	Ethnicity										

(continued)

Table 7.2 (continued)

Parameters		Brander (2003)	Lingard (2004)	Bourne (2007)	Escobar (2007)	Davis (2008)	Franklin (2008)	Nilsdotter (2008)	Rajgopal (2008)	Dowsey (2010)	Bourne (2010)
Quality assessment		Mod.	Mod.	Mod.	Mod.	Mod.	Low	Serious	Mod.	Mod.	Serious
Patient Reported Outcome Measures	Pain Catastrophizing Scale (PCS)										
	VAS pain	X									
	KSCR improvement		X	X							
	WOMAC Score	X			X	X			X		X
	WOMAC improvement			X					X		X
	SF12 PCS score						X			X	
	SF12 MCS score									X	
	SF12 PCS improvement		X	X			X			X	
	SF-36 Score				X					X	
	KSS score						X				
	KOOS Score							X			
	KOOS Improvement										
	IKS Score									X	
	IKS improvement									X	
	OKS Score										
	OKS improvement										
	EQ-5D score										
	EQ-5D improvement										
	Satisfaction										
	Post op ROM										
	Revision risk										

Table 7.2 (continued)

Parameters		Blackbum (2012)	Judge (2012)	Baker (2012)	Schnurr (2013)	Barlow (2014)	Lungu (2014)	Sueyoshi (2015)	Huijbregts (2015)	Maratt (2015)	Feldmann (2015)	Maempel (2016)	Van Onsem (2016)
Quality assessment		Mod.	Serious	Mod.	Mod.	Serious	Serious	Mod.	Mod.	Mod.	Serious	Low	Mod.
Preoperative predictive factors	Pre-op VAS Pain								SA				SA
	Pre-op pain medication												
	Neurological disease / Backpain												
	Pre-op KOOS score		SA										SA
	Pre-op KSS score												
	Pre-op WOMAC						SA			SA			SA
	Pre-op SF-12 PCS/SF-36					NA			SA				IA
	Pre-op SF-12 MCS								SA				
	Pre op OKS Score		SA	SA		NA			SA			SA	
	Pre-op EQ5D VAS			SA						SA			
	Pre-op ROM								IA			SA	
	Joint comorbidity/ Previous knee surgery		SA			NA		SA					
	Severity osteoarthritis (Kellgren)				SA								
	Pre-op knee alignment				IA			SA					IA
	Quadriceps strength												
	Depression/ Anxiety	SA	SA	SA		NA							SA
	Ability to cope												SA
	Allergy (>1 self-reported)												
	Medical co-morbidities / ASA score			SA					NA	NA			
	BMI		NA			NA		NA	NA	NA		SA	
	Gender		IA						NA	NA		SA	IA
	Age		IA	SA		NA		IA	SA	NA	IA	SA	IA
	Geography (UK vs US/AUS)												
	Income												
	Decreased social support					NA							
	Education / Socioeconomic status (SES)										SA		
	Smoking / Drinking												
	Employment status												
	Expectation									NA			
	Ethnicity									NA			

Table 7.2 (continued)

Parameters		Blackbum (2012)	Judge (2012)	Baker (2012)	Schnurr (2013)	Barlow (2014)	Lungu (2014)	Sueyoshi (2015)	Huijbregts (2015)	Maratt (2015)	Feldmann (2015)	Maempel (2016)	Van Onsem (2016)
Quality assessment		Mod.	Serious	Mod.	Mod.	Serious	Serious	Mod.	Mod.	Mod.	Serious	Low	Mod.
Patient Reported Outcome Measures	Pain Catastrophizing Scale (PCS)										X		X
	VAS pain												
	KSCR improvement												
	WOMAC Score					X	X			X	X		
	WOMAC improvement						X			X			
	SF12 PCS score												
	SF12 MCS score												
	SF12 PCS improvement												
	SF-36 Score					X							
	KSS score							X					X
	KOOS Score									X			X
	KOOS Improvement												
	IKS Score									X			
	IKS improvement												
	OKS Score	X	X	X		X			X				X
	OKS improvement			X									
	EQ-5D score			X									X
	EQ-5D improvement			X									
	Satisfaction				X				X				X
	Post op ROM											X	
	Revision risk												

SA Strong association, *IA* Inconsistent association, *NA* No association, *Mod.* Moderate, *VAS* Visual Analogic Scale, *PROM* Patient-Reported Outcome Measures, *KOOS* Knee injury and Osteoarthritis Outcome Score, *OKS* Oxford Knee Score, *EQ-5D* Euro QOL score, *KSS* Knee Society Score, *WOMAC* Western Ontario and McMaster Universities Osteoarthritis Index, *ROM* Range Of Motion, *BMI* Body Mass Index

Table 7.3 Different predictive factors and the strength of their correlation with TKA outcomes, for each included study

Parameters		Giurea (2016)	Hinarejos (2016)	Kremers (2017)	Jain (2017)	Sanchez Santos (2018)	Clement (2018)	Van Onsem (2018)	Clement (2018)	Abrecht (2019)
	Quality assessment	Mod.	Mod.	Serious	Serious	Low	Mod.	Serious	Mod.	Mod.
Preoperative predictive factors	Pre-op VAS Pain			NA						SA
	Pre-op pain medication									
	Neurological disease / Backpain						SA		IA	
	Pre-op KOOS score				IA			SA		
	Pre-op KSS score			NA				SA		
	Pre-op WOMAC score						SA			
	Pre-op SF-12 PCS/SF-36						SA			
	Pre-op SF-12 MCS						SA			
	Pre op OKS score					SA		SA		
	Pre-op EQ5D VAS									
	Pre-op ROM					SA		SA		
	Joint comorbidity/ Previous knee surgery					SA				IA
	Severity osteoarthritis (Kellgren)									
	Pre-op knee alignment									
	Quadriceps strength							SA		
	Depression/ Anxiety	SA				SA			IA	IA
	Ability to cope	SA				SA				
	Allergy (>1 self-reported)		SA							
	Medical co-morbidities / ASA score					SA	SA		NA	
	BMI	NA			NA	SA		NA	NA	SA
	Gender	NA			NA	SA		SA	NA	SA
	Age	NA			NA	IA	IA	NA	NA	SA
	Geography (UK vs US/AUS)									
	Income					SA				
	Decreased social support	NA								
	Education / Socioeconomic status (SES)									
	Smoking / Drinking									
	Employment status									
	Expectation				IA					

(continued)

Table 7.3 (continued)

Parameters		Giurea (2016)	Hinarejos (2016)	Kremers (2017)	Jain (2017)	Sanchez Santos (2018)	Clement (2018)	Van Onsem (2018)	Clement (2018)	Abrecht (2019)
	Quality assessment	Mod.	Mod.	Serious	Serious	Low	Mod.	Serious	Mod.	Mod.
Patient Reported Outcome Measures	Pain Catastrophizing Scale (PCS)									
	VAS Pain									X
	KSCR improvement									
	WOMAC Score		X				X			
	WOMAC improvement						X			
	SF12 PCS score				X		X			
	SF12 MCS score				X		X			
	SF12 PCS improvement						X			
	SF-36 Score									
	KSS score		X					X		
	KOOS Score				X			X		
	KOOS Improvement									
	IKS Score									
	IKS improvement									
	OKS Score					X		X		
	OKS improvement					X				
	EQ-5D score									
	EQ-5D improvement									
	Satisfaction	X					X		X	
	Post op ROM									
	Revision risk			X						

Table 7.3   (continued)

Parameters		Calkins (2019)	Twiggs (2019)	Tolk (2019)	Zabawa (2019)	Kunze (2019)	Clement (2019)	Ramkumar (2019)	Pua (2019)	Xu (2019)	Vissers (2020)	Kunze (2020)	Belford (2020)
Quality assessment		Serious	Low	Mod.	Mod.	Mod.	Mod.	Low	Mod.	Mod.	Mod.	Mod.	Mod.
Preoperative predictive factors	Pre-op VAS Pain				SA								SA
	Pre-op pain medication		NA										
	Neurological disease / Backpain		SA				SA						
	Pre-op KOOS score	NA	SA	SA									
	Pre-op KSS score				SA	SA						SA	
	Pre-op WOMAC score						SA						SA
	Pre-op SF-12 PCS/SF-36	NA					SA						
	Pre-op SF-12 MCS	NA					SA			SA			
	Pre op OKS score			SA							SA		SA
	Pre-op EQ5D VAS			SA									
	Pre-op ROM					SA			SA				
	Joint comorbidity/ Previous knee surgery		NA			SA							
	Severity osteoarthritis (Kellgren)					NA					SA		
	Pre-op knee alignment		NA			NA							
	Quadriceps strength												
	Depression/ Anxiety				SA		IA			SA			SA
	Ability to cope												
	Allergy (>1 self-reported)					SA						SA	
	Medical co-morbidities / ASA score					SA	NA	SA	IA		NA	SA	SA
	BMI	SA	SA	IA	SA	SA	NA		IA		NA		
	Gender	NA	NA	SA	SA		NA		IA		NA		
	Age	NA	NA	IA			NA		IA		NA	SA	
	Geography (UK vs US/AUS)												
	Income				NA								
	Decreased social support		NA										
	Education / Socioeconomic status (SES)				NA				NA				
	Smoking / Drinking		NA			SA							
	Employment status		NA										
	Expectation												

(continued)

Table 7.3 (continued)

Parameters		Calkins (2019)	Twiggs (2019)	Tolk (2019)	Zabawa (2019)	Kunze (2019)	Clement (2019)	Ramkumar (2019)	Pua (2019)	Xu (2019)	Vissers (2020)	Kunze (2020)	Belford (2020)
Quality assessment		Serious	Low	Mod.	Mod.	Mod.	Mod.	Low	Mod.	Mod.	Mod.	Mod.	Mod.
Patient Reported Outcome Measures	Pain Catastrophizing Scale (PCS)												
	VAS Pain								X				
	KSCR improvement												
	WOMAC Score						X			X			X
	WOMAC improvement												
	SF12 PCS score												
	SF12 MCS score												
	SF12 PCS improvement												
	SF-36 Score												
	KSS score	X			X	X						X	
	KOOS Score			X							X		
	KOOS Improvement		X										
	IKS Score												
	IKS improvement												
	OKS Score			X							X		X
	OKS improvement												
	EQ-5D score			X							X		
	EQ-5D improvement												
	Satisfaction					X	X						
	Post op ROM								X				
	Revision risk												

SA Strong association, *IA* Inconsistent association, *NA* No association, *Mod.* Moderate, *VAS* Visual Analogic Scale, *PROMs* Patient-Reported Outcome Measures, *KOOS* Knee injury and Osteoarthritis Outcome Score, *OKS* Oxford Knee Score, *EQ-5D* Euro QOL score, *KSS* Knee Society Score, *WOMAC* Western Ontario and McMaster Universities Osteoarthritis Index, *ROM* Range Of Motion, *BMI* Body Mass Index

preoperative WOMAC (Western Ontario and McMaster Universities Osteoarthritis Index) and SF-12 scores in pain, function, and stiffness were independent predictors of improvement in the same scores at 1-year postoperatively [31, 32]. Maratt et al. have defined the MCIDs (minimally clinically important differences) for the WOMAC pain score, WOMAC stiffness score, and WOMAC function score at 2 years after TKA and have assessed several parameters as predictive factors [33]. The preoperative WOMAC score and EQ5D score were the strongest predictive factors for improvement in postoperative WOMAC (pain, stiffness, and function) scores in a cohort of 2350 TKAs. In another study, the preoperative physical SF-12 score is also strongly associated with the OKS score at 1 year after TKA [25]. A one-point increase in preoperative physical SF-12 score resulted in a 0.38-point increase in 1-year OKS scores.

- Mental health

Anxiety and depression prior to surgery are frequently identified as risk factors for lower patient-reported outcomes after TKA [29], in particular, with regard to patient dissatisfaction [19, 27, 28, 32, 34, 35], knee pain [20], and walking limitations [18, 36]. Blackburn et al. described the severity of preoperative anxiety and depression as being associated with higher levels of knee disability postoperatively (Pearson correlation coefficient $-0.409, p = 0.009$) [5].

Predictive Factors with an Inconsistent Association with Outcomes

- Demographic characteristics

  Huijbregts et al. reported an inverse correlation between age and satisfaction with knee surgery: for each year of increasing age, the odds of dissatisfaction (Likert scale) at 3 months postoperative decreased by 4% and increased the change in OKS (Oxford Knee Scores) score by 0.12 points [25, 37]. Other authors have reported similar findings relative to age and satisfaction [25]. With respect to functional results, older age was found to be associated with a greater range of motion [38] in one paper, and Pua et al. noted age to be a predictive feature for walking limitation at 6 months after TKA, but not for postoperative range of motion or knee pain [36, 39]. However, age was not a highly predictive factor in all studies, and some authors did not find a correlation between age and clinical outcomes [27, 32, 40–42].

  With respect to sex, several studies have suggested that residual pain and stiffness [38], and consequently dissatisfaction, were more prevalent in female patients [28, 36]. Nevertheless, currently, there is not enough evidence to consider sex as a predictive feature of patient satisfaction [27, 40, 42].

  Body Mass Index (BMI) is a statistically significant predictor of satisfaction [KSS (Knee Society Score) subscale] [27, 43], of postoperative PROM scores [39, 44], and of postoperative range of motion [38]. Dowsey et al. described poorer functional outcomes (knee and function KSS) in morbidly obese patients (BMI > 40 kg/m^2) compared to the non-obese or obese (BMI $\leq$ 40 kg/m^2) [45]. Nevertheless, this correlation is not consistently demonstrated by all authors [41, 42]. Rajgopal et al. reported that morbidly obese patients received the same benefit after TKA as other patients. Indeed, the morbidly obese group had a slightly greater improvement in their WOMAC score [46].

  Some studies have grouped several demographic parameters (age, female gender, and BMI) to create a single demographic criterion. This "block" model correlated to average pain scores and opioid consumption in the early period after TKA ($p < 0.001$) [26]. A predictive model for postoperative PROM scores found a significant correlation between age and gender and OKS [44]. For example, younger women (age < 60 years old) had better OKS outcomes than men; but in the oldest age group (age 80 years old or more) women had worse outcomes than men [44].

- Clinical Comorbidities

  Several studies identified clinical comorbidities as significant predictive factors of poor outcomes after TKA [29]. Diabetes [32, 40] or allergies (to medication or environmental) [47, 48] were singled out. However, several studies did not find significant correlation between medical comorbidities or ASA scores and TKA outcomes [25, 31, 33, 34].

  Back pain is also correlated with poorer patient-reported outcomes after TKA [22], increased dissatisfaction, and persistent pain [32, 34].

- Osteoarthritis Severity

  In a retrospective cohort study of 996 TKAs, Schnurr et al. reported that the severity of preoperative osteoarthritis was the only feature that inversely correlated with patient satisfaction, after adjusting for confounding variables, at a mean follow-up of 2.8 years [42]. In comparison to severe arthritis Kellgren Lawrence grade IV, the risk for dissatisfaction was 2.6-fold higher for arthritis grade III ($p < 0.001$) and 3.0-fold higher for grade II ($p = 0.001$). However, the correlation of osteoarthritis severity with functional outcomes remains unclear [28, 40].

- Surgical History

  In one study, the number of previous knee surgeries was correlated to postoperative outcomes in some patients [40]. While the number of prior interventions was not specified, this feature was strongly correlated with immediate postoperative pain during the hospitalization ($p < 0.002$) [26]. Twiggs et al. are more unsure about the impact of previous knee surgeries on TKA outcomes [49].

- Preoperative knee alignment

  The impact of the preoperative knee alignment on the outcome after TKA is uncertain but the preponderance of articles suggests there is little correlation with outcomes. Sueyoshi et al. described a significant association between preoperative varus greater than 5° and postoperative pain ($p = 0.0096$) [41]. However, Twiggs et al. found no correlation between preoperative knee alignment and pain scores at 12 months [49] and other authors also failed to demonstrate a significant correlation between alignment before surgery and postoperative satisfaction [28, 40, 42].

- Preoperative range of motion

  Similarly, preoperative range of motion (ROM) has an uncertain impact on postoperative clinical outcomes after TKA despite having a direct correlation with postoperative ROM [36, 38, 50]. When looking specifically at pain and preoperative ROM, Sueyoshi et al. did not find a significant association between preoperative flexion contracture and postoperative knee pain [41].

Predictive Factors with a Low Association with Clinical Outcomes

Some features were not identified as significant predictors of clinical outcomes. For example, hypertension is not a predictive feature in studies with low or moderate risks. Features related to education, socioeconomic status, smoking and alcohol habits, and patient expectations were not found to be predictive of outcomes or pain after TKA [26, 27, 49, 51, 52]. Preoperative pain medication use was not a significant predictive factor of postoperative satisfaction at a mean follow-up of 2.8 years after TKA [42]. Surgical time and tourniquet time were not clearly identified as independent predictors of postoperative pain after TKA [26]. These features were not found to be predictive of postoperative outcomes in the literature reviewed and are unlikely to contribute to a predictive model.

Patient-Reported Outcome Measures

Twenty-three different outcome measurement parameters were found in the included studies. These parameters could be grouped as follows: (1) postoperative validated measures (further subdivided into specific to the knee, and those related to more general outcomes), (2) patient satisfaction measures, and (3) pain measures. Further, a separate group of variables can be defined as (4) improvement in PROM, where the change in a measure over time is the variable in question rather than the absolute value of the PROM at a given time point. Several predictive models have been developed to estimate various measures of postoperative outcome after TKA based on these measures (Supplementary Table). The main characteristics of these predictive models are described later.

Postoperative PROM (Specific to the Knee or General)

Some predictive models have focused on postoperative knee PROM or particular items reported as part of the PROM. Sanchez-Santos et al. described a predictive model for the postoperative OKS questionnaire at 12 months after TKA using data from a cohort of 1649 patients [44]. Tolk et al. estimated the probability of residual symptoms after TKA based on individual PROM questions and PROM total scores (KOOS physical function short form, EQ-5D, NRS pain and satisfaction, OKS) [30]. The predictive algorithm for residual symptoms concerning rising from a chair, stair negotiation, walking, and treatment success showed acceptable discriminative values. Predictive models regarding kneeling, squatting, pain, and satisfaction showed less favorable results on discrimination [30, 44]. However, the use of these models in clinical practice is neither intuitive nor practical. Furthermore, these models are built on relatively small data sets and may have inherent data bias and may not have wide applicability.

Lungu et al. described a predictive model to determine if a patient is at risk for poor outcomes after TKA relative to the 6-month WOMAC score [9]. The variables included in the prediction rule were five questions taken from the preoperative WOMAC score. This model had a sensitivity of 82.1%, a specificity of 71.7%, and a positive likelihood ratio of 2.9.

Patient Satisfaction

Patient satisfaction is frequently reported as the combined score for a standardized outcomes' questionnaire. Van Onsem et al. have established a predictive model for postoperative patient satisfaction at 3 months after TKA based on a cohort of 113 primary TKAs [28]. They created an algorithm that included patient age, gender, and various items combined from the KSS, KOOS, and WOMAC scores. A multivariate analysis was performed to determine the relevant predictive factors. The preoperative features selected included pain, stiffness, knee feeling, gender, age, patient anxiety, and patient history of depression. The algorithm allowed the classification of patients into either "satisfied" or "dissatisfied" at 3 months.

In a cohort of 484 patients, Kunze et al. have developed a preoperative knee survey score to predict patient outcome and satisfaction at 1 year after TKA [40]. The knee survey score (maximum possible score: 110 points) included several parameters (Table 7.4). The assessed parameters were 1-year improvements in the KSS and KSS Function (KKS-F) score, knee flexion, and patient satisfaction. They concluded that a knee survey score of 96.5 would confer a 97.5% sensitivity and 95.7% negative predictive value for satisfaction, and a knee survey score of less than or equal to 96.5 increased the probability of experiencing postoperative dissatisfaction.

Patient Pain

Some algorithms have been developed to facilitate patient selection for TKA during the surgical consultation. From a cohort of 4026 patients operated for primary TKA, Pua et al. developed a preoperative predictive model designed to determine the expected knee range of motion, knee pain, and walking limitations of a patient 6 months postoperatively [36]. They created a web application to facilitate the use of this model in clinical practice (https://sgh-physio.shinyapps. io/predicTKR/). The application shows the expected distribution of these three TKA outcomes for individual patients based on their preoperative demographic and clinical characteristics. However, no study has assessed the predictive value of this model.

Twiggs et al. created an algorithm designed to predict a patient's knee pain score 12 months after TKA [49]. The algorithm is based on a preoperative self-administered questionnaire and predicts the likelihood that a patient's change in the pain score will be equal to or greater than the minimum clinically important difference (MCID) in the PROM score being used for reference, in this case, 10 points for the KOOS pain score. The use of the MCID allows the patient and the surgeon to know during the preoperative consultation whether the patient will likely experience a clinically significant improvement in pain after a TKA. For example, when predicted to be at risk of not improving, 27% of patients did not improve; but if patients were predicted to be likely to improve, 98.6% went on to improve.

PROM Improvement

The most commonly used measurement to assess outcome after TKA is the improvement seen between results collected prior to surgery and postoperative data collected using validated instruments or objective measures such as range of motion [31].

Table 7.4 Studies reporting a predictive model for TKA outcomes

Study	Year	Sample size	Location	Predictive factors	Outcome measurement parameters	Delay	Predictive model
Judge et al.	2012	1991	UK	Age, gender, BMI, primary diagnosis, ASA score, Index of multiple deprivation, OKS, EQ5D	Satisfaction, OKS	6 months	N/A
Lungu et al.	2014	141	Canada	Five preoperative WOMAC questions: difficulty in taking off socks, getting on/off the toilet, performing light domestic duties, and rising from bed as well as degree of morning stiffness after the first wakening	WOMAC	6 months	Predictive rule, based on five preoperative WOMAC questions
Van Onsem et al.	2016	113	Belgium	Questions' selections based on KOOS, OKS, PCS, EQ-5D, KSS, age, and gender	KSS satisfaction subscore	3 months	Algorithm: Satisfaction at $M3 = 26.10 + 2.3*gender + 0.13*age + 1.58*Q3 - 1.40*Q4 - 1.08*Q5 - 0.75*Q6 - 1*Q7 - 1.12*Q8 - 0.88*Q9 - 1.10*Q10$
Sanchez et al.	2018	1649 (External validation on 595)	UK	Age, gender, marital status, index of multiple deprivation, BMI, anxiety/depression, OKS, ASA score, etiology, previous knee arthroscopy, flexion contracture, ACL status	OKS	12 months	N/A
Van Onsem et al.	2018	57	Belgium	Preoperative ROM, quadriceps and hamstring force, sit-to-stand test, 6-min walk test	KOOS, KSS, OKS	6 months	N/A
Twiggs et al.	2019	330 (two external validations)	USA/Australia	Age, gender, KOOS items, back pain, occurrence of hip pain, occurrence of falls in past year	Knee pain MCID = 10 points of KOOS pain score	12 months	Predictive model with a web application
Tolk et al.	2019	7071	NL	Age, gender, ASA score, BMI, smoking, previous knee surgery, Charnley score, KOOS-PS, OKS, EuroQoL 5D-3L, NRS	Residual symptoms (pain at rest and activity, sit-to-stand movement, stair negotiation, walking, performance of activities of daily living, kneeling, and squatting)	6 and 12 months	Predictive model for residual symptoms

Kunze et al.	2019	484	USA	BMI, drug allergies, osteophytes, soft-tissue thickness, flexion contracture, diabetes, opioid use, comorbidity, previous knee surgery, surgical indication, smoking	Patient-reported health state, KSS, ROM, satisfaction ≥ Knee survey score	12 months	Knee survey score on 110 patients. Four risks of experiencing postoperative dissatisfaction: score 96.5–110 = low risk score 75–96.4 = mild risk score 60–74.9 = medium risk score < 60 = high risk
Ramkumar et al.	2019	171,025	USA	Age, gender, ethnicity, emergency department, risk of mortality, severity of illness, comorbidity, weekend admission, hospital type, income	LOS charges/cost, discharge disposition		Model code (https://github.com/JaretK/NeuralNetArthroplasty)
Pua et al.	2019	4026	Singapore	Age, gender, race, educational level, diabetes, preoperative gait aids, contralateral knee pain, psychological distress	Knee extension, knee flexion, knee pain, walking limitation	6 months	Prediction model with a web application (https://sgh-physio.shinyapps.io/predicTKR/)

KOOS Knee injury and Osteoarthritis Outcome Score, *OKS* Oxford Knee Score, *PCS* Pain Catastrophizing Scale, *EQ-5D* Euro QOL score, *KSS* Knee Society Score, *WOMAC* Western Ontario and McMaster Universities Osteoarthritis Index, *ROM* Range Of Motion, *LOS* Length Of Stay

Discussion

The aim of this chapter was to identify and group the preoperative predictive factors and outcome measurement parameters that have been found to be predictive of clinical outcomes following total knee arthroplasty in the current literature. This compendium identifies those variables that are the most likely to be useful features in the context of predictive algorithms for clinical outcomes following TKA. These features are summarized in Table 7.5.

The challenge of developing useful predictive algorithms is twofold: (1) choosing the right predictive factors and (2) selecting those outcomes that are both "predictable" and useful measures of clinical satisfaction [9, 30]. Indeed, in several studies, predictive factors and outcomes are correlated independently of patient variables, because the same questions, the same scores, and the same parameters are assessed before and after TKA. Furthermore, many of the output variables (subscores) created in the PROM are interrelated. For this reason, multiple variable analysis is essential in order to assess the independent contribution of each feature to the prediction of postoperative outcomes. If the measured outcomes are similar to the predictive features, the outcomes will be strongly correlated with the limited preoperative parameters available [36]. For example, a patient with a preoperative fixed flexion deformity has a higher risk of having a postoperative fixed flexion deformity, or a patient with limited walking capacity preoperatively has a higher risk of having ongoing walking limitation at 6 months postoperatively [36]. Therefore, these parameters should be used independently. Ideally, we would create a reliable predictive model that could take into independent consideration the most relevant parameters. In this context, the improvement in PROM scores can be very useful to assess TKA outcomes. The clinical relevance of the improvements can be quantified by the MCID. Unfortunately, MCIDs are not universally valid across populations and cultures and vary by instrument.

Another challenge of using predictive models built and validated with data from one population

Table 7.5 Summary of the main preoperative predictive factors and outcome measurement parameters

	Predictive factors	Outcome measurement parameters	Delay

Strong correlation	• Pain
	  – VAS pain
	  – Back pain
	• Knee-specific PROMs
	  – KOOS
	  – WOMAC
	• Knee characteristics
	  – ROM
	• General PROMs
	  – EQ-5D
	• Mental health
	  – Anxiety/depression
	  – SF-12
		• Improvement of knee-specific PROMs
		  – OKS
		  – KOOS
		  – WOMAC
		• Satisfaction
		  – Self-assessment of improvement
		  – KSS satisfaction subscale
		• Pain
		- VAS pain
		- WOMAC pain
		- Persistent pain
			6 and 12 months

Inconsistent correlation	• Comorbidities/ASA score
	• BMI
	• Gender
	• Age
	• Previous knee surgery
	• Severity of osteoarthritis
	• Preoperative knee alignment
		• Knee-specific PROMs
		  – OKS
		  – KOOS
		  – WOMAC
		  – SF-36
		• General PROMs	

VAS Visual Analogic Scale, *PROM* Patient-Reported Outcome Measures, *KOOS* Knee injury and Osteoarthritis Outcome Score, *WOMAC* Western Ontario and McMaster Universities Osteoarthritis Index, *OKS* Oxford Knee Score, *EQ-5D* Euro QOL score, *KSS* Knee Society Score, *ROM* Range Of Motion, *BMI* Body Mass Index

is extrapolating the results of the algorithm using data from other populations. For example, Zabawa [27] and Calkins [43] did not support the validity of the Van Onsem prediction tool [28]. These differences can have several explanations. First, the populations under study can be very different from one country to another. For example, the mean BMI may vary considerably between two populations and if this parameter is identified as a predictive factor in the algorithm, the model may simply be inaccurate in the second population. Second, the indications for TKA can change between countries or between centers in the same country, particularly relative to age, BMI, and OA stage. Thus, the result from the model for a given patient may meet threshold criteria in one country/center but not in another. For this reason, predictive models using data from very large populations numbering in the hundreds of thousands, including several centers or countries, are more relevant and reliable than those built on limited data sets [30]. In some cases, however, the algorithm is based on features that are applicable outside of the data set from which they were derived. For example, Sanchez-Santos performed an external validation of his predictive model in an extended population [44]. The optimized model showed better discriminatory ability than the model that had been internally validated on the smaller data set. Further, re-calibration of the algorithm showed less sensitive predictive values. Indeed, in work done outside of orthopedics, it is common to use models trained on large public data sets and optimize them on much more specific and limited data sets.

It is also worth noting that while some correlations were identified between preoperative variables and postoperative clinical outcomes, the strength of even the best correlations was underwhelming. While it is possible that larger and more accurate data sets may increase the validity and predictive value of the algorithms, it is also possible that entirely different end points will be required. The existing "gold standard" PROM are now several decades old, and measured outcomes that were tied to problems faced by implant technology and surgical techniques that are now antiquated. Whereas, in the latter twentieth century, the primary concern was with implant survivorship of TKA, in the first two decades of the twenty-first century, attention has turned to functional outcomes following that procedure. However, the functional aspect of most scoring systems sets a reasonably low bar for success such as standing up from a chair rather than playing a round of golf. This is one reason so many PROM have well-defined ceiling effects [53–56].

With few exceptions, traditional PROM were validated at 1 year. Validation was performed at 1 year largely because improvements following TKA were found to largely plateau at 1 year. This latter point, validation, the practice of testing the assumption that the change measured by the instrument reflects an actual change in clinical outcomes, means that only variations between preoperative data and 1 year reported outcomes data have any meaning. Scores based on data collected at any time before one year (or the reference validation time frame of the study in question) have no validity. It is important, therefore, to understand that using predictive algorithms to predict PROM calculated using outcomes calculated at any other time than the validated time frame is likely to fail.

In terms of a modeling technique, a substantial number of publications relied on traditional regression models, which are robust and provide a quantitative assessment of the predictor's relationship with the output through the investigation of the model's coefficients [22, 30, 32, 41, 42]. However, machine-learning techniques have been shown to outperform linear regression models in specific tasks, such as the prediction of post-TKA EQ-5D-3L visual analog scale [57], estimating the risk of total joint replacement [58], and, more recently, length of stay prediction after TKA [59]. Therefore, we expect their level of adoption to increase in light of the promising results reported in some of the publications reviewed herein [51]. We hope that future research in this field will adopt the best practice of benchmarking different algorithms to a given prediction problem as we clearly have seen that there is no "one-size-fits-all" best solution in predictive modeling for TKA clinical outcomes.

Our findings should be considered in light of the key limitations of the data set. First, the inclusion criteria, such as English language or the requirement of full-text access, may have excluded relevant research. Second, the methodology score has known limitations with regard to the type of studies included (predictive cohort-based studies) and the difficulties in assessing the validity of the analyses conducted without having access to the raw data. Third, there was an important variability between the studies with respect to the type of predictive features studied, the type of outcome measurement parameters used, the follow-up period, the patient population and cohorts evaluated, and the analyses performed. This heterogeneity limits the possibility of performing a true meta-analysis of the results obtained when using predictive models in total knee arthroplasty. Lastly, the accuracy of predictive algorithms is derived from two critical aspects of the data set on which they are constructed: their size and the accuracy and completeness of the data sets within them. Generally, the number of individuals required to derive meaningful associations between variables and outcomes increases with the complexity of the relationship between variables. The larger the number of variables that can influence an outcome and the more complex the interaction between these variables, the larger the data set needs to be in order to discern and predict these complex interactions.

The indications for TKA are complex and multifactorial. Selecting patients for surgery based strictly on the prediction of clinical outcomes alone is probably not reasonable, particularly when the positive and negative predictive values of currently published algorithms are not particularly accurate. However, predictive models can communicate information and insight to both patients and surgeons that can be included in a shared decision-making process. Such tools should provide outputs that are easily integrated into clinical workflows. The output of these algorithms might one day be expanded from simply predicting outcomes to providing a stratification in the variation of possible outcomes based on the pursuit of different surgical strategies. In this scenario, the surgeon and patient would essentially customize the procedure to optimize the likelihood of meeting the patient's needs thus bringing orthopedics one step closer to providing "precision medicine." Examples include the decision between partial and total knee replacement or the choice of a cruciate retaining or cruciate sacrificing TKA. The "best" outcome is likely to be impacted by age, profession, obesity, anatomy, surgeon, implant, hospital, and country. By feeding results back to the data set, the models evolve and improve over time and become increasingly accurate (Fig. 7.2). We expect that such predictive models, when trained with appropriate and accurate data sets, could become an important adjunct to daily clinical practice in the near future.

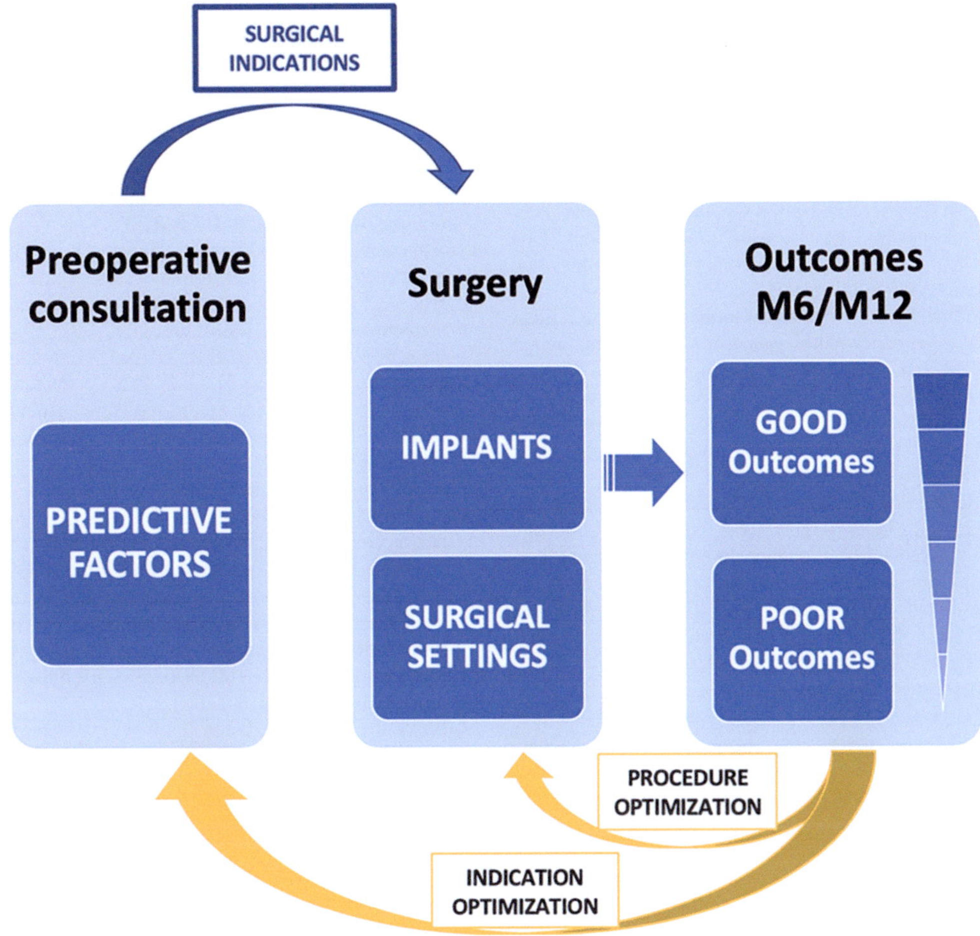

Fig. 7.2 Diagram explaining the correlation between predictive factors and outcomes in a predictive model

Conclusion

The existing literature on the predictive modeling of clinical outcomes following total knee arthroplasty has identified preoperative variables that have at least some correlation with clinical results. Functional features such as pain, PROM scores or mental health were highly predictive for clinical outcomes following TKA. Some variables such as demographics data, surgical history, or knee alignment were less strongly correlated with TKA outcomes. The challenge of developing useful predictive algorithms is further complicated by the need to select the most appropriate measurement parameters of TKA outcomes such as improvement in PROM, patient satisfaction, or postoperative pain. Creating accurate and reproducible predictive algorithms may one day provide advanced tools for shared decision-making relative to surgical indications and expected outcomes. However, the data gathered also suggested that work is still required to define outcome measures that correlate more accurately with preoperative variables and reflect patient satisfaction better.

References

1. Kurtz S, Ong K, Lau E, Mowat F, Halpern M. Projections of primary and revision hip and knee arthroplasty in the United States from 2005 to 2030. J Bone Joint Surg Am. 2007;89(4):780–5. https://doi.org/10.2106/JBJS.F.00222.
2. Bourne RB, Chesworth BM, Davis AM, Mahomed NN, Charron KD. Patient satisfaction after total knee arthroplasty: who is satisfied and who is not? Clin Orthop Relat Res. 2010;468(1):57–63. https://doi.org/10.1007/s11999-009-1119-9.
3. Beswick AD, Wylde V, Gooberman-Hill R, Blom A, Dieppe P. What proportion of patients report long-term pain after total hip or knee replacement for osteoarthritis? A systematic review of prospective studies in unselected patients. BMJ Open. 2012;2(1):e000435. https://doi.org/10.1136/bmjopen-2011-000435.
4. Baker PN, Rushton S, Jameson SS, Reed M, Gregg P, Deehan DJ. Patient satisfaction with total knee replacement cannot be predicted from pre-operative variables alone: a cohort study from the National Joint Registry for England and Wales. Bone Joint J. 2013;95-B(10):1359–65. https://doi.org/10.1302/0301-620X.95B10.32281.
5. Blackburn J, Qureshi A, Amirfeyz R, Bannister G. Does preoperative anxiety and depression predict satisfaction after total knee replacement? Knee. 2012;19(5):522–4. https://doi.org/10.1016/j.knee.2011.07.008.
6. Barlow T, Dunbar M, Sprowson A, Parsons N, Griffin D. Development of an outcome prediction tool for patients considering a total knee replacement—the Knee Outcome Prediction Study (KOPS). BMC Musculoskelet Disord. 2014;15:451. https://doi.org/10.1186/1471-2474-15-451.
7. Singh JA, Lewallen DG. Underlying diagnosis predicts patient-reported outcomes after revision total knee arthroplasty. Rheumatology (Oxford). 2014;53(2):361–6. https://doi.org/10.1093/rheumatology/ket357.
8. Williams DP, O'Brien S, Doran E, et al. Early postoperative predictors of satisfaction following total knee arthroplasty. Knee. 2013;20(6):442–6. https://doi.org/10.1016/j.knee.2013.05.011.
9. Lungu E, Desmeules F, Dionne CE, Belzile EL, Vendittoli PA. Prediction of poor outcomes six months following total knee arthroplasty in patients awaiting surgery. BMC Musculoskelet Disord. 2014;15:299. https://doi.org/10.1186/1471-2474-15-299.
10. Bini SA, Shah RF, Bendich I, Patterson JT, Hwang KM, Zaid MB. Machine learning algorithms can use wearable sensor data to accurately predict six-week patient-reported outcome scores following joint replacement in a prospective trial. J Arthroplasty. 2019;34(10):2242–7. https://doi.org/10.1016/j.arth.2019.07.024.
11. Shahid N, Rappon T, Berta W. Applications of artificial neural networks in health care organizational decision-making: a scoping review. PLoS One. 2019;14(2):e0212356. https://doi.org/10.1371/journal.pone.0212356.
12. Suk HI, Lee SW, Shen D, Alzheimer's Disease Neuroimaging Initiative. Latent feature representation with stacked auto-encoder for AD/MCI diagnosis. Brain Struct Funct. 2015;220(2):841–59. https://doi.org/10.1007/s00429-013-0687-3.
13. Amarasingham R, Moore BJ, Tabak YP, et al. An automated model to identify heart failure patients at risk for 30-day readmission or death using electronic medical record data. Med Care. 2010;48(11):981–8. https://doi.org/10.1097/MLR.0b013e3181ef60d9.
14. Zhang W, Li R, Deng H, et al. Deep convolutional neural networks for multi-modality isointense infant brain image segmentation. Neuroimage. 2015;10(8):214–24. https://doi.org/10.1016/j.neuroimage.2014.12.061.
15. Raghupathi W, Raghupathi V. Big data analytics in healthcare: promise and potential. Health Inf Sci Syst. 2014;2:3. https://doi.org/10.1186/2047-2501-2-3.
16. Bini SA. Artificial intelligence, machine learning, deep learning, and cognitive computing: what do these terms mean and how will they impact health care? J Arthroplasty. 2018;33(8):2358–61. https://doi.org/10.1016/j.arth.2018.02.067.
17. Baker PN, van der Meulen JH, Lewsey J, Gregg PJ, National Joint Registry for England and Wales. The role of pain and function in determining patient satisfaction after total knee replacement. Data from the National Joint Registry for England and Wales. J Bone Joint Surg Br. 2007;89(7):893–900. https://doi.org/10.1302/0301-620X.89B7.19091.
18. Baker PN, Deehan DJ, Lees D, et al. The effect of surgical factors on early patient-reported outcome measures (PROMS) following total knee replacement. J Bone Joint Surg Br. 2012;94(8):1058–66. https://doi.org/10.1302/0301-620X.94B8.28786.
19. Judge A, Arden NK, Cooper C, et al. Predictors of outcomes of total knee replacement surgery. Rheumatology (Oxford). 2012;51(10):1804–13. https://doi.org/10.1093/rheumatology/kes075.
20. Brander VA, Stulberg SD, Adams AD et al. Predicting total knee replacement pain: a prospective, observational study. Clin Orthop Relat Res. 2003;(416):27–36. https://doi.org/10.1097/01.blo.0000092983.12414.e9.
21. Wylde V, Rooker J, Halliday L, Blom A. Acute postoperative pain at rest after hip and knee arthroplasty: severity, sensory qualities and impact on sleep. Orthop Traumatol Surg Res. 2011;97(2):139–44. https://doi.org/10.1016/j.otsr.2010.12.003.
22. Escobar A, Quintana JM, Bilbao A, et al. Development of explicit criteria for prioritization of hip and knee replacement. J Eval Clin Pract. 2007;13(3):429–34. https://doi.org/10.1111/j.1365-2753.2006.00733.x.
23. Riddle DL, Perera RA, Jiranek WA, Dumenci L. Using surgical appropriateness criteria to examine outcomes

of total knee arthroplasty in a United States sample. Arthritis Care Res (Hoboken). 2015;67(3):349–57. https://doi.org/10.1002/acr.22428.

24. Sterne JA, Hernan MA, Reeves BC, et al. ROBINS-I: a tool for assessing risk of bias in non-randomised studies of interventions. BMJ. 2016;355:i4919. https://doi.org/10.1136/bmj.i4919.

25. Huijbregts HJ, Khan RJ, Fick DP, Jarrett OM, Haebich S. Prosthetic alignment after total knee replacement is not associated with dissatisfaction or change in Oxford Knee Score: a multivariable regression analysis. Knee. 2016;23(3):535–9. https://doi.org/10.1016/j.knee.2015.12.007.

26. Abrecht CR, Cornelius M, Wu A, et al. Prediction of pain and opioid utilization in the perioperative period in patients undergoing primary knee arthroplasty: psychophysical and psychosocial factors. Pain Med. 2019;20(1):161–71. https://doi.org/10.1093/pm/pny020.

27. Zabawa L, Li K, Chmell S. Patient dissatisfaction following total knee arthroplasty: external validation of a new prediction model. Eur J Orthop Surg Traumatol. 2019;29(4):861–7. https://doi.org/10.1007/s00590-019-02375-w.

28. Van Onsem S, Van Der Straeten C, Arnout N, Deprez P, Van Damme G, Victor J. A new prediction model for patient satisfaction after total knee arthroplasty. J Arthroplasty. 2016;31(12):2660–2667.e2661. https://doi.org/10.1016/j.arth.2016.06.004.

29. Lewis GN, Rice DA, McNair PJ, Kluger M. Predictors of persistent pain after total knee arthroplasty: a systematic review and meta-analysis. Br J Anaesth. 2015;114(4):551–61. https://doi.org/10.1093/bja/aeu441.

30. Tolk JJ, Waarsing JEH, Janssen RPA, van Steenbergen LN, Bierma-Zeinstra SMA, Reijman M. Development of preoperative prediction models for pain and functional outcome after total knee arthroplasty using the Dutch arthroplasty register data. J Arthroplasty. 2020;35(3):690–698.e692. https://doi.org/10.1016/j.arth.2019.10.010.

31. Clement ND, Merrie KL, Weir DJ, Holland JP, Deehan DJ. Asynchronous bilateral total knee arthroplasty: predictors of the functional outcome and patient satisfaction for the second knee replacement. J Arthroplasty. 2019;34(12):2950–6. https://doi.org/10.1016/j.arth.2019.06.056.

32. Clement ND, Walker LC, Bardgett M, et al. Patient age of less than 55 years is not an independent predictor of functional improvement or satisfaction after total knee arthroplasty. Arch Orthop Trauma Surg. 2018;138(12):1755–63. https://doi.org/10.1007/s00402-018-3041-7.

33. Maratt JD, Lee YY, Lyman S, Westrich GH. Predictors of satisfaction following total knee arthroplasty. J Arthroplasty. 2015;30(7):1142–5. https://doi.org/10.1016/j.arth.2015.01.039.

34. Clement ND, Bardgett M, Weir D, Holland J, Gerrand C, Deehan DJ. Three groups of dissatisfied patients exist after total knee arthroplasty: early, persistent, and late. Bone Joint J. 2018;100-B(2):161–9. https://doi.org/10.1302/0301-620X.100B2.BJJ-2017-1016.R1.

35. Giurea A, Fraberger G, Kolbitsch P, et al. The impact of personality traits on the outcome of total knee arthroplasty. Biomed Res Int. 2016;52:82–160. https://doi.org/10.1155/2016/5282160.

36. Pua YH, Poon CL, Seah FJ, et al. Predicting individual knee range of motion, knee pain, and walking limitation outcomes following total knee arthroplasty. Acta Orthop. 2019;90(2):179–86. https://doi.org/10.1080/17453674.2018.1560647.

37. Bourne RB, McCalden RW, MacDonald SJ, Mokete L, Guerin J. Influence of patient factors on TKA outcomes at 5 to 11 years followup. Clin Orthop Relat Res. 2007;46(4):27–31. https://doi.org/10.1097/BLO.0b013e318159c5ff.

38. Maempel JF, Clement ND, Brenkel IJ, Walmsley PJ. Range of movement correlates with the Oxford knee score after total knee replacement: a prediction model and validation. Knee. 2016;23(3):511–6. https://doi.org/10.1016/j.knee.2016.01.009.

39. Franklin PD, Li W, Ayers DC. The Chitranjan Ranawat award: functional outcome after total knee replacement varies with patient attributes. Clin Orthop Relat Res. 2008;466(11):2597–604. https://doi.org/10.1007/s11999-008-0428-8.

40. Kunze KN, Akram F, Fuller BC, Zabawa L, Sporer SM, Levine BR. Internal validation of a predictive model for satisfaction after primary total knee arthroplasty. J Arthroplasty. 2019;34(4):663–70. https://doi.org/10.1016/j.arth.2018.12.020.

41. Sueyoshi T, Lackey WG, Malinzak RA, et al. Predicting pain in total and partial knee arthroplasty. Open J Orthop. 2015;5:151–6.

42. Schnurr C, Jarrous M, Gudden I, Eysel P, Konig DP. Pre-operative arthritis severity as a predictor for total knee arthroplasty patients' satisfaction. Int Orthop. 2013;37(7):1257–61. https://doi.org/10.1007/s00264-013-1862-0.

43. Calkins TE, Culvern C, Nahhas CR, et al. External validity of a new prediction model for patient satisfaction after total knee arthroplasty. J Arthroplasty. 2019;34(8):1677–81. https://doi.org/10.1016/j.arth.2019.04.021.

44. Sanchez-Santos MT, Garriga C, Judge A, et al. Development and validation of a clinical prediction model for patient-reported pain and function after primary total knee replacement surgery. Sci Rep. 2018;8(1):3381. https://doi.org/10.1038/s41598-018-21714-1.

45. Dowsey MM, Liew D, Stoney JD, Choong PF. The impact of pre-operative obesity on weight change and outcome in total knee replacement: a prospective study of 529 consecutive patients. J Bone Joint Surg Br. 2010;92(4):513–20. https://doi.org/10.1302/0301-620X.92B4.23174.

46. Rajgopal V, Bourne RB, Chesworth BM, MacDonald SJ, McCalden RW, Rorabeck CH. The impact of morbid obesity on patient outcomes after total knee

arthroplasty. J Arthroplasty. 2008;23(6):795–800. https://doi.org/10.1016/j.arth.2007.08.005.

47. Hinarejos P, Ferrer T, Leal J, Torres-Claramunt R, Sanchez-Soler J, Monllau JC. Patient-reported allergies cause inferior outcomes after total knee arthroplasty. Knee Surg Sports Traumatol Arthrosc. 2016;24(10):3242–6. https://doi.org/10.1007/s00167-015-3837-8.

48. Kunze KN, Polce EM, Sadauskas AJ, Levine BR. Development of machine learning algorithms to predict patient dissatisfaction after primary total knee arthroplasty. J Arthroplasty. 2020;35:3117. https://doi.org/10.1016/j.arth.2020.05.061.

49. Twiggs JG, Wakelin EA, Fritsch BA, et al. Clinical and statistical validation of a probabilistic prediction tool of total knee arthroplasty outcome. J Arthroplasty. 2019;34(11):2624–31. https://doi.org/10.1016/j.arth.2019.06.007.

50. Van Onsem S, Verstraete M, Dhont S, Zwaenepoel B, Van Der Straeten C, Victor J. Improved walking distance and range of motion predict patient satisfaction after TKA. Knee Surg Sports Traumatol Arthrosc. 2018;26(11):3272–9. https://doi.org/10.1007/s00167-018-4856-z.

51. Davis ET, Lingard EA, Schemitsch EH, Waddell JP. Effects of socioeconomic status on patients' outcome after total knee arthroplasty. Int J Qual Health Care. 2008;20(1):40–6. https://doi.org/10.1093/intqhc/mzm059.

52. Nilsdotter AK, Toksvig-Larsen S, Roos EM. Knee arthroplasty: are patients' expectations fulfilled? A prospective study of pain and function in 102 patients with 5-year follow-up. Acta Orthop. 2009;80(1):55–61. https://doi.org/10.1080/17453670902805007.

53. Lim CR, Harris K, Dawson J, Beard DJ, Fitzpatrick R, Price AJ. Floor and ceiling effects in the OHS: an analysis of the NHS PROMs data set. BMJ Open. 2015;5(7):e007765. https://doi.org/10.1136/bmjopen-2015-007765.

54. Hamilton DF, Giesinger JM, MacDonald DJ, Simpson AH, Howie CR, Giesinger K. Responsiveness and ceiling effects of the Forgotten Joint Score-12 following total hip arthroplasty. Bone Joint Res. 2016;5(3):87–91. https://doi.org/10.1302/2046-3758.53.2000480.

55. Lyman S, Lee YY, Franklin PD, Li W, Mayman DJ, Padgett DE. Validation of the HOOS, JR: a short-form hip replacement survey. Clin Orthop Relat Res. 2016;474(6):1472–82. https://doi.org/10.1007/s11999-016-4718-2.

56. Steinhoff AK, Bugbee WD. Knee injury and osteoarthritis outcome score has higher responsiveness and lower ceiling effect than Knee Society Function Score after total knee arthroplasty. Knee Surg Sports Traumatol Arthrosc. 2016;24(8):2627–33. https://doi.org/10.1007/s00167-014-3433-3.

57. Huber M, Kurz C, Leidl R. Predicting patient-reported outcomes following hip and knee replacement surgery using supervised machine learning. BMC Med Inform Decis Mak. 2019;19(1):3. https://doi.org/10.1186/s12911-018-0731-6.

58. Qiu R, Jia Y, Wang F, et al. Predictive modeling of the total joint replacement surgery risk: a deep learning based approach with claims data. AMIA Jt Summits Transl Sci Proc. 2019. p. 562–571.

59. Li H, Jiao J, Zhang S, Tang H, Qu X, Yue B. Construction and comparison of predictive models for length of stay after total knee arthroplasty: regression model and machine learning analysis based on 1,826 cases in a single Singapore center. J Knee Surg. 2022;35:7. https://doi.org/10.1055/s-0040-1710573.

Updates on Computer-Assisted Navigation in Unicompartmental Knee Arthroplasty (UKA) and Total Knee Arthroplasty (TKA)

Kawsu Barry, Julius K. Oni, Ajit J. Deshmukh, and Savyasachi C. Thakkar

Learning Objectives

- Understanding the technological basis of the various computer-assisted orthopedic surgery (CAOS) systems and their objectives.
- Attain familiarity with the main CAOS systems currently in use.
- Understanding the current literature on the outcomes of CAOS in total and unicompartmental knee arthroplasty.

K. Barry (✉)
Department of Orthopedic Surgery, The Johns Hopkins University, Baltimore, MD, USA

The Iowa Clinic, Orthopaedic Surgery, West Des Moines, IA, USA
e-mail: kbarry16@jhmi.edu

J. K. Oni
Department of Orthopedic Surgery, The Johns Hopkins University, Baltimore, MD, USA
e-mail: joni1@jhmi.edu

A. J. Deshmukh
Department of Orthopaedic Surgery, Hospital for Joint Diseases, New York, NY, USA
e-mail: ajit.deshmukh@nyulangone.org

S. C. Thakkar
Adult Reconstruction Division, Department of Orthopaedic Surgery, The Johns Hopkins University, Columbia, MD, USA
e-mail: savya@jhmi.edu

Introduction

Computer-assisted surgery was first developed in the field of neurosurgery in 1908 by Horsely and Clark [1] and has evolved over the past few decades to become a mainstay in orthopedic surgery and knee arthroplasty surgery in particular. The first in vitro computer-assisted orthopedic surgery (CAOS) was performed by Nolte in 1991, inserting a pedicle screw in a sawbones vertebra [2]. Leading up to the mid-90s, the pioneering efforts of Saragaglia and Picard in France led to the first CAOS in total knee arthroplasty (TKA) procedure in a patient on January 21, 1997. The procedure was successfully completed in 2 h and 15 min. They subsequently went on to perform more similar procedures over the years that followed, many of them as part of a prospective randomized controlled trial, comparing it against conventional TKA. The prototype CAOS system used in the study became the basis of the OrthoPilot™ (B-Braun-Aesculap, Tuttlingen, Germany) model, an imageless system, which was introduced in 1999 [3]. The technology has continued to evolve in more than two decades since, leading to the development of a diverse array of CAOS modalities and systems with applications ranging from arthroplasty to oncological surgery.

Despite the long-standing availability and maturity of CAOS technology, its adoption has been rather modest and significant variability

© The Author(s), under exclusive license to Springer Nature Switzerland AG 2023
A. J. Deshmukh et al. (eds.), *Surgical Management of Knee Arthritis*,
https://doi.org/10.1007/978-3-031-47929-8_8

rates exist between countries. The reported usage is 2–5% in the United States and United Kingdom, 10% in France, and 20% in Germany and Australia [3]. The reasons for this will be explored later in the chapter.

The primary objective of CAOS in knee arthroplasty is to attain greater accuracy and precision of component positioning, to allow for consistent and reproducible restoration of limb alignment. The technology relies on computer tracking systems to accomplish this goal. This technology lends itself readily to the field of orthopedic surgery due to the stable and consistent spatial and temporal relationship between bony structures and adjacent anatomical structures. CAOS can be broadly classified into three categories: image-based, imageless, and handheld. Regardless of the modality used, three basic steps are involved: (1) data acquisition through fluoroscopy, computed tomography (CT), magnetic resonance imaging (MRI), or by imageless means, (2) registration of the data, which involves associating the acquired images to the intraoperative anatomic structures—it may involve the placement of "fiduciary markers" within the bone, and (3) tracking, which is the real-time feedback provided to the surgeon pertaining to the orientation and positioning of the instrumentation relative to the underlying bony anatomy. With appropriate execution of these steps, the surgeon is provided with concrete guidance on levels and magnitude of bony resection and even real-time ligamentous balance that will ultimately yield precise and accurate component positioning in the case of knee arthroplasty. In the following sections, a description of the different CAOS modalities will be provided.

Image-Based Computer-Assisted Orthopedic Surgery

In image-based CAOS systems, images of the surgical limb are acquired either preoperatively or intraoperatively. The imaging modalities most commonly used are CT or MRI; fluoroscopy is more commonly utilized in the intraoperative navigation setting. When CT or MRI are utilized, the images obtained are processed by software,

converting the two-dimensional slices into a three-dimensional model. This data is then superimposed on the patient's anatomy intraoperatively which, upon successful registration, allows for real-time tracking of the bony anatomy and surgical instruments to provide guidance on appropriate femoral and tibial cut parameters. This modality, although still utilized, has become less and less popular in comparison to imageless CAOS. The reasons for this include the additional time and expense of obtaining a CT or MRI preoperatively along with the exposure of patients to additional radiation in the case of CT scans, especially considering that obtaining such advanced imaging is not routine for patients undergoing knee arthroplasty during the preoperative course. The primary advantage of image-based CAOS is the accurate representation of the specific anatomy of patients, which can be very useful in complex deformity cases. An example of this is its utilization in patients who have significant extra-articular deformity. The placement of intramedullary guides, commonly a key step in conventional TKA, can often be precluded in patients with extra-articular deformity for a variety of reasons—these include the presence of irremovable hardware, sclerosis of the medullary canal, or severe angular deformity leading to an alteration of the mechanical axis. In such cases, CAOS has proved to be very useful in providing a reliable definition of the mechanical axis without the need for intramedullary instrumentation, hence allowing for precise intra-articular bony resection, leading to accurate and reproducible component positioning.

Imageless Computer-Assisted Navigation

This is the most popular modality of CAOS currently utilized in knee arthroplasty. Given its relative popularity, it will be described in greater detail. Most modern imageless navigation systems utilize predefined morphological statistical models that are typically derived from preexisting volumetric image datasets or alternatively on three-dimensional topographic scans of cadaveric bone specimens; intraoperative anatomic and kinematic data obtained from the patient are then registered to this statistical model to create a virtual three-dimensional knee model. This process constructs a frame of reference within which the navigation of any object in relation to the patient's anatomy occurs. Logistically, the components required for successful navigation are trackers, probes, a localizer, a computer, a graphical interface, and a control system. The trackers allow for the localization of any part of the patient's anatomical structures of interest. The means by which they achieve this is by their interaction with a localizer, which detects electromagnetic waves (usually infrared) emitted by the sensors installed on the trackers. The configuration of the sensors is such that it allows for the detection of the trackers as they move in space. The trackers, also called "fiduciary markers," are usually rigidly affixed to the bone, such as with pins or screws. A probe is a stylus-like object that contains sensors, similar to the trackers. Once calibrated, the stylus can be directed, by pointing with the tip, to specific anatomic reference points with submillimeter accuracy. A localizer detects signals from trackers to determine their spatial position with significant accuracy. The most common tracking system currently in use is optical, which uses cameras to detect infrared wave signals emitted by the trackers. Depending on the distance between the trackers and the localizer, a very high degree of accuracy can be achieved—for most cameras, for example, a less than 0.1 mm accuracy can be realized at a distance of 2 m. Newer tracking systems, such as accelerometer-based systems, are also gaining popularity. The computer is the central component that coordinates the input from all the other components of the system and records and generates data, ultimately providing actionable information to the surgeon. This information is presented in an easily digestible format by way of a graphical interface, which is displayed on the computer screen. It guides the surgeon on the exact steps to perform, providing real-time feedback on the consequences of potential actions along with guidance parameters for appropriate decision-making. A control system, much like a television remote control, allows the surgeon to execute actions on the program, thereby directing the workflow. It is commonly in the form of a foot pedal but it can also be a manual trigger on the probe or even a sterile touch screen.

With regard to operating room setup and workflow, the patient's position is identical to non-CAOS knee arthroplasty. The computer and localizer (camera) are usually positioned contralateral to the operative extremity. The surgical incision and exposure will then proceed as usual, followed by the fixation of the trackers to the femur and tibia; they should be positioned in such a way that they are within the field of view of the cameras and that they face the cameras so that their signals can be easily detected. These preceding steps collectively comprise the setup. This is followed by the registration step. This entails obtaining patient-specific anatomic and kinematic data to establish a frame of reference. The calibrated probe is used to acquire the anatomical landmarks by touching on specific predefined anatomic structures on the prompt. The kinematic landmarks are acquired by manipulation of the operative limb. Once registered, the surgeon is allowed to accurately assess parameters such as knee range of motion, limb alignment, and varus-valgus alignment. After successful registration, the planning phase is commenced. This involves pinning the tibial jig at the appropriate position with the guidance of the graphical interface, which displays numbers on the depth of resection as well as varus-varus angulation. The surgeon uses this information, integrating it with patient-specific parameters, to position the tibial jig where it is deemed to be most reasonable. With the tibial jig positioned, attention can then be turned to the femur. Prior to committing to any cuts, tracked tools designed to fit the femur allow for the calculation of sizing and verifying acceptable overall alignment of anticipated component positions. This is then followed by the assessment of gaps and component rotation before committing to final parameters. At every step, the graphical interface displays these data points on the screen, allowing the surgeon to tinker with them with immediate feedback until acceptable parameters are achieved. The execution step then follows, which entails performing the tibial and femoral cuts that were committed to in the planning phase. If patella resurfacing is indicated, it is commonly done in a

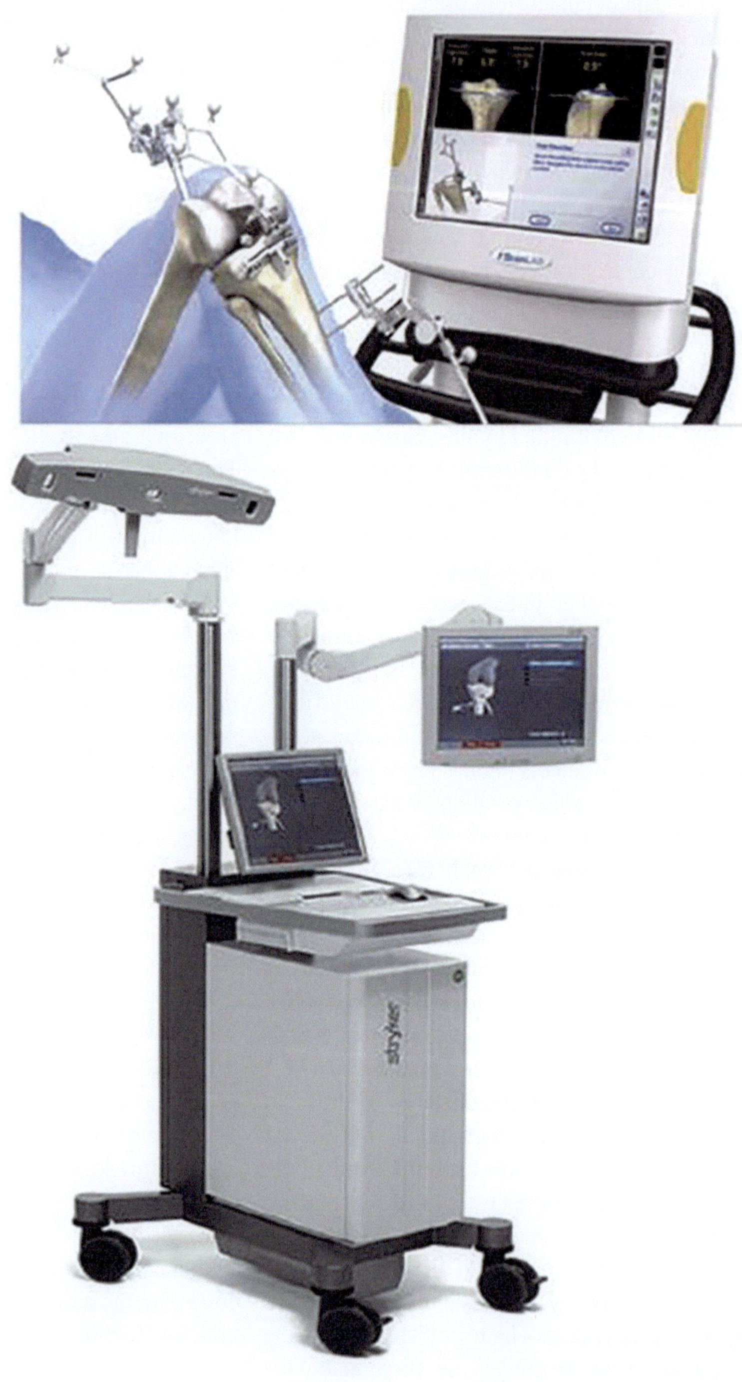

Fig. 8.1 Large-console image-based (top schematic) and imageless (bottom schematic) computer navigation systems [5]

non-navigated fashion, usually freehand or with a cutting guide. Once all the cuts are made, the graphical interface once again displays the resultant coronal and sagittal plane alignment, providing a final check for trialing and definitive implant placement [4]. Figure 8.1 shows the typical setup of large-console image-based and imageless CAOS systems.

Handheld Computer-Assisted Navigation

Both the aforementioned image-based and imageless CAOS systems can also be categorized as large-console navigation systems in that they require a computer monitor separate from the operative field with which the surgeon interacts over the course of CAOS. Handheld CAOS, as the name suggests, are portable systems whose components are all contained within the operative field and are small enough to fit in the palm of the surgeon's hands. This technology is the most recent of all the systems and has been made possible with the rapid technological advancements that have occurred in the past few decades. The most popular technology underlying handheld CAOS is accelerometer-based. An accelerometer is a device that measures forces of acceleration (the rate of change of an object's velocity) acting on an object, allowing it to determine the position of the object in space and track the object's movement. This sensing technology is exploited to great benefit in many industries. For example, in automobile collision safety systems, accelerometers sense when a sudden powerful force (collision) acts on a car, causing it to rapidly decelerate, which then sends an electric signal to a built-in computer, leading to the deployment of the airbags. Most accelerometers are extremely tiny in dimension and are very affordable, which has made their utilization ubiquitous in a multitude of handheld devices, such as video game controllers, smartphones, and tablets. The accelerometers utilized in portable CAOS are triaxial, allowing them to precisely measure motion parameters relative to a three-dimensional axis. The basic components of the accelerometer-based CAOS system are the display console, the reference sensor, and the jigs for the femur and tibia. The display console and reference sensor are each equipped with triaxial accelerometers that communicate wirelessly with each other. The jigs also typically comprise two parts that articulate with each other—a fixed part and a mobile part. The fixed component is affixed to the respective bone (femur or tibia), to which the sensor is attached, while the display console is attached to the mobile component, allowing for guidance on the proper orientation of the jig prior to committing to making bony cuts. With regard to the typical surgical workflow, it deviates minimally from the routine workflow for knee arthroplasty without the use of navigation. The navigation system can be set up and calibrated prior to the start of the procedure. After the initial exposure per routine, the fixed component of the femoral jig is inserted, usually in the anatomic center of the femur, similar to an intramedullary guide placement. The mobile component of the jig will then be attached to the fixed component. The sensor and display console are then attached to their respective jigs. This is then followed by the registration step, which entails moving the limb in a predefined sequence to allow for the definition of the mechanical axis (center of hip to center of knee). After successful registration, the surgeon is then able to adjust the jig until the desired varus-valgus and flexion-extension parameters are obtained—these parameters are displayed in real time on the display console instantaneously and with great precision. Once satisfied with the desired jig position, the distal femoral cutting block is placed, followed by the distal femur cut. A similar process is then undertaken on the tibial side—affixing the stationary jig to the center of the knee, registering through a set of predefined actions to define the tibial mechanical axis, and then making adjustments on the mobile jig with the feedback obtained from the navigation console to set the appropriate varus-valgus and posterior slope angles as well as depth of resection. The remainder of the surgery is then carried out per routine. Figure 8.2 shows a schematic representation of the typical setup of a handheld computer-assisted navigation system. Figure 8.3 shows intraoperative photographs of the OrthoAlign system in use.

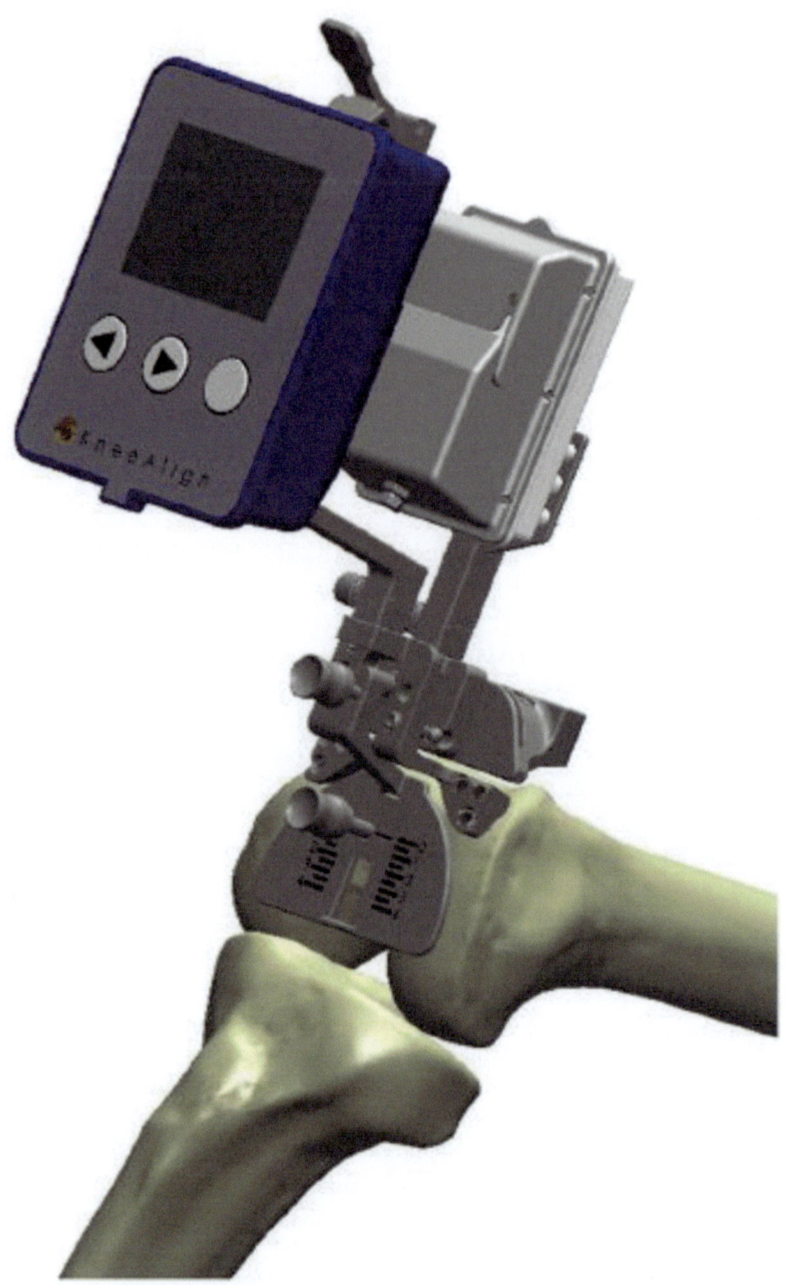

Fig. 8.2 Handheld computer-assisted navigation system [5]

Outcomes of Computer-Assisted Orthopedic Surgery in Unicompartmental and Total Knee Arthroplasty

The primary objective of knee arthroplasty, partial or total, is the stable implantation of components in such a way as to restore the mechanical alignment of the lower extremity, confer stability through adequate soft tissue balancing, with an excellent rate of survival while simultaneously providing its recipients a pain-free and highly functional knee. This is an objective that has mostly been met with modern knee arthroplasty implant designs and refined surgical techniques, even before the advent of CAOS. As previously

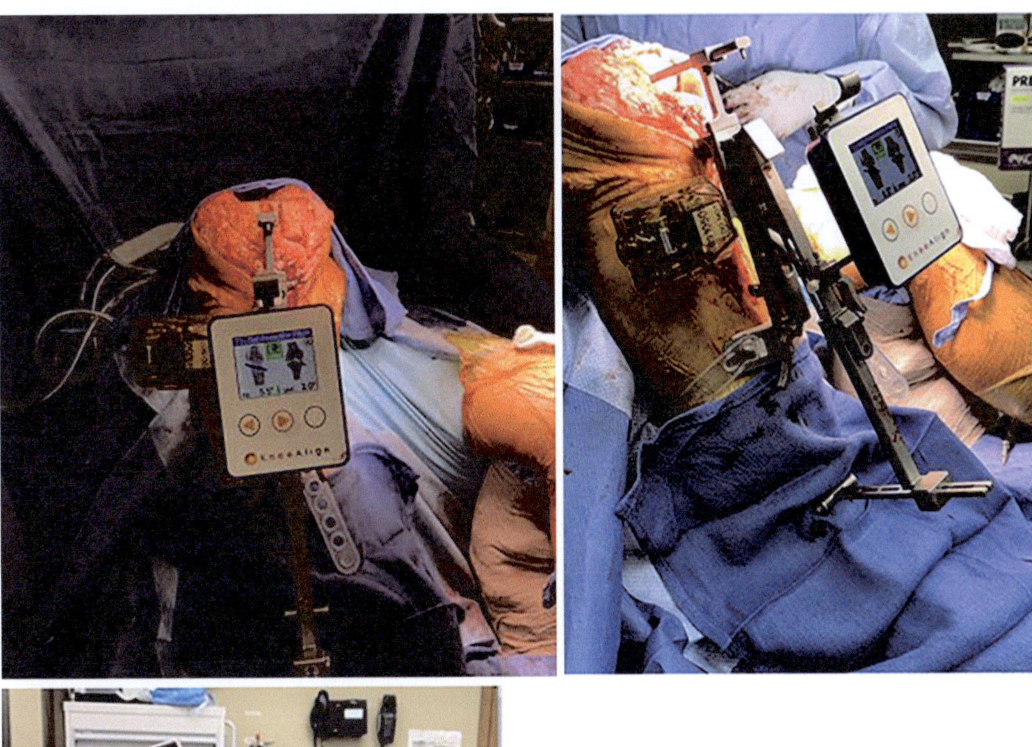

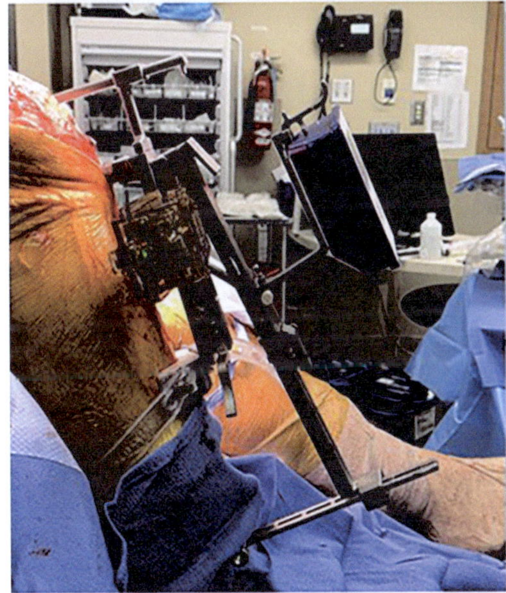

Fig. 8.3 Intraoperative photographs showing the OrthoAlign system in use during a TKA (Printed with permission from Thakkar 2022)

mentioned, the primary goal of CAOS in knee arthroplasty is to attain greater accuracy and precision of component positioning to allow for consistent and reproducible restoration of limb alignment. This is a goal that has also been realized to a great extent. Although the literature continues to be updated, the preponderance of the evidence to date has demonstrated that CAOS achieves superior postoperative alignment over conventional unicompartmental knee arthroplasty (UKA) and total knee arthroplasty (TKA). In a meta-analysis of 41 randomized controlled trials

(RCTs) and quasi-RCTs by Cheng et al. that compared CAOS TKA to conventional TKA, they showed that there were statistically significant reductions in the rate of coronal and sagittal plane malalignment in the CAOS group [6]. In a 2011 study of Asian patients with bilateral knee osteoarthritis with varus deformity who underwent staged bilateral TKA, randomized to undergo CAOS TKA in one knee and conventional TKA in the other, no significant differences with respect to radiographic accuracy of component placement and lower extremity alignment were observed when the preoperative varus deformity was less than 10°. However, when the preoperative varus deformity exceeded 20°, they found that the CAOS knees had reconstructed mechanical axes significantly closer to normal as well as femoral valgus and flexion angles [7]. An Austrian RCT comparing conventional TKA to CAOS TKA published in 2017 showed slightly contrasting results; at a mean of 12-year follow-up, the CAOS cohort had better radiographic limb alignment than the conventional cohort, but it was nonsignificant. In addition to these results, they also found no difference in long-term survival or patient-reported outcome measures [8]. Song et al. showed in a prospective study comparing conventional UKA to navigated UKA that at an average of 9-year follow-up, the navigated cohort demonstrated better component coronal alignment and fewer outliers radiographically [9]. In a meta-analysis published in 2013 comparing CAOS UKA versus conventional UKA, the use of CAOS was shown to result in more precise radiographic component positioning; the study also showed that the average operating time was approximately 15 min longer in the CAOS group [10].

Although there is abundant literature in support of the claim that CAOS allows for consistently accurate and precise component positioning in TKA and UKA, the popular argument against their mainstream adoption is that the superiority in accuracy and precision does not translate to superior clinical outcomes, especially considering the significant cost of these technologies and the added operative time. The overwhelming majority of studies over the past decade have demonstrated this lack of clinical superiority but it continues to be a hot topic of investigation and more studies will be published over the coming years. In a prospective randomized French study published in 2018 comparing conventional TKA to CAOS TKA, Ollivier et al. showed no difference in survivorship, rates of aseptic loosening, passive range of motion, and patient-reported outcome measures at 10 years [11]. A similar study performed in Italy demonstrated similar results [12]. A recent meta-analysis of nine RCTs comparing CAOS to conventional TKA demonstrated that at mean follow-up durations greater than 8 years, there were no significant differences in long-term functional outcomes and survivorship between them [13]. The aforementioned prospective study published in 2016 by Song et al. that compared conventional UKA to navigated UKA showed that at an average 9-year follow-up, the navigated cohort had better knee range of motion and patient-reported outcome scores but similar estimated 10-year survival rates [9]. Another similarly performed German study that compared minimally invasive conventional UKA to minimally invasive CAOS UKA showed that there was no significant difference in radiographic component position or in Knee Society Scores (KSS) but the navigation cohort operative time was 17 min longer on average [14]. A randomized controlled trial by Thiengwittayaporn et al. that compared minimally invasive TKA performed with and without handheld navigation demonstrated that handheld navigation resulted in fewer outliers in all coronal alignment parameters on both the tibial and femoral sides as well as better tibial slope angles; it also interestingly demonstrated that the operative time and bone cutting time were not different between the two cohorts [15].

One interesting area of CAOS application is in kinematically aligned TKAs. The conventional mechanical alignment technique establishes a neutral lower limb axis by performing bony cuts, soft tissue releases, and ultimately prosthetic implantation such that the hip-knee-ankle centers are coaxial. Kinematic alignment technique, on the other hand, preserves the native anatomy of patients by making bony cuts that do not alter the tibiofemoral alignment axis, which often minimizes the amount of ligament releases necessary to attain a balanced knee. The common means by which the kinematic alignment technique is achieved is by way of patient-specific instrumentation (PSI), which requires the acquisition of advanced imaging such as a CT or MRI and is also associated with increased overall cost relative to conventional knee arthroplasty procedures [16]. CAOS offers a great potential alternative to achieve kinematically aligned knee arthroplasty in that it allows for an accurate determination of the patients' native anatomy and provides the feedback to make the bony cuts and appropriately position the prostheses. In a retrospective case series of 100 kinetically aligned TKAs performed using navigation, Hutt et al. demonstrated satisfactory results both in terms of the reproducibility of the technique and functional outcome measures at 2.4 years follow-up [16]. More prospective studies are needed with longer-term follow-up to support the feasibility of the mainstream adoption of utilizing CAOS for kinematic alignment technique in knee arthroplasty.

The cost of adopting a CAOS system by a particular organization is one of its prohibitive factors. The upfront cost of incorporating a lot of the CAOS platforms can be quite substantial; furthermore, additional expenses are required for integrating these systems into the operating room workflow as well as their maintenance. Although multiple studies have been undertaken to investigate the cost-effectiveness of CAOS, they have mostly been based on theoretical models. A recent review that looked at only primary studies of cost-effectiveness analyses of CAOS since 2000 concluded that in the current practice atmosphere, the cost-effectiveness of CAOS is uncertain as it is associated with marginal increase in quality-adjusted life years at additional cost [17].

Given the substantial investment industry has made and continues to make in the development and advancement of CAOS, it hints at the reality that the technology is here to stay and that its widespread adoption is likely on the horizon. It will, however, hinge on increasing efforts to make the technology more efficiently and seamlessly integrated into practice settings along with increasing affordability and access. Although it is reasonable to anticipate that once CAOS becomes mainstream, the majority of primary TKAs and UKAs will be done utilizing them, it is in cases that involve complex deformities, revision surgeries, and minimally invasive surgery that the value of CAOS would be most optimized. Further, the advancement of robotic technology in the field of surgery in general is revolutionizing it and total joint arthroplasty is one of the niches at the forefront in regard to its application. Robot-assisted navigation is gaining popularity as it marries the aforementioned advantages of navigation to the automaticity of robotics, which holds the promise of even enhanced standardization of optimally positioned prostheses and the hope that it ultimately leads to superior long-term outcomes.

Summary

Computer-assisted orthopedic surgery in TKA and UKA has a proven track record of providing surgeons with a powerful tool to reproducibly implant well-aligned components with a high degree of accuracy and precision. The widespread adoption of the technology has been met with hesitation, however, with wide variability in the technology's adoption between countries around the world. The United States has been one of the slow adopters. One of the major prohibitive factors to the adoption of the technology is that of the cost. Another prohibitive factor is that of the additional operating room time incurred by procedures utilizing navigation, which also accounts for additional indirect cost. Accelerometer-based navigation may ameliorate some of these hindrances, however, given their substantially lower cost, portability, versatility, and favorable additional operating room time. Given that it is a more novel system, however, more data in the upcoming years will be telling and influential in the rate of its adoption. The lack of superiority with respect to clinical outcomes and survivorship of CAOS technology over conventional knee arthroplasty is perhaps the strongest argument against its mainstream adoption.

As longer-term outcomes data become available, it will be interesting to see if this phenomenon changes.

Disclosures Julius K. Oni: AAOS disclosures. AAOS: Board or committee member. American Association of Hip and Knee Surgeons: Board or committee member. Zimmer: Paid consultant. Savyasachi C. Thakkar: AAOS disclosures. AAOS: Board or committee member. American Association of Hip and Knee Surgeons: Board or committee member. Depuy Synthes: Paid consultant.

References

1. Karkenny AJ, Mendelis JR, Geller DS, Gomez JA. The role of intraoperative navigation in orthopaedic surgery. J Am Acad Orthop Surg. 2019;27:e849–58.
2. Deep K, Shankar S, Mahendra A. Computer assisted navigation in total knee and hip arthroplasty. SICOT J. 2017;3:50.
3. Saragaglia D, Rubens-Duval B, Gaillot J, Lateur G, Pailhé R. Total knee arthroplasties from the origin to navigation: history, rationale, indications. Int Orthop. 2019;43:597–604.
4. Picard F, Deep K, Jenny JY. Current state of the art in total knee arthroplasty computer navigation. Knee Surg Sports Traumatol Arthrosc. 2016;24: 3565–74.
5. Jones CW, Jerabek SA. Current role of computer navigation in total knee arthroplasty. J Arthroplasty. 2018;33(7):1989–93.
6. Cheng T, Zhao S, Peng X, Zhang X. Does computer-assisted surgery improve postoperative leg alignment and implant positioning following total knee arthroplasty? A meta-analysis of randomized controlled trials? Knee Surg Sports Traumatol Arthrosc. 2012;20(7):1307–22.
7. Huang TW, Hsu WH, Peng KT, Hsu RW, Weng YJ, Shen WJ. Total knee arthroplasty with use of computer-assisted navigation compared with conventional guiding systems in the same patient: radiographic results in Asian patients. J Bone Joint Surg Am. 2011;93(13):1197–202.
8. Cip J, Obwegeser F, Benesch T, Bach C, Ruckenstuhl P, Martin A. Twelve-year follow-up of navigated computer-assisted versus conventional total knee arthroplasty: a prospective randomized comparative trial. J Arthroplasty. 2018;33(5):1404–11.
9. Song EK, N M, Lee SH, Na BR, Seon JK. Comparison of outcome and survival after unicompartmental knee arthroplasty between navigation and conventional techniques with an average 9-year follow-up. J Arthroplasty. 2016;31(2):395–400.
10. Weber P, Crispin A, Schmidutz F, Utzschneider S, Pietschmann MF, Jansson V, Müller PE. Improved accuracy in computer-assisted unicondylar knee arthroplasty: a meta-analysis. Knee Surg Sports Traumatol Arthrosc. 2013;21(11):2453–61.
11. Ollivier M, Parratte S, Lino L, Flecher X, Pesenti S, Argenson JN. No benefit of computer-assisted TKA: 10-year results of a prospective randomized study. Clin Orthop Relat Res. 2018;476(1):126–34.
12. d'Amato M, Ensini A, Leardini A, Barbadoro P, Illuminati A, Belvedere C. Conventional versus computer-assisted surgery in total knee arthroplasty: comparison at ten years follow-up. Int Orthop. 2019;43(6):1355–63.
13. Rhee SJ, Kim HJ, Lee CR, Kim CW, Gwak HC, Kim JH. A comparison of long-term outcomes of computer-navigated and conventional total knee arthroplasty: a meta-analysis of randomized controlled trials. J Bone Joint Surg Am. 2019;101(20):1875–85.
14. Weber P, Utzschneider S, Sadoghi P, et al. Navigation in minimally invasive unicompartmental knee arthroplasty has no advantage in comparison to a conventional minimally invasive implantation. Arch Orthop Trauma Surg. 2012;132:281–8.
15. Thiengwittayaporn S, Fusakul Y, Kangkano N, et al. Hand-held navigation may improve accuracy in minimally invasive total knee arthroplasty: a prospective randomized controlled trial. Int Orthop. 2016;40:51–7.
16. Hutt JR, LeBlanc MA, Massé V, Lavigne M, Vendittoli PA. Kinematic TKA using navigation: surgical technique and initial results. Orthop Traumatol Surg Res. 2016;102(1):99–104.
17. Trieu J, Schilling C, Dowsey MM, Choong PF. The cost-effectiveness of computer navigation in primary total knee replacement: a scoping review. EFORT Open Rev. 2021;6(3):173–80.

Smart Tibial Trays

9

John Krumme, Amy Zhao, and Gregory J. Golladay

Introduction

Total knee arthroplasty (TKA) has become one of the most successful surgeries in orthopaedic surgery with a projection that 1,921,000 and 3,416,000 will be performed annually in the United States by 2030 and 2040, respectively [1]. As this number continues to climb, decreasing complications and failures as well as improving patient satisfaction becomes more important. Indications for revision TKA have been examined with the most common causes being aseptic loosening, infection, instability, periprosthetic fractures, and arthrofibrosis [2–4]. Patient satisfaction has remained consistent with as many as one in five not being satisfied with their outcome [5] (Fig. 9.1) [6]. Efforts are being concentrated to improve operative techniques to increase satisfaction and decrease complications. Both of these

can be accomplished potentially by improving ligamentous balancing [7].

Two consequences of poor balancing, instability and arthrofibrosis, have been implicated as an indication for revision total joint arthroplasty in 5–29% and 3–15% of revision cases performed, respectively [3]. These indications are directly related to poor soft-tissue balancing, and traditional gap balancing or measured resection methods offer no quantitative measure of force or tension [8]. This leads to an unbalanced knee in up to 50% of cases (Fig. 9.2) [7]. Similarly, patient satisfaction is also noted to be better when appropriate balancing is achieved and the two previously mentioned complications are avoided [6, 7]. Thus, a technical solution that can improve upon the deficiencies of measured resection and gap-balancing techniques could decrease revision surgeries and improve satisfaction.

Several technological solutions have been proposed to solve this problem and assist the surgeon in balancing. These have included patient-specific instrumentation [9], computer navigation [10], robotic arm-assisted surgery [11], and intra-operative sensors [7, 12–14] which have been extensively reviewed [15]. Of the mentioned solutions, intraoperative sensors that assist the surgeon with quantitative measurements for ligamentous balancing may be the easiest to implement into the flow of the TKA surgery [8]. The sensor is substituted for standard polyethylene trials during the balancing portion of the proce-

J. Krumme
Kansas City Orthopedic Alliance, Leawood, KS, USA

A. Zhao
Department of Orthopaedic Surgery, George Washington University, Washington, DC, USA
e-mail: zhaoa@gwmail.gwu.edu

G. J. Golladay (✉)
Department of Orthopaedic Surgery, Virginia Commonwealth University, Richmond, VA, USA
e-mail: gregory.golladay@vcuhealth.org

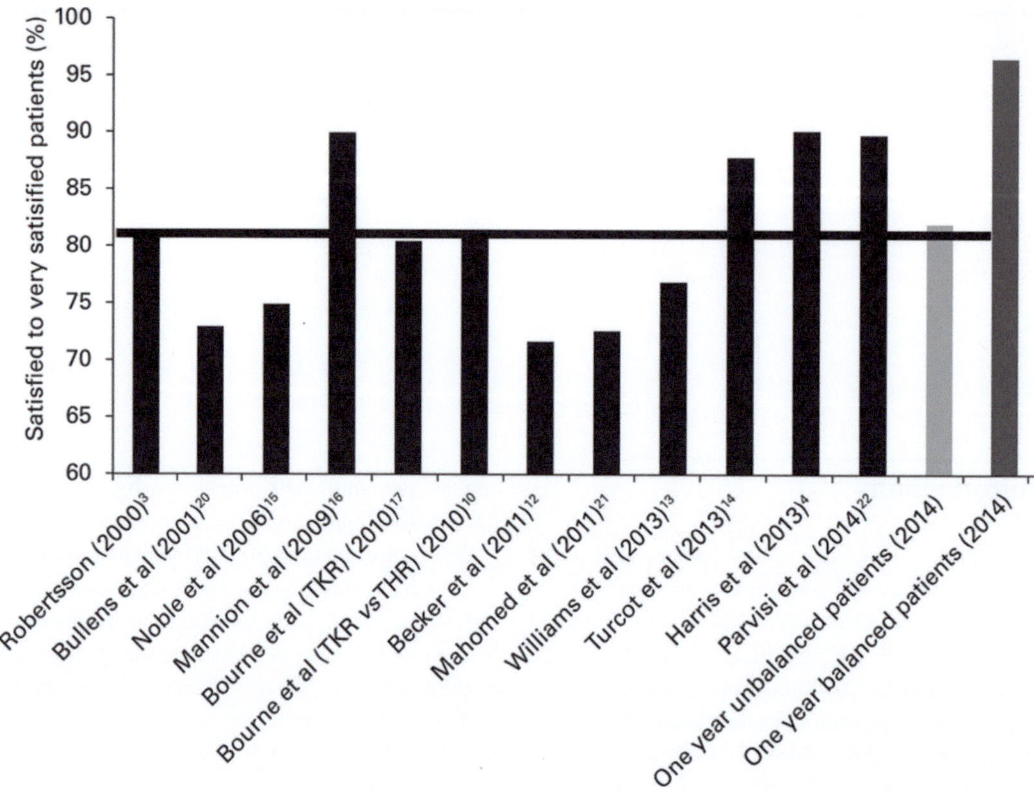

Fig. 9.1 From Gustke et al. [6] showing TKA satisfaction studies from 2000 to 2014. The far right shows balanced and unbalanced patients following utilization of a tibial smart tray

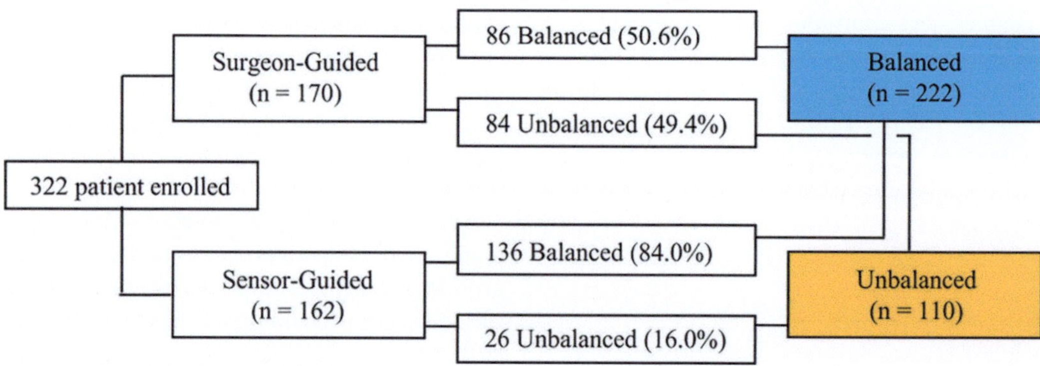

Fig. 9.2 From Golladay et al. [7] showing the rate of balanced and unbalanced TKA procedures performed with the smart tray and without the smart tray. The rate is significantly improved with the use of the smart tray

dure to provide quantitative feedback to the surgeon, and has been shown to provide quantitative data for balancing, improved short-term outcome scores, and decreased early complication rates, specifically for one specific leading reason for revision, arthrofibrosis.

Design and Materials

The purpose of the sensor in the tibial tray is to measure axial load distributions among different quadrants of the baseplate [16]. This device is a wireless and disposable unit [17]. Current

Unbalanced Condition   Balanced Condition

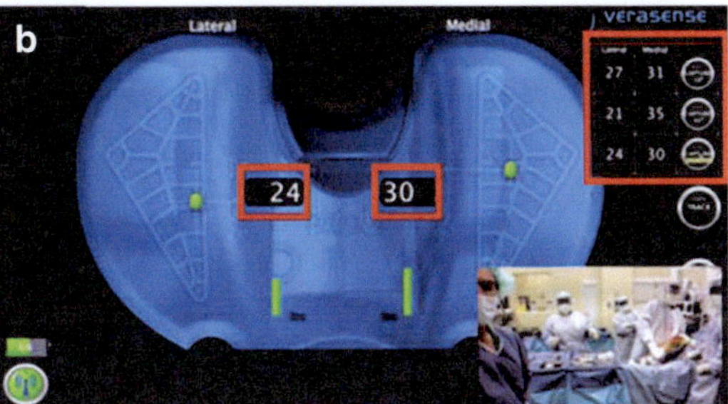

Fig. 9.3 Figure one from Golladay et al. [7] noting the unbalanced knee that requires adjustment on the left and the balanced knee on the right with pressure readings less than 40 and difference in pressures less than 15

utilization generally involves intraoperative guidance only [18], though there are reports of sensors utilized in final implanted prostheses [19]. The intraoperative sensor involves the use of piezoelectric ceramics that can transmit force data to a monitor in the operating room that allows the surgeon to visualize the forces and pressures acting on the sensors [16, 20]. Figure 9.3 shows the device that is commercially available and is compatible with multiple total joint implant vendors. The device will provide data for the medial and lateral compartment pressures in various degrees of flexion, and quantitative values have been determined that are considered acceptable for a quantitatively balanced TKA.

Intraoperative Technique for Application of Smart Tibial Trays

The implant is designed to not impede the usual flow of the arthroplasty procedure. The sensor is utilized during the trial implant portion of the case. The patella should be reduced to its anatomic position and the extensor mechanism held reduced with towel clips. The implant is inserted with the knee in full extension and the approximate slope is registered. Neutral rotation is perceived, and the tray is rotated so that the medial and lateral contact points are roughly equidistant to the anterior tibial cortex. The contact point rotation value is registered, and the knee is then flexed until the sensor indicates that it is in the appropriate position. The hip and ankle are then positioned so the device can register the mechanical alignment of the leg. Should the alignment be undesirable, the bones can be recut.

The joint is then taken through flexion and extension from 10, 45, and 90° with pressure readings obtained. These should be between 20 and 30 PSI with no larger than a 15 PSI difference between compartments for optimal results [21] as determined by a multicenter trial [7]. Should the number be greater than 15 PSI, further adjustments can be made with bone recuts or soft-tissue release. In general, bony resections are more powerful adjustments than soft-tissue releases. When the pressure difference is between 15 and 40, a soft-tissue release can be performed. When the difference is greater than 40 PSI or one compartment has an absolute pressure of greater than 60 PSI, a bony recut is required [8]. The cut should be taken from the tibia if the increase is in both flexion and extension and the femur if it is in flexion or extension alone.

This method provides direct quantitative feedback to the surgeon and allows adjustments to be made based on measurements rather than feel alone. An example of the balanced and unbalanced knee readings is shown in Fig. 9.3. A balancing matrix has also been published to assist the surgeon in decision making and whether to perform additional bony cuts or perform soft-tissue releases (Fig. 9.4) [13]. Surgeons should expect to perform further balancing following their initial assessment as balanced knees were only noted 35.7% of the time, with kinematically

BALANCING MATRIX	ASYMMETRICAL Imbalance MEDIAL Compartment	SYMMETRICAL (MEDIAL & LATERAL)	ASYMMETRICAL Imbalance LATERAL Compartment
EXTENSION ONLY	Evaluate MCL: -Palpate fibers of MCL to assess tension. Release posterior fibers of MCL (both deep and superficial). Evaluate Medial Posterior Capsule: -If MCL does not fully correct excess tension, release medial posterior capsule and/or semimembranosus at tibial attachment site.	<u>Condition 1. Loads 20 - 40lbf.</u> Release posterior capsule <u>Condition 2. Loads > 40 lbf.</u> If necessary, consider recutting distal femur	Evaluate Lateral Posterior Capsule & Arcuate: -Palpate the lateral posterior capsule and/or the arcuate ligament to assess tension; release as necessary. If lateral posterior capsule / arcuate does not fully address tension, consider releasing tight fibers of the IT band.
FLEXION AND EXTENSION	<u>Condition 1. Loads 20 – 40 lbf.</u> **Extension Balancing:** -Posterior MCL fibers released if in tension; recheck loads -Posterior medial capsule checked for tension and released, if needed; loads rechecked - If necessary, semimembranosus can be released **Flexion Balancing:** -Anterior MCL fibers released if in tension; loads rechecked <u>Condition 2. Load > 40 lbs.</u> If loads beyond 40 lbs. are displayed, consider recutting the tibia plateau to add more varus alignment.	Increase TIBIA RESECTION (or...Decrease shim thickness)	<u>Condition 1. Loads 20 – 40 lbs.</u> **Extension Balancing:** -Release posterior lateral corner; recheck loads -Release posterior lateral capsule and arcuate complex; recheck loads. - Consider releasing tight fibers of IT band, if necessary **Flexion Balancing:** -If excessive loads are still uncorrected, then popliteus tendon is checked for tension and released <u>Condition 2. Load > 40 lbs.</u> If necessary, you may recut tibia plateau to add more valgus alignment.
FLEXION ONLY	<u>Condition 1: Evaluate MCL</u> -Palpate fibers of MCL to assess tension. Release anterior fibers of MCL (both deep and superficial). <u>Condition 2: Evaluate PCL</u> -If medial femoral contact point exhibits excessive tension and posterior positioning, release anterolateral bundle PCL fibers.	<u>Condition 1. Loads > 40 lbf.</u> (excessive posterior rollback with visible anterior lift off) -Add more tibial slope. <u>Condition 2. Loads < 10lbf.</u> -Increase insert thickness	Evaluate Popliteus: -Release tight fibers of the popliteus tendon.

Fig. 9.4 From Gustke et al. [13] Guidelines in order to gain balance while using a smart tibial tray

aligned knees demonstrating higher rates of balancing than mechanically aligned knees (80% versus 35%) [17, 22]. Additionally, bony recuts may be necessary, with studies finding up to 9% of kinematically aligned and 49% of mechanically aligned knees requiring additional bone resection [22].

Surgeon Success of Predicting Quantitative Balance

Multiple evaluations have been performed to evaluate the surgeon's ability to determine the quantitative balance of the knee without a tibial smart tray as compared to with the tray. Sensitivity and specificity data were determined by MacDessi et al. on 322 TKA procedures [8]. They determined sensitivities from 78.2 to 85.7%, specificities from 24.8 to 53.5%, and accuracies of 57.5–65.8% in the three regions of flexion utilized for testing of 10, 45, and 90 (Fig. 9.5). Accuracy was also evaluated by Golladay et al. and found to be similar with 50.6% of the knees tested following surgeon-defined balancing meeting the quantitative balancing standards with the use of a sensor in the tibial tray [7]. However, a study by Meneghini et al. [23] showed that they only met the force difference of less than 15 PSI in 15.3% of their 207 TKAs. These data reliably

Flexion Angle Differences in Surgeon-Defined Assessment.

Statistical Measures of Performance	10° Flexion Mean (95% CI)	45° Flexion Mean (95% CI)	90° Flexion Mean (95% CI)	P Values
Sensitivity	78.2% (70.1%-84.6%)	79.3% (72.4%-84.8%)	85.7% (80.4%-89.8%)	.95 (10°-45°) .12 (10°-90°) .13 (45°-90°)
Specificity	53.5% (46.6%-60.3%)	34.8% (27.8%-42.5%)	24.8% (17.5%-33.9%)	.0004[a] (10°-45°) <.0001[a] (10°-90°) .10 (45°-90°)
Accuracy	63% (57.8%-68.3%)	57.5% (52.1%-62.9%)	65.8% (60.6%-71%)	.17 (10°-45°) .51 (10°-90°) .034[a] (45°-90°)
PPV	51.3% (44.2%-58.4%)	55.8% (49.4%-62.1%)	70.2% (64.7%-75.7%)	.41 (10°-45°) <.0001[a] (10°-90°) .001[a] (45°-90°)
NPV	79.7% (72.9%-86.5%)	61.8% (51.7%-71.9%)	45.6% (32.7%-58.5%)	.006[a] (10°-45°) <.0001[a] (10°-90°) .08 (45°-90°)

CI, confidence interval; PPV, positive predictive value; NPV, negative predictive value.

[a] Significant P values.

Fig. 9.5 From MacDessi et al. [8] Test reliability comparing surgeon-defined balance with quantitative balancing using the smart tibial tray

demonstrate that surgeons utilizing feel through measured resection or gap-balancing techniques do not tend to have largely reproducible results as it relates to intraoperative compartment pressures measured utilizing a smart tibial tray.

Outcomes

Since the device's approval in 2009 and clinical use starting in 2011, studies have only examined short-term outcomes data, and have overall shown improvements in patient satisfaction scores and decreases in early complications.

In a multicenter randomized controlled trial of 222 balanced knees and 110 unbalanced knees, Golladay et al. found that at 6 weeks and 6 months, quantitatively balanced knees performed better than unbalanced knees based on Knee Society Scores (KSS) for patient expectations and satisfaction and Forgotten Joint Scores (FJS) [7]. Similarly, a prospective cohort study by Gustke et al. demonstrated that at 1 year of follow-up for 135 knees, KSS and Western Ontario and McMaster University Osteoarthritis Index (WOMAC) scores were improved in the balanced knees as compared to unbalanced knees [6]. Amongst those with balanced knees, 94.1% reported satisfaction (127/135) (Fig. 9.1). In contrast, Meneghini et al. in a prospective cohort study with 4 months of follow-up found no significant difference in KSS when pressures varied in the compartments by more than 15 PSI. However, the authors show a difference in UCLA activity level when intercompartmental forces were less than 15 lbs as compared to greater than 60 lbs. [23]

Geller et al. evaluated 90-day rates of manipulation under anesthesia in 942 patients undergoing TKA, 690 performed without smart tibial trays and 252 with smart tibial trays. They found a statistically significant increased rate of manipulation in the non-sensor group compared to the sensory group (5% versus 1.6%, respectively) [24]. Ultimately, this retrospective study demonstrates that a quantitatively balanced knee has a decreased rate of repeat procedures with short-term follow-up.

Other short-term follow-up studies with intervals of within 2 years have been published [15]. With the exception of the Meneghini et al. study, these have concurred that during short-term follow-up of less than 2 years, there is a trend towards improvement in satisfaction and functionality scores. It should also be noted that only level one study on the topic showed an improvement in clinical outcome measures when total knees were quantitatively balanced. A summary of the outcomes data can be seen in Fig. 9.6 [15].

TABLE IV   Soft-Tissue Balancing Technology: Clinical Outcomes*

Study	Study Type	System	Industry Funding	No. of Sensor or Navigation Cases	No. of Conventional Cases	Follow-up (mo)	Conclusions	LOE
Lee[28] (2010)	RCT	CAN gap balancing	No	60	60 CAN measured resection	3	Navigated soft-tissue balanced TKA cohort had more accurate gap balancing than the conventional TKA group, but clinical outcomes postoperatively were similar for both groups	I
Pang[21] (2011)	RCT	CAN gap balancing	No	70	70	24	At 6-month follow-up, navigated cohort demonstrated better outcomes in Function Score (p = 0.040) and Total Oxford Score (p = 0.031); at the 2-year review, CAN had a better outcome in the Total Oxford Score (p = 0.030)	I
Singh[41] (2012)	RCT	CAN gap balancing	No	26	26 CAN measured resection	24	Patients who underwent navigated gap-balancing had nonsignificantly higher KSS (p = 0.46), KSSF (p = 0.44), and revised OKS (p = 0.12) at the 2-year follow-up	I
Golladay[71] (2019)	RCT	Intraoperative sensors	Yes	222 balanced TKAs	110 unbalanced TKAs	6	Patients with a quantitatively balanced TKA with the use of VERASENSE sensors had better validated FJS (p = 0.031) and 2011 KSS satisfaction and expectation (p = 0.011) at 6 weeks and 6 months compared with patients with quantitatively unbalanced knees	I
Han[42] (2008)	Case series	CAN gap balancing	No	100	—	28	The rectangular flexion and extension gaps were brought within 1 mm in about 70% of cases (72% in flexion, 74% in extension); a rectangular gap was achieved in 84% of all knees, with trapezoidal gaps achieved in the remaining 16%; there was no significant difference in range of motion (p = 0.528), KSS (p = 0.348), improvement of range of motion (p = 0.263), or restoration of limb alignment (p = 0.887) after TKA between the rectangular and trapezoidal groups	IV
Gustke[11] (2014)	Case series	Intraoperative sensors	Yes	176	—	6	There were 87% balanced patients and 13% unbalanced patients; the balanced cohort had better WOMAC (p < 0.001) and KSS (p < 0.001) at 6 months	IV

continued

Fig. 9.6 From Siddiqi et al. [15] outcomes of publications related to intraoperative sensors in TKA. All level 1–4 studies did show a difference with the exception of one level IV study by Meneghini et al.

Gustke[52] (2014)	Case series	Intraoperative sensors	Yes	135	—	12	135 patients from the other Gustke study[53] reported follow-up at 1 year; the balanced cohort continued to demonstrate superior scores in WOMAC (p < 0.085) and KSS (p < 0.001) at 1 year	IV
Meneghini[20] (2016)	Case series	Intraoperative sensors	No	189	—	4	No differences in KSSO, KSSS, KSSF, and EQ-5D health state scores based on intercompartmental load differences; however, improvement in UCLA activity level was noted when intercompartmental force differences were <15 lb (<6.8 kg) compared with force differences of >60 lb (>27 kg)	IV
Nodzo[67] (2017)	Case series	Intraoperative sensors	Yes	54	—	4.6	Sensor-guided TKA had improved KSS and functional scores at a mean 4.6-month follow-up	IV
Anderson[70] (2016)	Retrospective cohort	Intraoperative sensors	Yes	122	—	12	122 patients in a multicenter study underwent TKA based on a surgical algorithm using intraoperative sensors; the patient groups that followed the surgical algorithm appropriately reported significantly higher KSS and WOMAC scores and higher patient satisfaction at 1 year postoperatively	III

*LOE = Level of Evidence, RCT = randomized controlled trial, CAN = computer-assisted navigation, and TKA = total knee arthroplasty.

Fig. 9.6 (continued)

Future Directions

Given the device has only been utilized clinically since 2011, there remains a lack of long-term outcomes data involving smart tibial trays at the time of this publication. They are also utilized only intraoperatively, and the forces that are displaced by the tray in the operating room do not correspond to known forces with activities of daily living such as stair climbing. These two factors provide opportunities for future improvement and enhanced understanding of the benefits of a quantitatively balanced TKA.

First, long-term outcomes are necessary to determine the survivorship of quantitatively balanced total knees versus unbalanced knees. It is unknown if revision rates will remain the same or if they will decrease especially for rates of aseptic loosening. Future multidisciplinary trials are needed to elucidate long-term outcomes.

Second, permanently implanted sensors may provide a further understanding of the true balance of the knee following TKA. It is currently unknown if the current acceptable standard of a quantitatively balanced total knee applies to activities of daily living. The differences in the pressures seen intercompartmental when walking or climbing stairs may provide data that shows a better measurement for utilization and improvement in outcomes. These are two specific opportunities to better understand the technology and its role and application in TKA.

Conclusions

Smart tibial trays appear to be a useful technology which provides quantitative data to assist in balancing the TKA with only minimal disruption to the traditional flow of the operative procedure.

The technology provides a more consistent and reproducible methodology to the balancing portion of the procedure. As a result, knees that are quantitatively balanced demonstrate improved short-term outcomes, as represented by several clinical outcome and patient satisfaction scores. Further research is required to understand the effect of this technology on long-term outcomes and whether the intraoperative values truly correlate with quantitative balance for a knee when the patient returns to activities of daily living.

Key Study Points

- Decreased patient satisfaction and early complications including arthrofibrosis and instability may be related to poor intraoperative balancing technique.
- Of the technical assistive devices on the market for TKA, the smart tibial tray changes the surgical flow of TKA the least.
- Surgeons are poorly able to reproduce a quantitatively balanced knee without the use of smart tibial tray force measurements.
- A quantitatively balanced knee with compartmental pressures less than 40 PSI and intercompartmental force differences of less than 15 PSI may perform better than knees not quantitatively balanced.

References

1. Singh JA, Yu S, Chen L, Cleveland JD. Rates of total joint replacement in the United States: future projections to 2020–2040 using the national inpatient sample. J Rheumatol. 2019;46(9):1134–40. https://doi.org/10.3899/jrheum.170990. (This study uses the US National Inpatient Sample (NIS) combined with Census Bureau data to develop projections for primary THA and TKA from 2020 to 2040 using polynomial regression, ultimately projecting a 284% increase in THA and 401% increase in TKA by 2040. Level 4).
2. Bozic KJ, Kurtz SM, Lau E, et al. The epidemiology of revision total knee arthroplasty in the United States. Clin Orthop Relat Res. 2010;468(1):45–51. https://doi.org/10.1007/s11999-009-0945-0. (This study assessed the causes of failure and specific types of revision TKA procedures in the US and ultimately found that between October 2005 and December 2006, the most common causes of revision TKA were infection (25.2%) and implant loosening (16.1%). Level 3).
3. Lombardi AV, Berend KR, Adams JB. Why knee replacements fail in 2013: patient, surgeon, or implant? Bone Joint J. 2014;96B(11):101–4. https://doi.org/10.1302/0301-620X.96B11.34350. (This multi center evaluation of 844 revision TKAs from 2010 to 2011 demonstrated that aseptic loosening, instability, infection, wear, arthrofibrosis, and malalignment were the most common modes of failure. Level 3).
4. Sharkey PF, Lichstein PM, Shen C, Tokarski AT, Parvizi J. Why are total knee arthroplasties failing today-has anything changed after 10 years? J Arthroplasty. 2013;29(9):1774–8. https://doi.org/10.1016/j.arth.2013.07.024. (This retrospective study of 781 TKAs performed at one institution sought to determine the most common causes of TKA failure, ultimately finding that aseptic loosening, infection, instability, periprosthetic fracture, and arthrofibrosis were the most common causes. Level 3).
5. Bourne RB, Chesworth BM, Davis AM, Mahomed NN, Charron KDJ. Patient satisfaction after total knee arthroplasty: Who is satisfied and who is not? Clin Orthop Relat Res. 2010;468(1):57–63. https://doi.org/10.1007/s11999-009-1119-9. (This cross-sectional study examined patient satisfaction following 1703 primary TKAs and demonstrated that approximately one in five primary TKA patients were not satisfied with their outcome. The strongest predictors of patient dissatisfaction were unmet expectations, low 1-year WOMAC, preoperative pain at rest, and postoperative complication requiring hospital readmission. Level 3).
6. Gustke KA, Golladay GJ, Roche MW, Jerry GJ, Elson LC, Anderson CR. Increased satisfaction after total knee replacement using sensor-guided technology. Bone Joint J. 2014;96B(10):1333–8. https://doi.org/10.1302/0301-620X.96B10.34068. (This prospective multicenter study examined patient satisfaction after TKA performed with the aid of intraoperative sensors and found that 96.7% of patients who showed soft-tissue balance and 82.1% of patients who did not have soft-tissue balance demonstrated satisfaction one year post operatively. Level 2).
7. Golladay GJ, Bradbury TL, Gordon AC, et al. Are patients more satisfied with a balanced total knee arthroplasty? J Arthroplasty. 2019;34(7):S195–200. https://doi.org/10.1016/j.arth.2019.03.036. (This multicenter study examined post-operative patient satisfaction and joint awareness in TKA with and without a quantitatively balanced knee. The authors found that significantly more knees were balanced in the sensor-guided group, and patients with balanced knees demonstrated significantly better Forgotten Joint Score and Knee Society Satisfaction scores. Level 2).
8. MacDessi SJ, Gharaibeh MA, Harris IA. How accurately can soft tissue balance be determined in total knee arthroplasty? J Arthroplasty. 2019;34(2):290–294.e1. https://doi.org/10.1016/j.arth.2018.10.003. (This study aimed to examine the accuracy of surgeon-defined assessment of knee balance com-

pared to sensor data, ultimately finding that surgeon-defined assessment was a poor predictor of true soft tissue balance when compared to sensors. The authors also demonstrated that increased use of sensors did not improve surgeon capacity to determine balance. Level 2).

9. Gaukel S, Vuille-dit-Bille RN, Schläppi M, Koch PP. CT-based patient-specific instrumentation for total knee arthroplasty in over 700 cases: single-use instruments are as accurate as standard instruments. Knee Surgery, Sport Traumatol Arthrosc. 2020. https://doi.org/10.1007/s00167-020-06150-x (In this retrospective study examining the use of patient-specific instruments versus computer navigated and conventional techniques in demonstrating accuracy for correct leg axis found that more outliers occurred using standard instruments versus single-use instruments. Additionaly, use of CT-based patient-specific cutting block technique yielded high accuracy of knee angles and mechanical leg axes. Level 3).

10. Gothesen O, Skaden O, Dyrhovden G, Petursson G, Furnes O. Computerized navigation: a useful tool in total knee replacement. JBJS Essent Surg Tech. 2020;10(2):e0022. https://doi.org/10.2106/JBJS.ST.19.00022.

11. Mahoney O, Kinsey T, Sodhi BSNN, Chen AF, Orozco F, Hozack W. Improved component placement accuracy with robotic-arm assisted total knee arthroplasty. 2020;10075. (This nonrandomized prospective study aimed to compare the 3D accuracy of robotic-arm assisted TKA with conventional TKA for component positioning. Robotic-arm assisted TKA demonstrated greater accuracy for tibial component alignment, femoral component rotation, and tibial slope. Additionally, robotic-assisted demonstrated greater Knee Society functional scores, although found not to be statistically significant. Level 2).

12. Gustke KA, Golladay GJ, Roche MW, Elson LC, Anderson CR. Primary TKA patients with quantifiably balanced soft-tissue achieve significant clinical gains sooner than unbalanced patients. Adv Orthop. 2014;2014:628695. https://doi.org/10.1155/2014/628695. (This multicenter study evaluated 1-year follow up a previously reported group of patients who had sensor-assisted TKA and compared clinical outcomes of quantitatively balanced versus unbalanced knees. At 1 year, the balanced cohort showed improved Knee Society and WOMAC scores. Patients with balanced knees additionally participated in more activity. Level 3).

13. Gustke KA, Golladay GJ, Roche MW, Elson LC, Anderson CR. A targeted approach to ligament balancing using kinetic sensors. J Arthroplasty. 2017;32(7):2127–32. https://doi.org/10.1016/j.arth.2017.02.021. (This study examined intraoperative data to determine how targeted ligament releases affect intra-articular loading and ultimately found that loading across the joint became more symmetric after releases, and on average, 2–3 corrections were made in order to achieve ligament balance. Level 3).

14. Gustke KA, Golladay GJ, Roche MW, Elson LC, Anderson CR. A new method for defining balance: promising short-term clinical outcomes of sensor-guided TKA. J Arthroplasty. 2014;29(5):955–60. https://doi.org/10.1016/j.arth.2013.10.020. (This multicenter evaluation evaluated outcome measurements in patients with balanced knees. Ultimately, the authors found that 6 month outcomes were significantly improved amongst the balanced cohorts. Additionally, balanced joints were the most significant contributing factor to improved postoperative outcomes. Level 3).

15. Siddiqi A, Smith T, McPhilemy JJ, Ranawat AS, Sculco PK, Chen AF. Soft-tissue balancing technology for total knee arthroplasty. JBJS Rev. 2020;8(1):e0050. https://doi.org/10.2106/JBJS.RVW.19.00050.

16. Almouahed S, Gouriou M, Hamitouche C, Stindel E, Roux C. Design and evaluation of instrumented smart knee implant. IEEE Trans Biomed Eng. 2011;58(4):971–82.

17. Cho KJ, Seon JK, Jang WY, Park CG, Song EK. Objective quantification of ligament balancing using VERASENSE in measured resection and modified gap balance total knee arthroplasty. BMC Musculoskelet Disord. 2018;19(1):1–11. https://doi.org/10.1186/s12891-018-2190-8. (This study aimed to quantify the compartment pressure of the knee joint throughout motion during TKA using orthosensor, determine the usefulness of orthosensor, and evaluate the types and effectiveness of additional ligament balancing. With the orthosensor, the authors were able to obtain a 94% quantified balanced knee. Measurede resection TKA showed less balanced knee and also required more additionall procedures compared to modified gap-balancing TKA. Level 2).

18. Ibrahim A, Jain M, Salman E, Willing R, Towfighian S. A smart knee implant using triboelectric energy harvesters. Smart Mater Struct. 2019. https://doi.org/10.1016/j.physbeh.2017.03.040 (This study characterized a triboelectric energy harvester under body loads and aimed to additionally design electronics to digitize the load data.)

19. D'Lima DD, Fregly BJ, Colwell CW. Implantable sensor technology: measuring bone and joint biomechanics of daily life in vivo. Arthritis Res Ther. 2013;15(1):1–8. https://doi.org/10.1186/ar4138. (This review addresses and summarizes developments in sensors that measure strains in bone, intraarticular cartilage contact pressures, and forces in several joints).

20. Arami A, Vallet A, Aminian K. Accurate measurement of concurrent flexion-extension and internal-external rotations in smart knee prostheses. IEEE Trans Biomed Eng. 2013;60(9):2504–10. https://doi.org/10.1109/TBME.2013.2259489. (This study presents a system for integration into TKA prosethesis that accurately measures flexion-extension and internal-external rotations. In particular, the system places 2 magnets into the femoral and tibial parts of

the prosthesis and a sensor into the polyethylene component. Level 2).

21. Gustke KA. Soft-tissue and alignment correction: the use of smart trials in total knee replacement. Bone Joint J. 2014;96B(11):78–83. https://doi.org/10.1302/0301-620X.96B11.34339.

22. MacDessi SJ, Griffiths-Jones W, Chen DB, et al. Restoring the constitutional alignment with a restrictive kinematic protocol improves quantitative soft-tissue balance in total knee arthroplasty: a randomized controlled trial. Bone Joint J. 2020;102(1):117–24. https://doi.org/10.1302/0301-620X.102B1.BJJ-2019-0674.R2. (This randomized trial compares patients undergoing TKA using kinematic alignment versus mechanical alignment and found that restoring the constitutional alignment with kinematic alignment in TKA resulted in a statistically significant improvement in knee balance. Additionally, bone recuts were less likely in the kinematically aligned group. Level 2).

23. Meneghini RM, Ziemba-Davis MM, Lovro LR, Ireland PH, Damer BM. Can intraoperative sensors determine the "target" ligament balance? Early outcomes in total knee arthroplasty. J Arthroplasty. 2016;31(10):2181–7. https://doi.org/10.1016/j.arth.2016.03.046. (This multicenter retrospective study reviewed TKAs performed with standard surgical techniques and ligament releases with insertion of sensor-embedded smart tibial trays. The aim was to determine if patient outcomes were affected by ligament balance and to determine an optimal balance. Greater improvement in UCLA activity level was associated with a mediolateral force difference of under 60lbs. Knee Society scores were unrelated to balance. Level 3).

24. Geller JA, Lakra A, Murtaugh T. The use of electronic sensor device to augment ligament balancing leads to a lower rate of arthrofibrosis after total knee arthroplasty. J Arthroplasty. 2017;32(5):1502–4. https://doi.org/10.1016/j.arth.2016.12.019. (This study evaluated the incidence of arthrofibrosis before and after implementation of a sensor device and found that ligament balancing using sensor assistance resulted in a statistically significant decrease in manipulation under anesthesia following TKA. Level 3).

Advances in Medial Unicompartmental Knee Arthroplasty

10

Julius K. Oni and Wenzel Waldstein

Introduction

Unicompartmental knee arthroplasty (UKA) is a safe and effective treatment option for isolated end-stage unicompartmental (unicondylar) knee osteoarthritis (OA) [1]. Approximately 90% of UKA procedures are performed for medial compartment arthritis, thus the name medial UKA [2].

The possibility of a UKA was first theorized in the 1950s by McKeever as a metallic tibial component implanted in a knee with advanced unicompartmental OA [3]. The concept of a minimally invasive procedure that results in less soft tissue trauma and removal of bone than a total knee arthroplasty (TKA) took hold. Further developments over the next two decades resulted in the first modern implant design employing a flat polyethylene metal-backed tibial component and a metallic polyradial femoral counterpart [4]. However, in the 1980s, an increase in the understanding of OA led to an exponential rise in the interest in TKA and to the introduction of the Oxford Knee, whereas the interest in UKA stagnated [5].

Today, the advantages of UKA over TKA in isolated medial OA are abundant and include a faster recovery, lower cost, fewer major complications like thromboembolism, stroke and myocardial infarction, and ultimately lower mortality [2, 6], as well as superior patient-reported satisfaction and functional outcomes [2, 7–9]. The most significant disadvantage of UKA is the higher revision rates compared to TKA. The exact magnitude of increased revision rates is a topic of much controversy due to discrepancies in the data reported by national registries and cohort studies. Despite increasing evidence in its favor, many orthopaedic surgeons still consider UKA a highly specialized procedure for a very specific type of patient. A recent analysis of national joint registries demonstrated that more than 50% of knee surgeons in the UK, Australia, and New Zealand perform less than 5% of UKA yearly [10]. Globally, only 10% of orthopaedic surgeons perform UKA [11]. This rate of UKA utilization is pointedly low considering the potential advantages of this minimally invasive procedure. The established indications and patient selection criteria for UKA, in addition to discrepancies between the results of national registries and design-center cohort studies, have proven pivotal in contributing to the hesitancy to perform this procedure.

This chapter aims to elucidate the results of the latest studies and advances in the field of medial UKA as well as address the current dis-

J. K. Oni
Department of Orthopedic Surgery, Johns Hopkins Bayview Medical Center, Baltimore, MD, USA

W. Waldstein (✉)
Orthopedic Clinic Paulinenhilfe, Diakonie Klinikum, Stuttgart, Germany

A. J. Deshmukh et al. (eds.), *Surgical Management of Knee Arthritis*, https://doi.org/10.1007/978-3-031-47929-8_10

117

crepancies and debates for the benefit of the orthopaedic surgeon.

Indications and Contraindications for Medial UKA

Adequate patient selection is crucial for the long-term survival of UKA [3]. The debate on indications and contraindications has been ongoing for over 30 years [12]. Many surgeons [13, 14] still adhere to the selection criteria by Kozinn and Scott published in 1989 [15] who propose to perform a medial UKA only in patients with isolated medial compartment OA, with no lateral joint tenderness, no anterior knee pain, in patients over 60 years of age, under 82 kg of weight, with low physical demands, with a varus deformity of under 10°, no patellofemoral arthritis, a flexion contracture of under 5°, intact collaterals and no inflammatory conditions. If these strict indication criteria were applied, a maximum of 10% of patients with varus knee OA would be considered candidates for a medial UKA. Therefore, the indication criteria for medial UKA were extended and modified over the last 20 years.

The primary indication for medial UKA is isolated anteromedial osteoarthritis (AMOA) of the knee [16]. Typically, in AMOA of the knee, the anterior cruciate ligament (ACL) and medial collateral ligament (MCL) are functionally intact. There is no posterior wear on the tibia plateau and the intra-articular deformity is fully correctable. The cartilage in the lateral compartment is biomechanically intact [17] (Fig. 10.1).

Inactive osteonecrosis of the medial femoral condyle is another ideal indication for medial UKA [18]. Potential cysts and significant surrounding edema should be ruled out preoperatively due to concerns of implant fixation. Active osteonecrosis with significant edema may lead to higher rates of loosening. Full-thickness cartilage in the weight-bearing area of the lateral compartment is required for medial UKA [19, 20]. Patients with arthritis in the weight-bearing area of the lateral compartment should not be considered for medial UKA [21]. However, a full-thickness cartilage ulcer on the medial wall of the

lateral femoral condyle caused by impingement of the lateral femoral condyle on the lateral tibial spine is no contraindication [22]. Lateral-compartment osteophytes in varus knee OA may not be a contraindication. It has been shown that in varus knees, lateral osteophytes are not associated with biomechanically weaker cartilage, more advanced histological cartilage degeneration, lower cartilage volume or diminished cartilage thickness in the lateral compartment [23, 24]. Furthermore, it has been demonstrated that the presence of chondrocalcinosis does not affect the functional outcome or survival following UKA [25, 26].

In patients with isolated AMOA, the functional integrity of the ACL has historically been considered an essential requirement for UKA [27, 28]. Higher failure rates have been reported for UKA in patients with an insufficient ACL at the time of surgery [29] (Fig. 10.2). However, a recent meta-analysis reported no difference in the outcome of medial UKA with or without ACL deficiency [30]. In the young and active with symptomatic ACL insufficiency and AMOA, staged or simultaneous ACL reconstruction and UKA presents a possible but technically demanding treatment option [31]. In carefully selected older patients without preoperative instability, UKA without ACL reconstruction may be an option [31]. A recent study reports no significant differences in kinetics and kinematics between conventional UKA with an intact ACL, and an ACL-deficient UKA group in which the tibial component was implanted with a decreased slope [32]. However, these observations were made on a small sample size with no long-term follow-up.

Medial facet patellofemoral joint degeneration does not affect the outcome of medial UKA while caution is advised in patients with advanced lateral facet patellofemoral joint disease [33–36]. In the latter, a significantly worse outcome was reported in the literature [33, 34] and a total knee arthroplasty (TKA) might be the preferred treatment option. This was confirmed by Argenson et al. who consider extensive loss of cartilage in the patellofemoral joint to be a contraindication to fixed-bearing unicompartmental arthroplasty

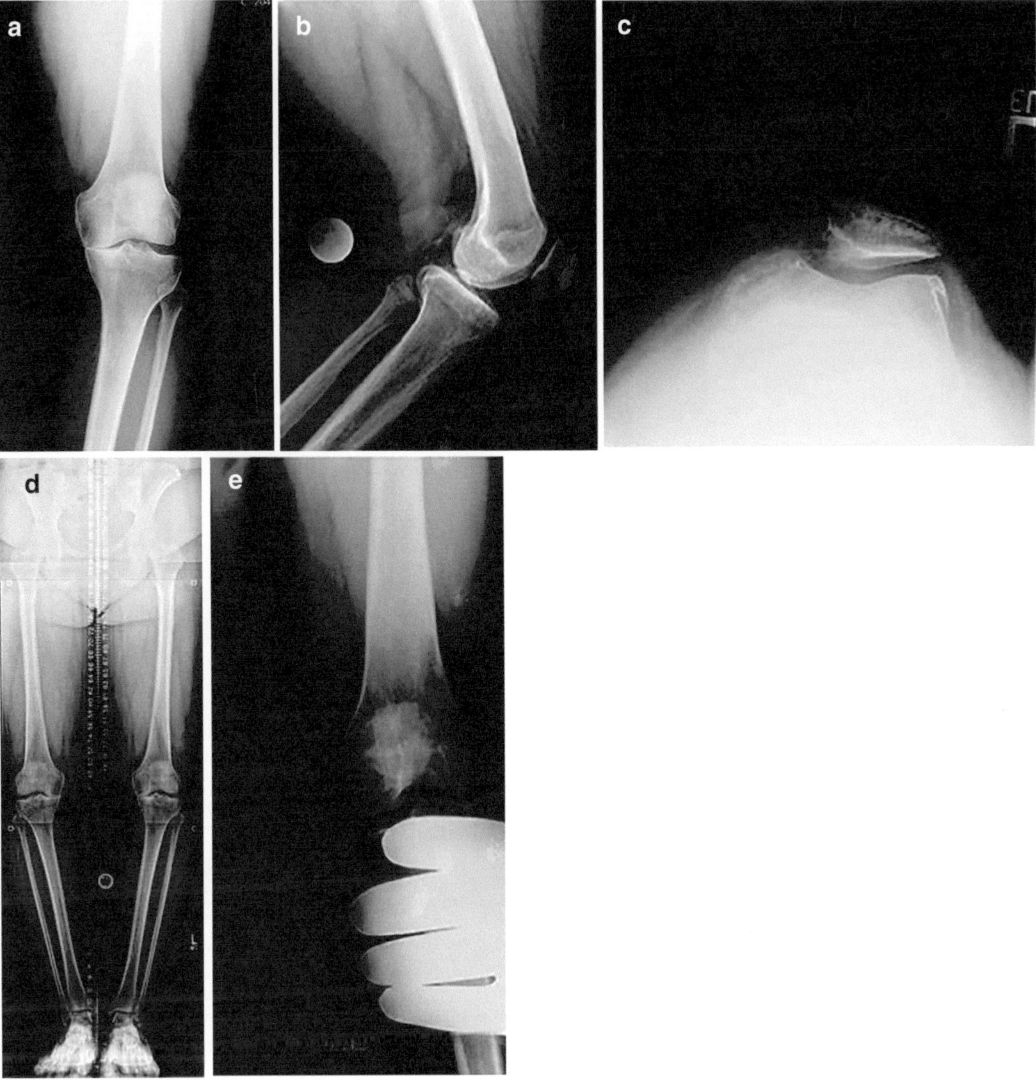

Fig. 10.1 Complete radiographic work-up in a candidate (62 years old, female) for medial UKA: (**a**) standing AP knee radiograph with bone-on-bone anteromedial osteoarthritis of the left knee, osteophytes in the lateral compartment can be ignored; (**b**) true lateral radiograph with no posterior tibial erosion suggestive of a functionally intact ACL; (**c**) skyline radiograph with no lateral facet patellofemoral arthritis, (**d**) standing long-leg radiographs with no extra-articular deformity and a mechanical varus deformity of 11° and (e) valgus stress radiograph obtained in 20° of flexion shows a fully correctable varus deformity with full-thickness lateral-compartment cartilage and re-establishment of lateral femorotibial joint congruency

[37]. Anterior knee pain is not a general contraindication for medial UKA.

Medial UKA is indicated in varus knees with a correctable intra-articular deformity after removal of medial osteophytes [38]. The cut-off of 10° preoperative varus deformity as proposed by Kozinn and Scott appears too generic, and does not take the concept of a constitutional varus into account. Particularly, as in some health care systems, preoperative standing long-leg radiographs are not routinely obtained and the overall alignment remains unknown [38]. However, the intra-articular deformity should be correctable which can reliably be assessed on preoperative valgus stress radiographs [39]. There is limited data on the outcome of medial UKA in patients

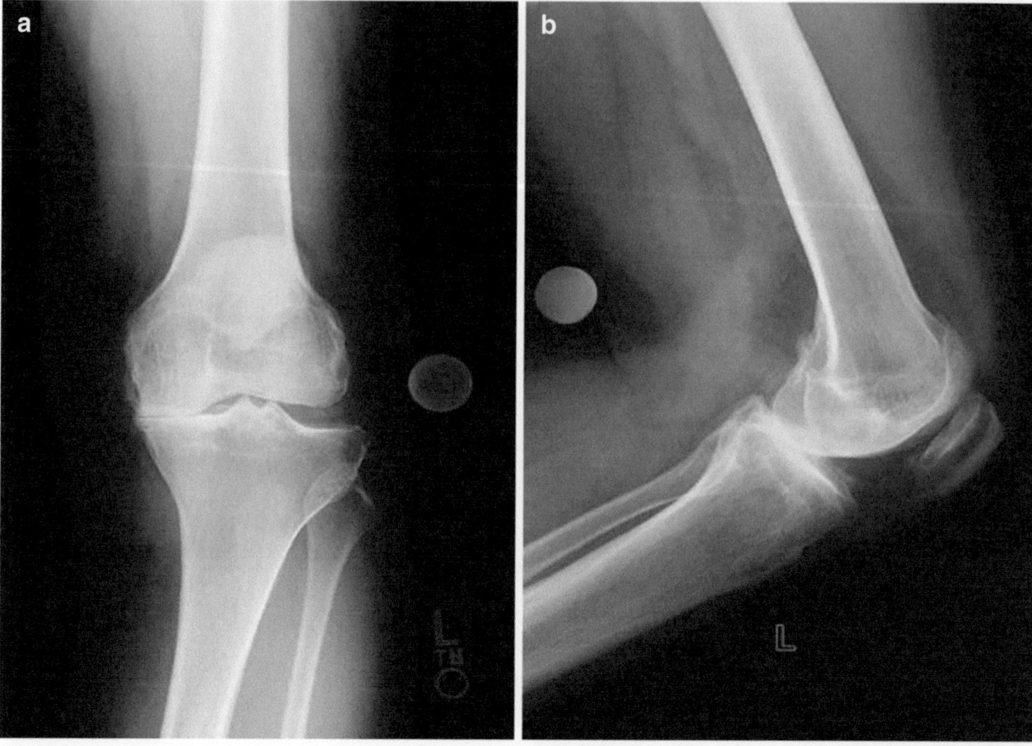

Fig. 10.2 Preoperative radiographs in a 61-year-old male patient with functional ACL insufficiency: (**a**) standing AP knee radiograph shows medial bone-on-bone OA with substantial coronal tibiofemoral subluxation; (**b**) lateral radiograph shows posterior tibial erosion as a sign of sagittal instability. Functional ACL insufficiency is a contraindication for medial UKA

with more advanced deformities [40, 41]. In this context, it should be noted that knees with more advanced varus deformities should always be critically evaluated for functional ACL insufficiency. Springer et al. reported that ACL insufficiency was observed in 33% of all arthritic knees with a varus deformity of >10° [42] (Fig. 10.2). With regard to flexion deformities, full extension should be achieved during surgery after removal of anterior and posterior osteophytes as postoperative fixed flexion deformities of >10° after UKA are associated with significantly poorer functional outcomes [43, 44].

Young age (<60 years) has long been a contraindication for UKA. Yet, it has been shown that younger patients below the age of 60 years will also benefit from UKA [45]. However, the patient's acceptance for an increased cumulative revision rate after UKA implantation has to be discussed as part of a shared decision-making process. The Australian, Swedish and UK joint registries suggest that the risk of revision surgery is substantially higher in younger patients (<55 years) [46, 47]. This has been confirmed by a meta-analysis reporting an increased likelihood for revision in younger patients [48]. In contrast, a large cohort study on mobile-bearing UKA showed no higher revision rates in younger patients at mean follow-up of 10 years [49, 50]. Similarly, for fixed-bearing UKA, a recent cohort study on patients younger than 55 years reported an all-cause unicompartmental to total knee arthroplasty revision rate of 10% at 10 years [51]. Older patients (>80 years) particularly benefit because of the smaller intervention and the known lower perioperative risks in comparison to TKA [6]. In general, patient age should not be considered a contraindication for UKA.

Many studies in the last few years have reported on the outcome of UKAs in obese patients with conflicting results. There is no consensus of whether obese patients really benefit from a UKA instead of a TKA. Some authors suggest that UKA can be safely offered to even the heaviest patients without concern for increased complications or inferior results [52–54]. In a cohort of 746 robotic-assisted UKAs with a mean BMI of 32 kg/m^2, BMI had no influence on clinical outcomes and readmission rates up to a mean follow-up of 35 months [54]. The Oxford group recommended that high BMI should not be a contraindication for UKA based on their promising results of patients with a BMI of >35 kg/m^2 at 10 years [53]. In a recent meta-analysis, no statistically significant difference in the revision rate of obese (BMI >30 kg/m^2) and non-obese patients was observed [55]. Others have also reported that a BMI >30 kg/m^2 does not influence the long-term rate of survival of UKA [48, 52]. In contrast, Xu et al. described obesity (BMI >30 kg/m^2) as a significant predictor of poorer improvement in clinical outcome and an increased rate of revision 10 years postoperatively [56]. In one of the few studies on patients with a BMI >40 kg/m^2, Nettrour et al. concluded that the rate of early major revision surgery in morbidly-obese patients undergoing UKA may be over five times greater than that of other patients [57]. Failure modes were predominantly disease progression in other compartments or mobile-bearing instability [57]. Traditionally, inflammatory forms of arthritis were seen as an absolute contraindication for UKA. Due to the development of new treatment options for patients with rheumatoid arthritis, the disease activity is nowadays much better controlled. In selected patients with low disease activity, good bone mineral density and AMOA, a medial UKA may be an option. However, disease activity should be closely monitored as higher inflammatory activity increases the risk of radiographic loosening in arthroplasty patients [58].

Radiographic Evaluation

Standardized preoperative radiographs are most of the time sufficient to indicate medial UKA [38]. Anteromedial bone-on-bone arthritis observed on standing anteroposterior (AP) knee radiographs is required for medial UKA. If no bone-on-bone OA is seen on standing AP views, a varus stress radiograph or an MRI may be performed to rule in patients with medial full-thickness cartilage wear. Assessment of overall mechanical alignment on standing long-leg radiographs allows for a differentiation between intra- and extra-articular deformity, and may be helpful for adjustments in the operative technique. True lateral radiographs are important to assess functional ACL integrity. Wear should be limited to the anterior portion of the tibia plateau. Lateral radiographs with posterior tibial erosion suggest functional ACL insufficiency which is a contraindication for medial UKA (Fig. 10.2). In cases in which the extent of posterior erosion on the lateral radiograph cannot be assessed with confidence, an MRI with assessment of both the ACL morphology and the underlying cartilage wear pattern on medial appears to provide additional clinical benefit [59]. The amount of coronal tibiofemoral subluxation on standing AP views should also be taken into consideration when assessing ACL sufficiency. It has been shown that with increasing tibiofemoral subluxation (>6 mm), functional ACL insufficiency becomes more likely [1].

Valgus stress radiographs are essential to assess lateral-compartment cartilage [38]. Valgus stress views are useful to preoperatively assess the correctability of the deformity. The coronal deformity should be reducible to pre-arthritic values. Non-correctable varus deformities are a contraindication. Furthermore, the reestablishment of lateral femorotibial joint congruency can be determined on stress films [1] (Fig. 10.1). Skyline radiographs should be performed to exclude advanced lateral facet patellofemoral arthritis. In patients with mild to moderate anterior knee pain, a normal skyline radiograph can rule out full-thickness cartilage defects of the lateral patellar with confidence [60]. In cases of radiographic abnormalities or severe anterior knee pain, an MRI allows for the most accurate assessment of the patellofemoral joint [60].

Implant Design Concepts

The MacIntosh and McKeever hemiarthroplasty were the first attempts for a unicompartmental knee arthroplasty dating back to the early 1950s [61, 62]. Implant designs and modes of fixation have evolved since then; the most substantial modifications over the last 30 years were the introduction of modular metal-backed tibial components, mobile-bearing designs, and cementless component fixation. Broadly, UKA designs can be categorized into modular metal-backed (MB) versus all-polyethylene (AP) tibia designs, cemented versus cementless fixation techniques, and fixed- versus mobile-bearing surfaces [3]. The inlay technique relies on minimal bone resection and subchondral bone support. The only technique is based on bone cuts performed with instrumentation similar to total knee arthroplasty, and implants that are placed on cortical and cancellous bone. The bearing surface can either be a modular polyethylene (PE) implant with a metal-backed (MB) tibial base plate or an all polyethylene (AP) tibial implant. Mobile-bearing or fixed-bearing (FB) design concepts have been developed for modular MB UKA.

All Polyethylene Versus Metal-Backed

Historical implants like the original Marmor prosthesis, the St. Georg sled (Waldemar Link, Hamburg, Germany), and the Repicci (Biomet, Warsaw, IN) are based on resurfacing of the tibia, and consist of an All Polyethylene (AP) cemented tibia and biconcave metal femoral component [63]. The proposed advantages of AP include greater bone preservation due to thin implants, low backside wear and reduced implant costs [64]. All Polyethylene designs have shown variable results in the literature [65]. However, for older patients (>70 years), an AP tibia might be a good treatment option with ten-year survivorship of up to 92% [66] (Fig. 10.3).

Metal-backed (MB) tibial components were developed to improve load transfer and ensure a more reliable cement fixation. MB implants have shown a more consistent survivorship, offer the benefit of more intraoperative options due to modularity; however, MB implants require more bone resection [65].

Cemented Versus Cementless

Most UKA designs use cement to fix the components to the bone. However, due to observations of high rates of misleading radiolucent lines with associated revisions there has been an increased interest in cementless fixation [67, 68]. In 2009, the Oxford group reported their encouraging one-year results for their cementless medial mobile-bearing UKA [69]. There have been observations of a higher tibial fracture rate in cementless

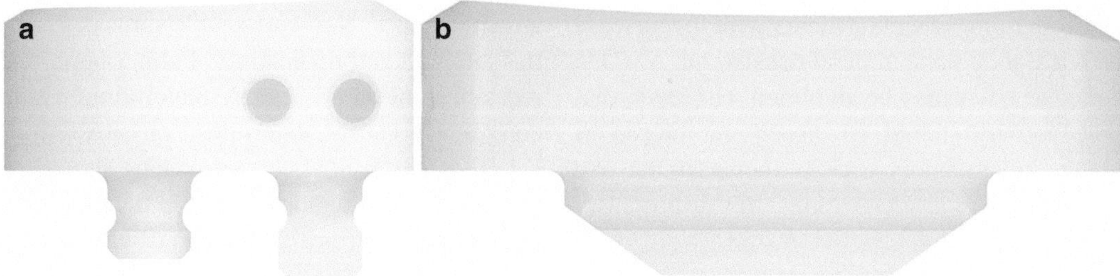

Fig. 10.3 The Sigma® Partial Knee is available with an all-polyethylene cemented tibial component: (**a**) front view, (**b**) side view (courtesy DePuy Synthes)

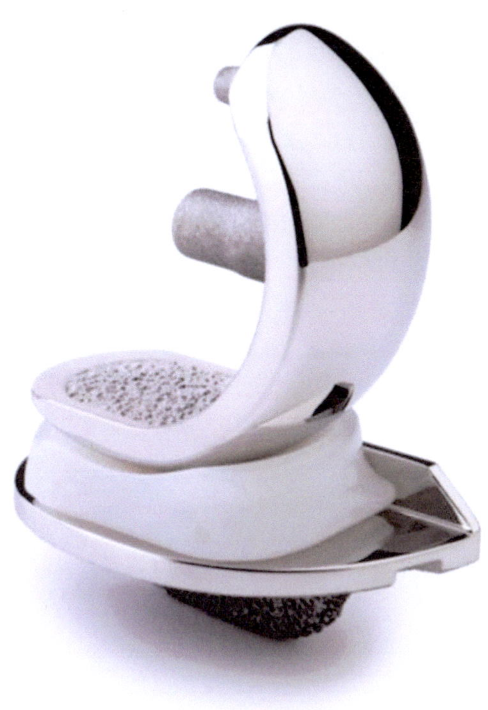

Fig. 10.4 The Oxford® Cementless Partial Knee allows for a cementless femoral and tibial fixation. (Courtesy ZimmerBiomet)

medial UKA with mechanically aligned Oxford tibial components. Suda et al. reported a significant reduction in the fracture risk when the tibial component is placed in slight varus which is now generally recommened [70]. The first cementless Oxford UKA had a porous titanium undersurface with a calcium hydroxyapatite coating. The femoral component was slightly modified with a cylindrical main femoral peg and an additional small anterior peg to enhance primary fixation [69] (Fig. 10.4).

Fixed-Bearing Versus Mobile-Bearing

In fixed-bearing MB implants, the PE insert is engaged into the locking mechanism of the tibial component. Mobile-bearing MB designs have a flat tibial baseplate, a spherical femoral component and a conforming PE insert that matches the curvature of the femoral component [4]. Mobile-

bearing UKA theoretically offers the advantage of reduced polyethylene wear due to increased conformity and diminished stresses on the PE insert, as well as more physiological kinematics [5]. However, ligament balancing is technically challenging leading to an increased risk of bearing dislocation and impingement [6]. Fixed-bearing MB implants on the other hand are technically more forgiving and may, therefore, be the better option to achieve higher survival rates for low-volume surgeons as mentioned by Bonutti [6] (Fig. 10.5).

Clinical Outcome and Revision Rates

The use of UKA varies among countries. According to the Australian Orthopaedic Association National Joint Replacement Registry (AOANJRR), UKA accounted for 5.6% of all knee procedures in 2019. The National Joint Registry annual report 2020 indicates a 11.5% share of UKA of all primary knee procedures. In the UK, 7.2% of all primary knee arthroplasty was cemented UKA and 4.3% was cementless UKA. Interestingly, the percentage of cemented FB UKA has constantly been growing from 0.8% in 2004 to 5.8% in 2019. Cementless mobile-bearing UKA is also becoming more popular in the UK with an increase from 0.7% in 2009 to 4.1% in 2019. Across registries, cemented FB implants and cementless mobile-bearing implants are currently the most frequently used designs [7, 8]. The AOANJRR reports a 15-year cumulative percent revision (CPR) of 22% for FB primary UKA and 23% for mobile-bearing primary UKA, respectively. Looking at the NJR data, the lowest cumulative revision rates at ten years were observed for cemented FB UKA (8.6%) and cementless mobile-bearing UKA (8.4%). However, cemented mobile-bearing UKA had a significantly higher cumulative revision rate of 12% at 10 years and 18.9% at 15 years [71]. The most frequent causes for revision were arthritis progression, aseptic loosening and pain for cemented FB designs and disease progression, bearing dislocation and aseptic loosening for cementless mobile-bearing designs, respectively [7]. Kannan et al. analyzed the survivorship of

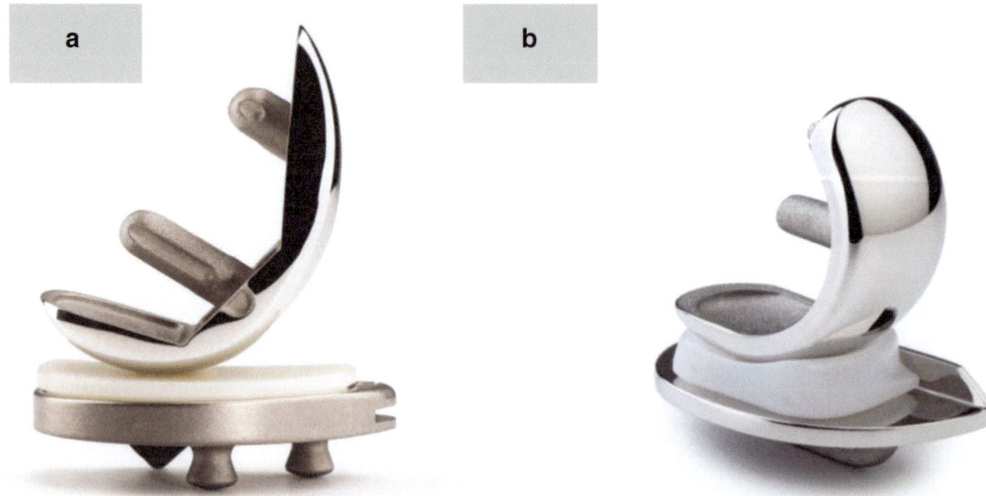

Fig. 10.5 (**a**) The Persona® Partial Knee (ZimmerBiomet) is an example for a modern cemented fixed-bearing metal-backed design, (**b**) The Oxford® Partial Knee is the most commonly used cemented mobile-bearing implant. (Courtesy ZimmerBiomet)

UKA depending on bearing surface using data from the AOANJRR [72]. The best survivorship of the current UKA designs at 15 years was reported for modular FB UKA with a CPR of 16% in comparison to 23% for mobile-bearing UKA [9]. However, it must be noted that cemented and cementless mobile-bearing designs were grouped into one category.

Various single center cohort studies reported excellent survivorship of 92–98% at ten years for cemented [73] and cementless [74] medial Oxford UKA, as well as for cemented FB designs [75]. Excellent patient satisfaction, pain relief, functional improvement and quality of life improvement can be achieved with mobile-bearing and FB implants [76]. In a recent meta-analysis, no differences in terms of revision rates, complications, and knee function were observed between mobile-bearing and FB UKA [77].

In summary, mobile-bearing UKA may better restore physiological knee kinematics; however, bearing dislocation remains a unique cause of failure with these designs. Overall, the functional outcomes and long-term survivorship of mobile-bearing and fixed-bearing UKAs are comparable, although registry data may show a potential advantage of fixed-bearing UKA with regard to revision rates.

Operative Techniques

In addition to the above implant design considerations, numerous operative-related factors have been proven to affect short- and long-term outcomes in UKA patients; these include caseload and surgeon experience, surgeon technical and non-technical skills, attitudes towards patient selection, surgical approaches used, component placement and alignment, as well as conventional versus technology-assisted options. The overall goal of medial UKA is to restore pre-arthritic anatomy. Below is a brief description of the established, conventional cemented medial UKA procedure derived from Campbell's Operative Orthopaedics with added emphasis on the potential pitfalls that require extra attention from the surgeon [78].

A longitudinal skin incision is made along the medial border of the patellar tendon. It must be large enough to sufficiently expose the knee joint but small enough to minimize the soft-tissue release. The capsular incision must not proceed superior to the vastus medialis. A Hohmann-type retractor is used to expose the femoral condyle by laterally levering away the patella while the knee is flexed [78]. The medial compartment is exposed by incising the coronary ligament, removing the medial meniscal anterior horn, and lifting the periosteal sleeve from the anteromedial tibia. Thorough inspection of the medial compartment is required to ensure the patient is indeed a suitable candidate for medial UKA. Removal of peripheral osteophytes will result in better exposure of the joint, intercondylar notch osteophyte removal will prevent cruciate ligament impingement and damage. Significant soft tissue balancing may be a result of a severe varus deformity or insufficient resection of bone. Using an extramedullary mechanical guide to align the proximal horizontal tibial cut with the midline of the ankle ensures the cut is perpendicular to the mechanical axis; a posterior tibial slope is also re-formed with a 2-mm deep resection or as otherwise stated by the implant instructions [78]. The proximal tibial cut should be as small as possible, enough to remove the arthritic surface whilst being in line with the posterior slope [79]. The sagittal tibial cut ought to be adjacent to the tibial spine to maximize the tibial surface area without affecting the anterior cruciate ligament [78, 79]. To avoid future fracture of the medial tibial plateau, the tibial cut should not penetrate the posterior cortex. A spacer block (typically 8 mm) is placed in the flexed knee to approximate the size of the gap for the smallest tibial resection. Once the knee is fully extended another spacer block is placed to approximate the distal femoral cut needed to balance the gaps in full extension and flexion.

A femoral cutting jig is placed to make the distal femoral resection, a femoral sizing guide is inserted, and an appropriately sized cutting block is chosen to make the posterior condylar resection and chamfer cut [78]. The medial meniscus is carefully resected, and all loose debris must be removed from the posterior recess of the knee. It is important to avoid overcorrecting the patient's varus deformity (aim to under-correct the mechanical axis by 2–3°) as overcorrection will lead to excessive load and wear in the lateral compartment, and excessive stress on medial soft-tissue structures. The trial implant is then inserted, and the knee joint is reduced to test for the following: alignment, extension, flexion to gravity, AP stability in flexion, varus and valgus stability in flexion, patellar tracking, and component rotation. Beware of an undersized tibial component as that can lead to excessive stress and potential tibial fracture or implant loosening [79].

The bone is prepared for a final time and the implants are cemented as per implant-specific instructions. It is important to avoid excessive force during tibial component impaction in order to minimize the risk of iatrogenic fractures. Femoral component placement should align with the center (or just lateral to it) of the medial femoral condyle to augment tracking with the tibial components [79]. Extra attention must be made to interdigitate the cement in the bone and to allow sufficient drying before the knee is mobilized. After cement hardening and prior to wound closure, all loose debris and cement in the joint should be removed [78].

Surgeon-Related Factors

Numerous operative-related factors have been proven to affect clinical outcomes in UKA patients; among the most important are the factors relating to the surgeon. There is strong evidence that TKA patients of higher caseload (volume) surgeons have better outcomes and less complications compared to their counterparts of lower-volume surgeons [80]. This difference is amplified in UKA, with revision rates for the highest-volume surgeons four times less than their lowest-volume colleagues [81]. Analyses of the UK National Joint Registry demonstrated that surgeons who performed UKA in 5% of their patients had poorer outcomes compared to their colleagues performing UKA in 40–60% of their patients [79, 82, 83]. Furthermore, implant survival rates at five years were 6% lower when performed by high-volume surgeons compared to those by low-volume surgeons [79, 82]. A 2017 study of 14,496 cemented medial Oxford III UKA in 126 hospitals demonstrated that lower-volume hospitals, and by extension lower-volume surgeons, had higher rates of revision and lower rates of implant survival than lower-volume hospitals [84]. A portion of this difference is expected to be due to lower-volume surgeons selecting healthier, younger patients with earlier-stage OA. However, the measurable disparities in patient characteristics were small and the likely factor behind these results is the broader selection criteria used by higher-volume surgeons in order to perform UKA on a larger proportion of their patients [81]. Additionally, lower-volume surgeons are more likely to perform UKA revisions without an objective cause of symptoms (i.e., unexplained pain) than their more experienced colleagues [85]. The relationship between usage and volume is further elucidated by a meta-analysis that established that the proportion of UKA (usage) was more significant than the mere number of procedures per year (volume). Regardless of volume, a usage rate of 20% or greater yielded a significantly lower rate of failure [86].

Importantly, the effect of caseload on outcomes is seen across every group of surgeons' UKA volume, with extra importance in the very low-volume surgeon group (less than five UKA per year). This group presents the greatest concern as they produce the worst results [81]. Liddle et al. argue that these surgeons can improve their results by performing a greater number of UKA to increase their usage or, if they are unable to do so, or modify their practice by ultimately retiring this procedure and referring those patients to their higher UKA-volume colleagues [81]. This school of thought has underpinned the debate on 'centralization' and 'regionalization' seen in the field of TKA, sparking a similar discussion for UKA with far-reaching socioeconomic consequences [80].

Although the differences in the outcomes of patients operated on by low-volume surgeons and high-volume surgeons can be partly explained by the patient selection criteria used, other factors may also be at play; these likely include surgical technique, stage of disease, surgeons' thresholds for revision. Ultimately, there is clear evidence that UKA volume and usage rates help determine

the survival and revision rates of UKA. The variables behind this are complex and future research will benefit from more in-depth intra-operative technique and post-operative radiograph studies in elucidating and determining these variables; particularly before any changes to clinical practice can be suggested.

Component Placement and Alignment

Post-operative knee kinematics play an important role in the clinical outcomes of a UKA. The return and maintenance of femorotibial geometry aids in avoiding common modes of failure. The parameters fundamental to this geometry include component size, placement, and divergence; the hip-knee-ankle axis; maintenance of joint line; and soft-tissue balancing [87].

The size and placement of the components are vital to the clinical outcomes and rate of failure in UKA, this is particularly evident of the tibial component. Surgeons must ensure the tibial component is appropriately sized as oversizing and tibial overhang of >3 mm results in worse clinical outcomes at 5 years [88]. Care must also be taken not to undersize the tibial component to avoid excessive stress and implant loosening [79]. Tibial placement orientation is a significant factor in knee kinematics and thus the longevity of the implant. Excessive varus angulation of >5° results in component subsidence and higher rates of failure in cemented UKA [89, 90]. The posterior tibial slope is another important variable in knee kinematics. An increase in the slope results in anterior tibial translation and thus an increase in the stress placed on the anterior cruciate ligament, a risk factor for ACL instability. A study of 100 UKA implants 16 years after the procedure found that a slope of >7° results in greater tibial component loosening [91]. It is suggested that the change in slope need not exceed >2° the original physiologic value in order to reduce the risk of premature failure [92]. Placement of the femoral component is central to inter-component divergence and geometry. The femoral component should form a 90° angle with its tibial counterpart. Deviations of >6° from this ideal inter-component alignment will result in worse outcomes and higher rates of failure [92]. Limb alignment is determined by the hip-knee-ankle mechanism axis, also known as Maquet's line, thus restoring this mechanical axis to its pre-arthritis form is one of the key aims in UKA. Intra-operatively, this axis is determined by the thickness of the tibial component, volume of tibial resection, ligament tension, and the extent of preoperative deformity [93]. Overcorrection of varus deformity will result in premature arthritic degeneration in the lateral compartment, and under-correction will result in premature implant wear and loosening [91]. Maintaining a post-operative varus angle of 1–4° will result in optimal outcomes [94, 95]. The knee joint line is directly affected by the post-operative joint space in the medial compartment. Disruption of the joint line has shown to lead to adverse outcomes in UKA as the subsequent joint incongruence results to pronounced changes in load transfer between the two compartments [96]. It is suggested to keep the change in the joint space height of the medical compartment within 3 mm of that of the lateral compartment [96, 97]. The above variables must be noted as they are the intra-operative factors that will lead to premature failure in medial UKA.

Minimally Invasive UKA

The discussion thus far has had a focus on the conventional surgical approach to a medial UKA (medial parapatellar arthrotomy). A minimally invasive surgical (MIS) approach has been developed for UKA with the aim of improving recovery and minimizing soft-tissue trauma. Currently three variations of a MIS approach exist: a midvastus approach in which a 20 mm incision is made in the vastus medialis, a quadricep-sparing approach in which the medial parapatellar incision does not proximally extend into the quadriceps, and a subvastus approach in which the medial parapatellar incision extends deep to the vastus medialis tendon.

Hamilton et al. and Scuderi et al. have indeed reported a faster recovery time, reduced postoperative pain, faster return of knee flexion with MIS compared to a conventional approach [98, 99]. Price et al. demonstrated small incision UKA patients had half the recovery time their conventional incision-matched counterparts had [100]. In an RCT by Riley et al., minimally invasive UKA resulted in faster discharge, less hospital occupancy, and cost savings of 27% compared to conventional UKA [101]. However, the added complexity of MIS is not without its drawbacks. In Hamilton et al.'s study some centers reported more aspetic loosening and substantially higher revision rates, as high as 11% at the two-year mark, in the MIS cohort. The underlying causes reported include retained debris, meniscal defects, lateral compartment chondral pathology, and wound complications [102]. On the other hand, Muller et al. saw improved functional outcomes in the MIS cohort compared to a conventional approach; however, suboptimal placement of the components were observed in the MIS group [103]. Another study also found greater tibial component varus misalignment in the minimally invasive UKA procedures [104].

A clear indication for the adoption of MIS is yet to be established due to the discrepancies in the literature's evidence. Current literature will benefit from multiple geographically diverse, large volume assessor-blind RCTs into MIS versus conventional surgical approaches to UKA and their effects on clinical outcomes and survivability.

Technology-Assisted UKA

As a technically challenging procedure, UKA suffers from very small tolerances to surgical errors. The smallest of component misplacement can lead to early failure of the implant [92]. As a result of this small margin for error and the ever-growing interface between technology and orthopaedic surgery, computer-assisted technologies have been developed for UKA. These procedures can be categorized as computer navigation UKA, robotic-assisted UKA, and patient-specific instrumentation.

The aim of computer navigation systems is to guide the surgeon by optimizing the precise placement of the implant components [105]. Computer navigation systems can be grouped by the prevailing modality employed: CT-guided, image-guided or image-free. In CT-guided computer-assisted UKA, a preoperative CT is obtained and uploaded to the computer to accurately model the anatomy of the bones. This type has become less popular due to the increased radiation exposure for the patient as well as cost.

Image-guided UKA employs intra-operative fluoroscopy to detect the key boney landmarks, but this also uses radiation. The increasingly popular type, image-free UKA, uses a digital stylus to mark the key boney landmarks. This in turn allows the computer to model the boney anatomy, limb geometry, and biomechanical axes, thus allowing greater precision in executing tibial and femoral cuts, limb alignment, component placement, and soft-tissue balancing [105]. Real-time information about the leg axis in computer navigation UKA reduces the risk of varus overcorrection compared with a conventional technique [103]. Furthermore, component placement is improved and there are no differences in failure rates at 9 years [105]. In UKA revision, computer navigation techniques result in more optimal results for less experienced surgeons [106].

Robot-assisted techniques have been developed to further enhance and improve surgical cutting accuracy and alignment. The most used robotic-assisted systems are the Navio Surgical System by Smith & Nephew, the Stryker/MAKO haptic-guided robot by MAKO Surgical Corp, and Acrobot by Acrobot Co. Ltd. As semi-active systems, surgeons retain full control of a robotic arm that integrates their commands with computerized navigational input. Through boney landmark mapping, continuous visual and tactile feedback, and target zone guidance, surgeons are provided with assistance regarding the volume and orientation of bone resection, component placement, and soft-tissue balancing [107, 108]. Studies comparing robotic-assisted UKA with conventional manual UKA have demonstrated improved cutting accuracy, limb alignment, component placement, and restoration of the native joint line [108–112]. Cobb et al.'s prospective randomized control study found that all robotic-assisted UKA had a mechanical axis within 2° of neutral [109]. Bell et al.'s echoed these findings in their post-operative CT study; they found that robotic-assisted UKA significantly reduced tibial and femoral component misplacement compared to conventional UKA [110]. Citak et al.'s cadaveric study reported greater accuracy in implant placement of both femoral and tibial components using the MAKO robotic-assisted system [113]. Plate et al.'s study demonstrated the MAKO robotic-assisted system achieved soft-tissue balancing accuracy of up to 0.53 mm within the preoperative plan and 83% of procedures were within 1.0 mm throughout the range of motion [107]. An additional advantage of robotic-assisted UKA is a shorter learning curve, allowing less experienced surgeons to achieve optimal results sooner in their careers [114].

Cobb et al. randomized control study of the Acrobot study found that the intra-operative advantages of a robotic-assisted system translated to improved clinical outcomes at 6- and 18-weeks follow-up compared to conventional UKA. The mean average increase from preoperative to post-operative levels in the American Knee Society Score was twice as large in the Acrobot system group 65.2 versus 32.5 in the conventional UKA group [109]. A statistically significant difference it supports the notion that accurate alignment affects clinical outcome. Pearle et al.'s multicenter study reported improved rates of survival and patient satisfaction at two-year follow-up [115].

Although these findings support robotic-assisted UKA's potential of improving short-term clinical outcomes, the literature lacks definitive evidence on long-term functional outcomes and survivorship, and thus further well-designed longitudinal studies and randomized control trials are required. Moreover, robotic-assisted UKA is not without its risks. CT- and image-guided computer navigation used in some robotic-assisted systems expose the patient to extra radiation. Some systems rely on optical-tracking array pin tracts, which increase the risk of stress fractures in cortical bone [116]. Additionally, these systems are costly and present increased expense to the patient and healthcare system. Moschetti et al. argue that robotic-assisted UKA is only cost-efficient compared to conventional UKA when annual UKA volume is 95 or greater [117]. A potential drawback of shortening the learning curve in robotic-assisted UKA may transfer the less experienced surgeon's learning from the operating room to the computer planning stage [93]. Cobb et al. noted the increased operating time in robotic-assisted UKA versus conventional [109]. Interestingly, new data from the Australian registry suggests higher rates of early revision for infection for robotically-assisted UKA which might be associated to the increased operating time [118]. Finally, valuable operating room area may be taken up by the large robotic machinery.

Patient-specific instrumentation (PSI) and the use of 3-D printing presents an exciting avenue in the field of UKA. The hypothesis states that patient-specific implants designed by computer-aided design will result in uniform load through the implant components and subsequently better outcomes. Van Den Heever et al. established lower and more even load distribution at tibial component in a PSI UKA than a conventional UKA [119]. Jaffry et al.'s study showed that PSI UKA resulted in similar component positioning to robotic-assisted UKA, and better component placement and alignment than conventional UKA [120]. However, Kerens et al. found no statistically significant difference in the component placement between PSI and conventional UKA in their study [121]. Similarly, Ollivier et al. could not justify PSI's improvement due to added cost and uncertainty [122].

Advances in technology continue to present an interesting, exciting, and ever-expanding frontier in the field of UKA; however, alongside advantages in component placement and short-term clinical outcomes, significant doubts regarding radiation hazard, resource allocation and cost-efficiency, and long-term outcomes arise. Further high-quality studies are needed to elucidate the true value of technology-assisted UKA.

Outcomes and Failure

Functional Outcomes

UKA and TKA are the most performed procedures for end-stage medial compartment OA. Often pitted against each other as alternatives, the surgeon must have a thorough understanding of their effects on patients' short- and long-term outcomes. For this reason, there is great interest in studies comparing the outcomes of UKA with TKA.

The short-term advantages of UKA over TKA include a shorter operative time; faster recovery; greater post-operative range of motion; greater activity at time of discharge; fewer major complications including blood loss, venous thromboembolism, cerebrovascular events, myocardial infarction, and deep infections; and ultimately, lower mortality [2, 6, 123]. Long-term benefits include lower morbidity, preservation of bone stock for future surgery, higher functional activity, greater joint forgettability, and generally, nut not always, superior patient-reported and functional outcome scores [2, 7–9, 124]. The improved patient-reported outcomes and joint forgetfulness in UKA compared to TKA are, in part, explained by intact ACLs, PCLs, and portion of the meniscus, as well as reduced rates of patella infera compared to TKA [124, 125]. Friesenbichler et al. found that UKA patients reported less knee pain and stiffness at 6 months post-operatively compared to their TKA counterparts; furthermore, UKA patients exhibited greater quadriceps strength and gait function

[126]. These studies' results contrast with the greater uncertainty and dissatisfaction of TKA patients [127].

Numerous scores have been developed and validated in order to accurately measure and quantify post-knee arthroplasty functional outcomes. The most common scores in the literature are the Knee Society Score (KSS), the Oxford Knee Score (OKS), the Western Ontario and McMaster Universities Osteoarthritis Index (WOMAC), the Bristol Knee Score (BKS), the Knee Injury and Osteoarthritis Score (KOOS), the Knee Outcome Surgery-Activities of Daily Living Scale (KOS-ADLS), and the High Activity Arthroplasty Score (HAAS). Six major prospect randomized control studies have elucidated the score differences in UKA versus TKA (Table 10.1). Newman et al. conducted a 15-year prospective randomized control trial of 102 patients culminating in 2009. They report 15-year post-operative BKS scores of 92 and 87.5 for UKA and TKA, post-operatively [128, 134]. Sun et al. compared MB UKA with FB TKA at an average 52 months of follow-up and found that UKA patients demonstrated an average KSS of 80.5 compared to TKA's KSS of 78.9. Additionally, UKA patients had 2° more range of motion compared to the TKA patients [129]. Costa et al. found equal KSS scores between EIUS/Zimmer UKA patients and Stryker Scorpio/NRG TKA patients at 5-year follow-up [130]. In 2017, Kulrestha et al. saw no significant difference between UKA and TKA in HAAS and KOS-ADLS at 2-year follow-up. However, they noted UKA patients had shorter recovery periods, less complications, and less

readmission rates [131]. In 2019, Beard et al.'s randomized control trial of 528 found UKA patients had an OKS of 38 at 5 years and TKA had an OKS of 37, in addition, mean HAAS was found to be 7.9 in UKA and 7.6 TKA patients. Despite not exhibiting statistically significant differences, Beard et al. found that UKA were more cost-effective despite having the same level of functional outcome [132]. They argue that increasing the proportion of UKA will benefit the healthcare system without detracting from patient outcomes.

Knifsund et al. in 2020 carried out the only double-blind, prospective, multicenter, randomized control trial of functional outcomes in UKA versus TKA. With a patient pool of 143, 2-year post-operative functional outcomes were recorded. They demonstrated an OKS of 41.2 in UKA versus 40.1 in TKA, KSS of 180.9 in UKA and 178.6 in TKA [133]. Like Beard et al.'s study, these differences are not statistically significant [132]. However, Knifsund et al. found significant improvement in post-operative recovery in UKA compared to TKA (statistically significant differences in OKS and KOOS at 2 and 12 months) [133].

Although an increase in functional outcome scores is seen in UKA compared to TKA, the literature disagrees as to whether these differences are significant or not, with higher-level evidence pointing towards the latter. Regardless, UKA has many proven short- and long-term benefits over TKA in a large majority of patients and should be viewed as a definitive treatment option for isolated medical compartment OA rather than an alternative treatment option.

Table 10.1 Randomized control trials comparing functional outcome scores between UKA and TKA

Study	Year	Blinding	Average follow-up (years)	Average functional scores	
				UKA	TKA
Newman et al. [128]	2009	Single	15	BKS 92	BKS 87.5
Sun et al. [129]	2010	Single	4	KSS F 80.5	KSS F 78.9
Costa et al. [130]	2011	Single	5	KSS K/F 96/91	KSS K/F 96/91
Kulshrestha et al. [131]	2017	Single	2	KOS-ADL 90.4	KOS-ADL 89.9
Beard et al. [132]	2019	Single	5	OKS 38 HAAS 7.9	OKS 37 HAAS 7.6
Knifsund et al. [133]	2020	Double	2	OKS 41.2	OKS 40.1

Table 10.2 Ten-year survival rates of unicompartmental knee arthroplasty from major level 4 cohort studies versus national registries

Cohort study	No. of UKA	Average follow-up (years)	Survival at 10 years
Pandit et al. [135]	1000	10.3	94%
Faour-Martin et al. [136]	511	10.4	94.5%
Emerson et al. [137]	213	10	90.6%
Kim et al. [138]	166	10	90.4%
Lisowski et al. [139]	138	11.7	91.6%
Foran et al. [140]	62	10	98%
National registry	**No. of UKA**	**Longest follow-up (years)**	**Survival at 10 years**
NJR [82]	75,719	13	87.8%
Australia [71]	46,094	15	85.4%
New Zealand [141]	9635	17	89%
Norway [142]	7648	12	79%

Table 10.3 Studies comparing the 10-year survivorship of UKA versus TKA

	No. of UKA		Average follow-up (years)		10-year survival, %	
Study	UKA	TKA	UKA	TKA	UKA	TKA
Sun et al. [129]	28	28	4	4	75	100
Weale et al. [125]	50	52	5	5	96	98
Amin et al. [143]	54	54	5	5	85	98
Costa et al. [130]	34	34	5	5	85	100
Lum et al. [144]	201	189	5.4	5.5	98.5	96.8
Ackroyd et al. [98]	408	531	6.4	5.7	87.5	89.6
Lyons et al. [82]	279	5606	7.1	6.5	90	95
Horikawa et al. [145]	28	50	9	10.5	84	92
Newman et al. [128]	52	50	15	15	89.8	78.7

Survivorship

One of the key measurements of an arthroplasty's success is how long the prosthetic joint survives before it needs revision, this is reported in the literature as a rate of survival/failure over time. Many evidence level 4 cohort studies demonstrated favorable survivability of UKAs (Table 10.2). In Pandit et al.'s study of 1000 UKAs, the post-operative 10-year rate of survival reported was 94% [135]. Similarly, Faour-Martin et al.'s study on 511 UKAs found a 94.5% rate of survival [136]. Emerson et al. saw survival rates of 90.6% at the 10-year mark [137]. Smaller studies have shown 10-year survival rates ranging from 90.4 to 98% [138–140].

National Registries vary greatly on the data they describe; however, they all generally rate lower rates of survival than the cohort studies (Table 10.1). The National Joint Registry of England and Wales (NJR) followed the outcomes of 75,719 UKAs, reporting 10-year survival rates of 89.2% for fixed-bearing UKAs and 87.6% for mobile-bearing UKAs [82]. The greatest risk factor for failure in this registry was younger age. The Australian registry of 46,094 UKAs reported a 10-year survival of 85.4% with the most common cause of failure being aseptic loosening (43.5%), OA progression (29.4%), and unexplained pain (9.5%). The greatest risk factors for failure were younger age (<55 years) and female gender [71]. The New Zealand registry of 9635 UKAs reported the greatest rate of survival at 89% with the uncemented Oxford UKA having the greatest survival (96%) [141]. The Norwegian registry reported the lowest rates of survival at 79% [142].

Numerous reviews in the literature have compared the survivorship of UKA with that of TKA (Table 10.3). The most significant disadvantage of UKA is the three times higher revision rates compared to TKA. Liddle et al. noted, "if 100 patients receiving TKA received UKA instead, the result would be around one fewer death and three more reoperations in the first 4 years after surgery" [6]. Data form the Norwegian Arthroplasty Register demonstrate a 10-year survival free from revision of 94% for TKA and 81% for UKA, respectively [45]. In a regional registry, a revision rate of 18% for UKA and 6%

for TKA has been reported at 15 years [146]. Based on numbers from the Australian Orthopaedic Association National Joint Replacement Registry, arthritis progression and component loosening are the commonest failure modes of UKA, irrespective of the implant design [72]. In a review of the Finnish registry, 5-year revision rates were 10.6% for UKA and 3.7% for TKA; 15-year revision rates were 30.4% and 11.3% for UKA and TKA, respectively. Even when both groups are matched for gender and age, UKA presented a higher risk for revision than TKA [147]. Data from the US Medicare database also echoed these findings; mean average 5-year survival of UKAs was 95.3% compared to TKA's 98% [148].

Lyons et al.'s cohort study found that survivorship the TKA with 5-year survival of 98% and 10-year survival of 95% for TKA and 5-year survival of 95% and 10-year survival of 90% for UKA [98]. Lim et al.'s cohort study also found lower survival rates in the UKA group (93.7%) than in the TKA group (97%). Other cohort studies saw no statistically significant differences in survivorship in the two groups. Randomized control trials also echoed these discrepancies; Sun et al.'s RCT of 56 patients found a 75% 10-year survial rate in their UKA groups versus the 100% 10-year survival for TKA [129]. Costa et al.'s RCT found a UKA versus TKA survival rate of 85% versus 100% [130]. However, Newman et al.'s 15-year RCT found a higher survival rate for UKA (89.8%) compared to TKA (78.7%) [128]. More importantly, Knifsund et al.'s double-blind RCT found no statistical difference in the number of revisions between the study groups [133].

Current literature poses a significant controversy which is the discrepancy between the results of national registries reporting lower survivability of UKA versus TKA and cohort and RCT studies from design-centers reporting no difference in survivability between UKA and TKA. The national registry data undoubtedly contributes to a lower usage of UKA by orthopaedic surgeons (5–11% usage when 47% of patients qualify for UKA) further exacerbating the problem as lower usage and volume surgeons see four times the revision rate compared to their higher usage and volume colleagues [6, 81, 149]. Some factors can be attributed to these discrepancies including a lower threshold for revising a UKA versus revising a TKA; the ease of revising a UKA compared to revising a TKA; a lower margin of component placement error in UKA compared to TKA; a younger, healthier patient base selected for UKA; more modes of failure in UKA; and the varying levels of UKA usage of surgeons.

There is a lower threshold for revising UKA than TKA. UKA revisions occur in 63% of poorly performing knees with OKS <20, whereas only 12% of TKAs are revised in that same group indicating a greater clinical sensitivity to UKA failure than TKA failure regardless of outcome [150]. Anecdotally, UKA revisions are deemed easier to perform than TKA revisions. Studies report that TKA revisions require greater metal augmentation, use of tibial stems and stabilized components [151]. Less experienced surgeons were more likely to revise UKA for unexplained pain than their more experienced colleagues. Furthermore, revised UKAs typically have better functional outcomes than revised TKAs [152]. The patient pool for TKA is generally older with reduced activities of daily living than the younger patient pool typically seen in UKA, thus more UKA revisions will be seen based on life expectancy alone. Additionally, joint replacement in early-stage arthritis is associated with poorer outcomes than in end-stage arthritis, hence the selection of younger patients with earlier-stage arthritis in UKA reflects that [153, 154]. UKAs are more sensitive to component misalignment than TKAs; overcorrection of varus deformity and deviations from the original joint line by only 3° lead to greater rates of failure in UKA than TKA [92, 155]. This is further compounded by UKA's longer learning curve, whereby the less experienced surgeon will make more component placement errors in their career. Progression of OA in the contralateral compartment is an important mode of UKA failure that does not exist for TKA, thereby increasing the number of mechanisms a UKA can fail [156].

As discussed above, the discrepancies on UKA's survivorship have contributed to lower usage by surgeons. However, usage directly and positively affects functional outcomes and implant survival, thus creating a perpetual positive-feedback loop of avoiding UKA in indicated patients [83]. Using survivorship rates of UKA versus TKA as a sole measure of success is inappropriate as the aforementioned variables mean that UKA and TKA's rates of survivorship cannot be directly compared. Ultimately, surgeons can optimize their patients' outcomes by increasing the proportion of UKAs they perform, this can be achieved by using broader indications and advocating for the procedure to suitable patients.

Modes of Failure

The failure of a UKA is multifactorial; however, primary mechanisms have been identified and classified as mode of failure by either cause or timing. As the field of UKA develops, stakeholders are keen on minimizing the occurrence and severity of the following mechanisms.

A 2016 systemic review by van der List et al. found aseptic loosening to be leading cause of UKA failure overall (36%), followed by progression of osteoarthritis (OA) in the contralateral compartment (20%), unexplained pain (11%), instability (6%), infection (5%), and polyethylene wear (4%) [157]. The most common reason for early failure (<5 years post-primary UKA) was aseptic loosening (25%); however, in late UKA revisions, the leading mode of failure is progression of OA (38%) [92]. Citak et al.'s study also confirmed these findings, reporting aseptic loosening and progression of OA as the most common causes of failure in medial UKA [158]. Epinette et al. in their multicenter study reported tibial loosening was more common than femoral loosening [159].

Progression of OA is generally the second most common mode of failure in UKA; it is exacerbated by suboptimal component placement and deviations from the neutral joint line. Restoring the preoperative joint line ensures equal load transfer between the medial and lateral compartments of the knee. An increase in the joint space gap in the medial compartment will increase the load and thus exacerbate the degeneration in the lateral compartment. A lowering of the joint line position is associated with increased risk of aseptic loosening [160].

Unexplained pain is the third most significant mode of failure affecting 11% (with a range of 4–23%) of UKA procedures [159]. Unexplained pain is defined as post-operative pain without an obvious reason delineated by physical examination or plain radiography. Park et al.'s MRI study demonstrated the effectiveness of MRI in identifying the underlying physical characteristics seen in the joints of patients with unexplained pain. Their most common findings included: osteolysis, loose bodies, tibial loosening, synovitis, stress fractures, and infections [161]. Polyethylene wear is an important mode of failure closely associated with varus undercorrection and fixed-bearing (FB) implant designs. FB implants generally see greater loads than when combined with their generally thinner polyethylene thickness due to a metal-backed tibial tray results in faster wear [25]. Current evidence does not support that polyethylene wear is associated with weight or gender [161].

The above are the most common modes of failure seen in literature and should be of note to surgeons performing UKA. In addition to these mechanisms, UKA can fail due to fractures and tibial component subsidence, instability, infection, and misalignment [100, 162].

Revision of a Medial UKA

UKA is reported to have higher revision rates than TKA; despite, a UKA's preservation of bone stock for future surgery, they are noted for some difficulties when revised. Wynn-Jones et al. found in their study of 80 UKAs that required revision, the median tibial component thickness was 15 mm and tibial weaknesses were common, leading to thicker revision components being used [163]. Chou et al.'s study confirmed that almost every case of UKA revision can be converted to TKA; however, the lack of anatomic landmarks resulted in increased technical difficulty and the need for additional constructs in two out of three cases [164].

Outcomes of a revised UKA may also be an area of concern. A review of a national registry found that rates of re-revision of UKA to TKA were four times that of primary TKA, and revision of failed UKA to a further UKA was 13 times higher. Oxford Knee Score was significantly lower in UKA to TKA revision (30.02) compared to primary TKA [165]. Hang et al.'s review of the Australian registry yielded similar findings. However, a much greater proportion of UKAs are revised compared to TKA in knees with poor outcomes (OKS <20), indicating a much lower threshold for UKA revision [166]. The complications rate between UKA revision and primary TKA were more comparable. Sierra et al.'s study of UKA to TKA revision yielded a complication rate of 13% (4.4% with aseptic loosening, 3.3% had stiffness, and 1.2% had deep infection). Comparable to primary TKA, UKA revision complication rates were found to be better than after TKA revision [167]. Functional outcomes scores were not significant different between UKA revision and TKA revision.

As interest in UKA increases, due to better outcomes than primary TKA, it must be noted that the literature points towards a higher revision rate in UKA compared to primary TKA. Functional outcomes and re-revision rates in revised UKA are worse than primary TKA, and this will influence the number of UKAs offered to younger patients. However, revisions of UKA have better outcomes and less complications than revisions of TKA. Ultimately, UKA should be considered an excellent treatment option for isolated medical compartment OA, and as the field advances outcomes in its revision will continue to improve.

Cost Efficiency of UKA

In a time of increasing hospital resource scarcity, surgical options for the same condition should be compared on a cost-efficient, value basis. A Markov analytical model of Sweden's national registry was used by Ghromrawi et al. to compare the costs of UKA and TKA. They found lower life-time costs (UKA: $35,000–$46,600 versus TKA: $42,000–47,600) and higher lifetime quality-adjusted life years for UKA patients older than 65 years compared to their TKA counterparts. These differences translate to potential societal savings of $84–$544 million [168]. The cost-effectiveness of UKA reduces when the patients are younger, owing to greater revision rates and worse functional outcomes, as well as when UKA patients require rehabilitation admission or rehabilitation costs of TKA decrease by 60%.

Shankar et al.'s hospital coding analyses demonstrated that UKA's reduced operative time, earlier recovery, fewer post-operative complications compared to TKA reduce costs by $4846 per patient. Furthermore, average implant component costs were $4149 for UKA and $5787 for TKA [169].

The literature supports the idea that UKA in suitable patients with isolated medial compartment OA is a significantly high-value, cost-effective treatment option with good clinical outcomes, increases in quality-adjusted life years, less post-operative complications, and reduced hospital stays. As UKA utilization increases, these benefits will only become more pertinent to healthcare stakeholders. However, clinical decision making will remain patient-centered with outcomes being the priority and financial efficiency a secondary consideration.

Post-operative Care

UKA is noted for faster recovery than TKA thanks to advances in anesthetic and pain management, but the post-operative protocol is similar [101]. Weight-bearing is recommended to improve range of motion and decrease the risk of complication such as PVT, PE, urinary retention, and chest infection. Reilly et al. reported less hospital-acquired infection and greater patient satisfaction due to earlier hospital discharge [101].

AP, lateral, and long leg plain radiographs should be obtained in 1.5, 6, and 12 months postoperatively to monitor mechanical axes, leg alignment, radiolucent lines, and progression of osteoarthritis in the lateral compartment. Radiolucent lines that are ≤ 2 mm in thickness, stable, and well-defined are physiological and commonly seen after UKA; radiolucent lines that are >2 mm thick, evolving, and lack definition are pathological signs of infection or component loosening [170, 171].

One of the biggest advantages of UKA over TKA presented to patients is an earlier recovery; thus, their expectations are tailored towards earlier post-operative. Witjes et al.'s systematic review reports that a greater proportion of UKA patients returned to sports after surgery than TKA patients [172]. Nearly 35% of UKA patients participated in the high-impact sports they were doing preoperatively, 100% participated in their intermediate-impact sports, and 93% returned to their low-impact sports [172]. Walton et al. echoed these findings by reporting that TKA patients were less likely to maintain their preoperative levels of physical activity compared to UKA patients. However, among the patients that did return to sports, they found no difference in timing between the UKA and TKA groups [173]. Ultimately, UKA patients enjoy a high level of success with their implants, with improved recovery, functional outcomes, alignment, and quadriceps strength; thus, with appropriately managed expectations, these patients can indeed lead very active and healthy lifestyle.

Future Perspectives

As the mean population age rises with increasing life expectancy, the prevalence of osteoarthritis will also increase. UKA presents itself as a safe and effective treatment option for isolated end-stage medial compartment OA. Currently, usage is approximated at 5–11% whilst 47% of patients are suitably indicated for UKA [11]. As evidence supports the correlation between usage (as well as caseload and experience) and clinical outcomes, the number of UKAs performed globally will also rise.

Advances in implant design and robotic-assisted surgery are pushing the frontier in the field of knee arthroplasty. Robotic-assisted UKA and personalized implants have resulted in greater precision of component placement, better patient-reported outcomes, and greater satisfaction by patient and surgeon [108, 110, 113]. Improvements in robotic-assisted UKA will likely focus on simplifying the process, shortening the learning curve for less experience surgeons, and improving image-free guidance modalities [116]. Although it is difficult to predict future technological innovations in implant designs, developments in polyethylene characteristics and kinematics will also help to improve clinical outcomes and reduce rates of failure [174]. Uncemented UKA is gaining popularity due to good functional outcomes and survivability, and this will only increase in the future [175]. Ultimately, advances in UKA will pique the interest of orthopaedic surgeons across the globe, and a noticeable rise in the number of UKAs performed will be seen.

Summary

Knee OA presents a large socioeconomic and healthcare burden globally, and this burden is only increasing. The supply of a safe, effective treatment will need to meet this increased demand. Despite good functional outcomes, reduced preoperative complications, and better cost-effectiveness in UKA, surgeons hesitate to offer this procedure to suitable patients due to a longer learning curve and a perceived higher rate of failure compared to TKA. As further research delineates and scrutinizes these discrepancies and advances in the procedure are made, a confident assumption can be made that UKA's place in unicompartmental OA will only grow.

The expansion of traditional indications, increasing surgeons' usage, use of validated technology adjuncts such as robotic-assistance, and improvements in implant design all contribute to UKA's good to excellent results, better outcomes compared to TKA, and to lowering UKA's rate of failure. After being initially overlooked, UKA is seeing a resurgence and future research has an abundance of exciting directions to pursue.

References

1. Heyse TJ, Khefacha A, Peersman G, Cartier P. Survivorship of UKA in the middle-aged. Knee. 2012;19(5):585–91.
2. Tay ML, McGlashan SR, Monk AP, Young SW. Revision indications for medial unicompartmental knee arthroplasty: a systematic review. Arch Orthop Trauma Surg. 2022;142(2):301–14.
3. McKeever DC. The choice of prosthetic materials and evaluation of results. Clin Orthop. 1955;6:17–21.
4. Marmor L. The modular knee. Clin Orthop Relat Res. 1973;94:242–8.
5. Goodfellow JW, Tibrewal SB, Sherman KP, O'Connor JJ. Unicompartmental Oxford meniscal knee arthroplasty. J Arthroplasty. 1987;2(1):1–9.
6. Liddle AD, Judge A, Pandit H, Murray DW. Adverse outcomes after total and unicompartmental knee replacement in 101,330 matched patients: a study of data from the National Joint Registry for England and Wales. Lancet. 2014;384(9952):1437–45.
7. Gill JR, Corbett JA, Wastnedge E, Nicolai P. Forgotten joint score: comparison between total and unicondylar knee arthroplasty. Knee. 2021;29:26–32.
8. Wilson HA, Middleton R, Abram SGF, Smith S, Alvand A, Jackson WF, Bottomley N, Hopewell S, Price AJ. Patient relevant outcomes of unicompartmental versus total knee replacement: systematic review and meta-analysis. BMJ. 2019;364:l352.
9. Zuiderbaan HA, van der List JP, Khamaisy S, Nawabi DH, Thein R, Ishmael C, Paul S, Pearle AD. Unicompartmental knee arthroplasty versus total knee arthroplasty: which type of artificial joint do patients forget? Knee Surg Sports Traumatol Arthrosc. 2017;25(3):681–6.
10. Klasan A, Parker DA, Lewis PL, Young SW. Low percentage of surgeons meet the minimum recommended unicompartmental knee arthroplasty usage thresholds: analysis of 3037 surgeons from three National Joint Registries. Knee Surg Sports Traumatol Arthrosc. 2022;30(3):958–64.
11. American Joint Replacement Registry. American Joint Replacement Registry—annual report 2014. 2014. http://www.ajrr.net/images/annual_reports/AJRR_2014_Annual_Report_final_11-11-15.pdf.
12. Pandit H, Jenkins C, Gill HS, Smith G, Price AJ, Dodd CA, Murray DW. Unnecessary contraindications for mobile-bearing unicompartmental knee replacement. J Bone Joint Surg Br. 2011;93(5):622.
13. Schindler OS, Scott WN, Scuderi GR. The practice of unicompartmental knee arthroplasty in the United Kingdom. J Orthop Surg (Hong Kong). 2010;18(3):312.
14. Berger RA, Meneghini RM, Sheinkop MB, Della Valle CJ, Jacobs JJ, Rosenberg AG, Galante JO. The progression of patellofemoral arthrosis after medial unicompartmental replacement: results at 11 to 15 years. Clin Orthop Relat Res. 2004;(428):92.
15. Kozinn SC, Scott R. Unicondylar knee arthroplasty. J Bone Joint Surg Am. 1989;71(1):145.
16. Pandit H, Jenkins C, Barker K, Dodd CA, Murray DW. The Oxford medial unicompartmental knee replacement using a minimally-invasive approach. J Bone Joint Surg Br. 2006;88(1):54.
17. Berend KR, Berend ME, Dalury DF, Argenson JN, Dodd CA, Scott RD. Consensus statement on indications and contraindications for medial unicompartmental knee arthroplasty. J Surg Orthop Adv. 2015;24(4):252.
18. Parratte S, Argenson JN, Dumas J, Aubaniac JM. Unicompartmental knee arthroplasty for avascular osteonecrosis. Clin Orthop Relat Res. 2007;464:37.
19. Goodfellow J. Unicompartmental arthroplasty with the Oxford knee. Oxford: Oxford University Press; 2006.
20. Murray DW, Liddle AD, Dodd CA, Pandit H. Unicompartmental knee arthroplasty: is the glass half full or half empty? Bone Joint J. 2015;97-B(10 Suppl A):3.
21. Berger RA, Della Valle CJ. Unicompartmental knee arthroplasty: indications, techniques, and results. Instr Course Lect. 2010;59:47.
22. Kendrick BJ, Rout R, Bottomley NJ, Pandit H, Gill HS, Price AJ, Dodd CA, Murray DW. The implications of damage to the lateral femoral condyle on medial unicompartmental knee replacement. J Bone Joint Surg Br. 2010;92(3):374.
23. Faschingbauer M, Renner L, Waldstein W, Boettner F. Are lateral compartment osteophytes a predictor for lateral cartilage damage in varus osteoarthritic knees?: data from the osteoarthritis initiative. Bone Joint J. 2015;97-B(12):1634.
24. Waldstein W, Kasparek MF, Faschingbauer M, Windhager R, Boettner F. Lateral-compartment osteophytes are not associated with lateral-compartment cartilage degeneration in arthritic varus knees. Clin Orthop Relat Res. 2017;475(5):1386.
25. Kumar V, Pandit HG, Liddle AD, Borror W, Jenkins C, Mellon SJ, Hamilton TW, Athanasou N, Dodd CA, Murray DW. Comparison of outcomes after UKA in patients with and without chondrocalcinosis: a matched cohort study. Knee Surg Sports Traumatol Arthrosc. 2017;25(1):319.
26. Moret CS, Iordache E, D'Ambrosi R, Hirschmann MT. Chondrocalcinosis does not affect functional outcome and prosthesis survival in patients after total or unicompartmental knee arthroplasty: a systematic review. Knee Surg Sports Traumatol Arthrosc. 2021;30:1039.
27. Goodfellow JW, O'Connor J, Dodd CA, Murray DW. Unicompartmental arthroplasty with the Oxford knee. Oxford: Oxford University Press; 2006.
28. Deschamps G, Chol C. Fixed-bearing unicompartmental knee arthroplasty. Patients' selection and

operative technique. Orthop Traumatol Surg Res. 2011;97(6):648.

29. Goodfellow J, O'Connor J. The anterior cruciate ligament in knee arthroplasty. A risk-factor with unconstrained meniscal prostheses. Clin Orthop Relat Res. 1992;(276):245.

30. Du G, et al. No difference unicompartmental knee arthroplasty for medial knee osteoarthritis with or without anterior cruciate ligament deficiency: a systematic review and meta-analysis. J Arthroplasty. 2023;38(3):586–593.e1.

31. Mancuso F, Dodd CA, Murray DW, Pandit H. Medial unicompartmental knee arthroplasty in the ACL-deficient knee. J Orthop Traumatol. 2016;17(3):267.

32. Suter L, Roth A, Angst M, von Knoch F, Preiss S, List R, Ferguson S, Zumbrunn T. Is ACL deficiency always a contraindication for medial UKA? Kinematic and kinetic analysis of implanted and contralateral knees. Gait Posture. 2019;68:244.

33. Beard DJ, Pandit H, Gill HS, Hollinghurst D, Dodd CA, Murray DW. The influence of the presence and severity of pre-existing patellofemoral degenerative changes on the outcome of the Oxford medial unicompartmental knee replacement. J Bone Joint Surg Br. 2007;89(12):1597.

34. Beard DJ, Pandit H, Ostlere S, Jenkins C, Dodd CA, Murray DW. Pre-operative clinical and radiological assessment of the patellofemoral joint in unicompartmental knee replacement and its influence on outcome. J Bone Joint Surg Br. 2007;89(12):1602.

35. Munk S, Odgaard A, Madsen F, Dalsgaard J, Jorn LP, Langhoff O, Jepsen CF, Hansen TB. Preoperative lateral subluxation of the patella is a predictor of poor early outcome of Oxford phase-III medial unicompartmental knee arthroplasty. Acta Orthop. 2011;82(5):582.

36. Liddle AD, Pandit H, Jenkins C, Price AJ, Dodd CA, Gill HS, Murray DW. Preoperative pain location is a poor predictor of outcome after Oxford unicompartmental knee arthroplasty at 1 and 5 years. Knee Surg Sports Traumatol Arthrosc. 2013;21(11):2421–6.

37. Argenson JN, Blanc G, Aubaniac JM, Parratte S. Modern unicompartmental knee arthroplasty with cement: a concise follow-up, at a mean of twenty years, of a previous report. J Bone Joint Surg Am. 2013;95(10):905.

38. Hamilton TW, Pandit HG, Lombardi AV, Adams JB, Oosthuizen CR, Clave A, Dodd CA, Berend KR, Murray DW. Radiological decision aid to determine suitability for medial unicompartmental knee arthroplasty: development and preliminary validation. Bone Joint J. 2016;98-B(10 Suppl B):3.

39. Waldstein W, et al. The value of valgus stress radiographs in the workup for medial unicompartmental arthritis. Clin Orthop Relat Res. 2013;471(12):3998–4003.

40. Seng CS, Ho DC, Chong HC, Chia SL, Chin PL, Lo NN, Yeo SJ. Outcomes and survivorship of unicondylar knee arthroplasty in patients with severe deformity. Knee Surg Sports Traumatol Arthrosc. 2017;25(3):639.

41. Kleeblad LJ, van der List JP, Pearle AD, Fragomen AT, Rozbruch SR. Predicting the feasibility of correcting mechanical axis in large varus deformities with unicompartmental knee arthroplasty. J Arthroplasty. 2018;33(2):372.

42. Springer B, et al. The functional status of the ACL in varus OA of the knee: the association with varus deformity and coronal tibiofemoral subluxation. J Arthroplasty. 2021;36(2):501–6.

43. Chen JY, Loh B, Woo YL, Chia SL, Lo NN, Yeo SJ. Fixed flexion deformity after unicompartmental knee arthroplasty: how much is too much. J Arthroplasty. 2016;31(6):1313.

44. Yeh JZY, Chen JY, Lim JW, Pang HN, Tay DKJ, Chia SL, Lo NN, Yeo SJ. Postoperative fixed flexion deformity greater than 10 degrees lead to poorer functional outcome 10 years after unicompartmental knee arthroplasty. Knee Surg Sports Traumatol Arthrosc. 2018;26(6):1723.

45. Pennington DW, Swienckowski JJ, Lutes WB, Drake GN. Unicompartmental knee arthroplasty in patients sixty years of age or younger. J Bone Joint Surg Am. 1968;85(10):2003.

46. Dyrhovden GS, Lygre SHL, Badawy M, Gøthesen Ø, Furnes O. Have the causes of revision for total and unicompartmental knee arthroplasties changed during the past two decades? Clin Orthop Relat Res. 1874;475(7):2017.

47. National Joint Registry. NJR annual report 2020. 2021. https://reports.njrcentre.org.uk/Portals/0/PDFdownloads/NJR%2017th%20Annual%20Report%202020.pdf.

48. van der List JP, Chawla H, Zuiderbaan HA, Pearle AD. The role of preoperative patient characteristics on outcomes of unicompartmental knee arthroplasty: a meta-analysis critique. J Arthroplasty. 2016;31(11):2617.

49. Kennedy JA, Matharu GS, Hamilton TW, Mellon SJ, Murray DW. Age and outcomes of medial meniscal-bearing unicompartmental knee arthroplasty. J Arthroplasty. 2018;33(10):3153.

50. Mohammad HR, Mellon S, Judge A, Dodd C, Murray D. The effect of age on the outcomes of cementless mobile bearing unicompartmental knee replacements. Knee Surg Sports Traumatol Arthrosc. 2022;30(3):928–38.

51. Calkins TE, Hannon CP, Fillingham YA, Culvern CC, Berger RA, Della Valle CJ. Fixed-bearing medial unicompartmental knee arthroplasty in patients younger than 55 years of age at 4-19 years of follow-up: a concise follow-up of a previous report. J Arthroplasty. 2021;36(3):917.

52. Cavaignac E, Lafontan V, Reina N, Pailhe R, Wargny M, Laffosse JM, Chiron P. Obesity has no adverse effect on the outcome of unicompartmental knee replacement at a minimum follow-up of seven years. Bone Joint J. 2013;95-B(8):1064.

53. Molloy J, Kennedy J, Jenkins C, Mellon S, Dodd C, Murray D. Obesity should not be considered a contraindication to medial Oxford UKA: long-term patient-reported outcomes and implant survival in 1000 knees. Knee Surg Sports Traumatol Arthrosc. 2019;27(7):2259.

54. Plate JF, Augart MA, Seyler TM, Bracey DN, Hoggard A, Akbar M, Jinnah RH, Poehling GG. Obesity has no effect on outcomes following unicompartmental knee arthroplasty. Knee Surg Sports Traumatol Arthrosc. 2017;25(3):645.

55. Musbahi O, Hamilton TW, Crellin AJ, Mellon SJ, Kendrick B, Murray DW. The effect of obesity on revision rate in unicompartmental knee arthroplasty: a systematic review and meta-analysis. Knee Surg Sports Traumatol Arthrosc. 2021;29(10):3467–77.

56. Xu S, Lim WJ, Chen JY, Lo NN, Chia SL, Tay DKJ, Hao Y, Yeo SJ. The influence of obesity on clinical outcomes of fixed-bearing unicompartmental knee arthroplasty: a ten-year follow-up study. Bone Joint J. 2019;101-B(2):213.

57. Nettrour JF, Ellis RT, Hansen BJ, Keeney JA. High failure rates for unicompartmental knee arthroplasty in morbidly obese patients: a two-year minimum follow-up study. J Arthroplasty. 2020;35(4): 989–96.

58. Bohler C, Weimann P, Alasti F, Smolen JS, Windhager R, Aletaha D. Rheumatoid arthritis disease activity and the risk of aseptic arthroplasty loosening. Semin Arthritis Rheum. 2020;50(2):245–51.

59. Waldstein W, Merle C, Monsef JB, Boettner F. Varus knee osteoarthritis: how can we identify ACL insufficiency? Knee Surg Sports Traumatol Arthrosc. 2015;23(8):2178.

60. Waldstein W, Jawetz ST, Farshad-Amacker NA, Merle C, Schmidt-Braekling T, Boettner F. Assessment of the lateral patellar facet in varus arthritis of the knee. Knee. 2014;21(5):920.

61. Emerson RH Jr, Potter T. The use of the McKeever metallic hemiarthroplasty for unicompartmental arthritis. J Bone Joint Surg Am. 1985;67(2):208.

62. MacIntosh DL, Hunter GA. The use of the hemiarthroplasty prosthesis for advanced osteoarthritis and rheumatoid arthritis of the knee. J Bone Joint Surg Br. 1972;54(2):244.

63. Jamali AA, et al. Unicompartmental knee arthroplasty: past, present, and future. Am J Orthop (Belle Mead NJ). 2009;38(1):17–23.

64. Saenz CL, McGrath MS, Marker DR, Seyler TM, Mont MA, Bonutti PM. Early failure of a unicompartmental knee arthroplasty design with an all-polyethylene tibial component. Knee. 2010;17(1):53.

65. Bonutti PM, Dethmers DA. Contemporary unicompartmental knee arthroplasty: fixed vs mobile bearing. J Arthroplasty. 2008;23(7 Suppl):24–7.

66. Bruce DJ, Hassaballa M, Robinson JR, Porteous AJ, Murray JR, Newman JH. Minimum 10-year outcomes of a fixed bearing all-polyethylene unicompartmental knee arthroplasty used to treat medial osteoarthritis. Knee. 2020;27(3):1018.

67. Lindstrand A, Stenström A, Egund N. The PCA unicompartmental knee. A 1-4-year comparison of fixation with or without cement. Acta Orthop Scand. 1988;59(6):695.

68. Saxler G, Temmen D, Bontemps G. Medium-term results of the AMC-unicompartmental knee arthroplasty. Knee. 2004;11(5):349.

69. Pandit H, Jenkins C, Beard DJ, Gallagher J, Price AJ, Dodd CA, Goodfellow JW, Murray DW. Cementless Oxford unicompartmental knee replacement shows reduced radiolucency at one year. J Bone Joint Surg Br. 2009;91(2):185.

70. Suda Y, et al. Varus placement of the tibial component of Oxford unicompartmental knee arthroplasty decreases the risk of postoperative tibial fracture. Bone Joint J. 2022;104-B(10):1118–25.

71. Australian Orthopaedic Association. Australian Orthopaedic Association national joint replacement registry annual report 2015. https://aoanjrr.sahmri.com/documents/10180/217745/HipandKneeArthroplasty. Accessed 28 Sept 2021.

72. Kannan A, et al. Do fixed or mobile bearing implants have better survivorship in medial unicompartmental knee arthroplasty? A study from the Australian Orthopaedic Association National Joint Replacement Registry. Clin Orthop Relat Res. 2021;479:1548.

73. Walker T, Hetto P, Bruckner T, Gotterbarm T, Merle C, Panzram B, Innmann MM, Moradi B. Minimally invasive Oxford unicompartmental knee arthroplasty ensures excellent functional outcome and high survivorship in the long term. Knee Surg Sports Traumatol Arthrosc. 2019;27(5):1658.

74. Mohammad HR, Kennedy JA, Mellon SJ, Judge A, Dodd CA, Murray DW. Ten-year clinical and radiographic results of 1000 cementless Oxford unicompartmental knee replacements. Knee Surg Sports Traumatol Arthrosc. 2020;28(5):1479.

75. Berger RA, et al. Results of unicompartmental knee arthroplasty at a minimum of ten years of follow-up. J Bone Joint Surg Am. 2005;87(5):999–1006.

76. Pronk Y, Paters AAM, Brinkman JM. No difference in patient satisfaction after mobile bearing or fixed bearing medial unicompartmental knee arthroplasty. Knee Surg Sports Traumatol Arthrosc. 2021;29(3):947–54.

77. Cao Z, Niu C, Gong C, Sun Y, Xie J, Song Y. Comparison of fixed-bearing and mobile-bearing unicompartmental knee arthroplasty: a systematic review and meta-analysis. J Arthroplasty. 2019;34(12):3114.

78. Azar FM, Beaty JH, Canale ST. Campbell's operative orthopaedics. 13th ed. Philadelphia: Elsevier; 2017. 442p.

79. Jennings JM, Kleeman-Forsthuber LT, Bolognesi MP. Medial unicompartmental arthroplasty of the knee. J Am Acad Orthop Surg. 2019;27(5):166–76. https://doi.org/10.5435/JAAOS-D-17-00690. PMID: 30407979.

80. Lau RL, Perruccio AV, Gandhi R, Mahomed NN. The role of surgeon volume on patient outcome

in total knee arthroplasty: a systematic review of the literature. BMC Musculoskelet Disord. 2012;13: 250.

81. Liddle AD, Pandit H, Judge A, Murray DW. Effect of surgical caseload on revision rate following total and unicompartmental knee replacement. J Bone Joint Surg Am. 2016;98(1):1–8.

82. National Joint Registry for England Wales and Northern Ireland 13th annual report. 2016. http://www.njrcentre.org.uk/njrcentre/Home/tabid/36/Default.aspx. Accessed 28 Sept 2021.

83. Liddle AD, Pandit H, Judge A, Murray DW. Optimal usage of unicompartmental knee arthroplasty: a study of 41,986 cases from the National Joint Registry for England and Wales. Bone Joint J. 2015;97-B(11):1506–11.

84. Badawy M, Fenstad AM, Bartz-Johannessen CA, Indrekvam K, Havelin LI, Robertsson O, W-Dahl A, Eskelinen A, Mäkelä K, Pedersen AB, Schrøder HM, Furnes O. Hospital volume and the risk of revision in Oxford unicompartmental knee arthroplasty in the Nordic countries—an observational study of 14,496 cases. BMC Musculoskelet Disord. 2017;18(1): 388.

85. Baker PN, Petheram T, Avery PJ, Gregg PJ, Deehan DJ. Revision for unexplained pain following unicompartmental and total knee replacement. J Bone Joint Surg Am. 2012;94(17):e126.

86. Hamilton TW, Rizkalla JM, Kontochristos L, et al. The interaction of caseload and usage in determining outcomes of unicompartmental knee arthroplasty: a meta-analysis. J Arthroplasty. 2017;32:3228.

87. Walker T, Zahn N, Bruckner T, Streit MR, Mohr G, Aldinger PR, Clarius M, Gotterbarm T. Mid-term results of lateral unicondylar mobile bearing knee arthroplasty: a multicentre study of 363 cases. Bone Joint J. 2018;100-B(1):42–9.

88. Chau R, Gulati A, Pandit H, Beard DJ, Price AJ, Dodd CA, Gill HS, Murray DW. Tibial component overhang following unicompartmental knee replacement—does it matter? Knee. 2009;16(5):310–3.

89. Barbadoro P, Ensini A, Leardini A, d'Amato M, Feliciangeli A, Timoncini A, Amadei F, Belvedere C, Giannini S. Tibial component alignment and risk of loosening in unicompartmental knee arthroplasty: a radiographic and radiostereometric study. Knee Surg Sports Traumatol Arthrosc. 2014;22(12):3157–62.

90. Collier MB, Eickmann TH, Sukezaki F, McAuley JP, Engh GA. Patient, implant, and alignment factors associated with revision of medial compartment unicondylar arthroplasty. J Arthroplasty. 2006;21:108–15.

91. Hernigou P, Deschamps G. Posterior slope of the tibial implant and the outcome of unicompartmental knee arthroplasty. J Bone Joint Surg Am. 2004;86(3):506–11.

92. Chatellard R, Sauleau V, Colmar M, Robert H, Raynaud G, Brilhault J. Medial unicompartmental knee arthroplasty: does tibial component position influence clinical outcomes and arthroplasty survival? Orthop Traumatol Surg Res. 2013;99(4 Suppl):S219–25.

93. Mittal A, Meshram P, Kim WH, Kim TK. Unicompartmental knee arthroplasty, an enigma, and the ten enigmas of medial UKA. J Orthop Traumatol. 2020;21(1):15.

94. Zuiderbaan HA, van der List JP, Chawla H, Khamaisy S, Thein R, Pearle AD. Predictors of subjective outcome after medial unicompartmental knee arthroplasty. J Arthroplasty. 2016;31(7):1453–8.

95. Vasso M, Del Regno C, D'Amelio A, Viggiano D, Corona K, Schiavone PA. Minor varus alignment provides better results than neutral alignment in medial UKA. Knee. 2015;22(2):117–21.

96. Kwon OR, Kang KT, Son J, Suh DS, Baek C, Koh YG. Importance of joint line preservation in unicompartmental knee arthroplasty: finite element analysis. J Orthop Res. 2017;35(2):347–52.

97. Mazas F. Arthroplastie unicompartimentaire du genou. Cahiers d'enseignement de la SOFCOT, vol. 34. Paris: Elsevier Masson; 1989. p. 113–23.

98. Ackroyd CE, Whitehouse SL, Newman JH, Joslin CC. A comparative study of the medial St Georg sled and kinematic total knee arthroplasties. Ten-year survivorship. J Bone Joint Surg Br. 2002;84:667–72.

99. Scuderi GR, Tenholder M, Capeci C. Surgical approaches in mini-incision total knee arthroplasty. Clin Orthop Relat Res. 2004;248:61–77.

100. Price AJ, Webb J, Topf H, Dodd CAF, Goodfellow JW, Murray DW. Rapid recovery after Oxford unicompartmental arthroplasty through a short incision. J Arthroplasty. 2001;16:970–6.

101. Reilly KA, Beard DJ, Barker KL, Dodd CA, Price AJ, Murray DW. Efficacy of an accelerated recovery protocol for Oxford unicompartmental knee arthroplasty. A randomised controlled trial. Knee. 2005;12:351–2.

102. Hamilton WG, Ammeen D, Engh CA, Engh GA. Learning curve with minimally invasive unicompartmental knee arthroplasty. J Arthroplasty. 2010;25:735–40.

103. Muller PE, Pellengahr C, Witt M, Kircher J, Refior HJ, Jansson V. Influence of minimally invasive surgery on implant positioning and the functional outcome for medial unicompartmental knee arthroplasty. J Arthroplasty. 2004;19:296–301.

104. Dalury DF, Dennis DA. Mini-incision total knee arthroplasty can increase risk of component malalignment. Clin Orthop Relat Res. 2005;440:77–81.

105. Konyves A, Willis-Owen CA, Spriggins AJ. The long-term benefit of computer-assisted surgical navigation in unicompartmental knee arthroplasty. J Orthop Surg Res. 2010;31:94.

106. Saragaglia D, Picard F, Chaussard C, et al. Mise en place des prothèses totales du genou assistée par ordinateur: comparaison avec la technique conventionnelle. Rev Chir Orthop. 2001;87:18–28.

107. Plate JF, Mofidi A, Mannava S, Smith BP, Lang JE, Poehling GG, Conditt MA, Jinnah RH. Achieving accurate ligament balancing using robotic-assisted

unicompartmental knee arthroplasty. Adv Orthop. 2013;2013:837167.

108. Lonner JH, John TK, Conditt MA. Robotic arm-assisted UKA improves tibial component alignment: a pilot study. Clin Orthop Relat Res. 2010;468:141–6.

109. Cobb J, Henckel J, Gomes P, Harris S, Jakopec M, Rodriguez F, Barrett A, Davies B. Hands-on robotic unicompartmental knee replacement: a prospective, randomised controlled study of the acrobot system. J Bone Joint Surg Br. 2006;88(2):188–97.

110. Bell SW, Anthony I, Jones B, MacLean A, Rowe P, Blyth M. Improved accuracy of component positioning with robotic-assisted unicompartmental knee arthroplasty: data from a prospective, randomized controlled study. J Bone Joint Surg Am. 2016;98(8):627–35.

111. van der List JP, Chawla H, Joskowicz L, Pearle AD. Current state of computer navigation and robotics in unicompartmental and total knee arthroplasty: a systematic review with meta-analysis. Knee Surg Sports Traumatol Arthrosc. 2016;24(11):3482–95.

112. Herry Y, Batailler C, Lording T, Servien E, Neyret P, Lustig S. Improved joint-line restitution in unicompartmental knee arthroplasty using a robotic-assisted surgical technique. Int Orthop. 2017;41(11):2265–71.

113. Citak M, Suero EM, Citak M, et al. Unicompartmental knee arthroplasty: is robotic technology more accurate than conventional technique? Knee. 2013;20(4):268–71.

114. Pearle AD, O'Loughlin PF, Kendoff DO. Robot-assisted unicompartmental knee arthroplasty. J Arthroplasty. 2010;25:230–7.

115. Pearle AD, van der List JP, Lee L, Coon TM, Borus TA, Roche MW. Survivorship and patient satisfaction of robotic-assisted medial unicompartmental knee arthroplasty at a minimum two-year follow-up. Knee. 2017;24(2):419–28.

116. Lonner JH, Moretti VM. The evolution of image-free robotic assistance in unicompartmental knee arthroplasty. Am J Orthop. 2016;45:249–54.

117. Moschetti WE, Konopka JF, Rubash HE, Genuario JW. Can robot-assisted unicompartmental knee arthroplasty be cost-effective? A Markov decision analysis. J Arthroplasty. 2016;31(4):759–65.

118. St Mart JP, et al. The three-year survivorship of robotically assisted versus non-robotically assisted unicompartmental knee arthroplasty. Bone Joint J. 2020;102-B(3):319–3.

119. Van Den Heever DJ, Scheffer C, Erasmus PJ, Dillon EM. Contact stresses in a patient-specific unicompartmental knee replacement. Conference proceedings: annual international conference of the IEEE Engineering in Medicine and Biology Society. IEEE Engineering in Medicine and Biology Society. Conference 2010;2010:5113–5116.

120. Jaffry Z, Masjedi M, Clarke S, Harris S, Karia M, Andrews B, Cobb J. Unicompartmental knee arthroplasties: robot vs. patient specific instrumentation. Knee. 2014;21(2):428–34.

121. Kerens B, Schotanus MG, Boonen B, Kort NP. No radiographic difference between patient-specific guiding and conventional Oxford UKA surgery. Knee Surg Sports Traumatol Arthrosc. 2015;23(5):1324–9.

122. Ollivier M, Parratte S, Lunebourg A, Viehweger E, Argenson JN. The John Insall award: no functional benefit after unicompartmental knee arthroplasty performed with patient-specific instrumentation: a randomized trial. Clin Orthop Relat Res. 2016;474(1):60–8.

123. Wiik AV, Manning V, Strachan RK, Amis AA, Cobb JP. Unicompartmental knee arthroplasty enables near normal gait at higher speeds, unlike total knee arthroplasty. J Arthroplasty. 2013;28(9 Suppl):176–8.

124. Hopper GP, Leach WJ. Participation in sporting activities following knee replacement: total versus unicompartmental. Knee Surg Sports Traumatol Arthrosc. 2008;16(10):973–9.

125. Weale AE, Murray DW, Newman JH, Ackroyd CE. The length of the patellar tendon after unicompartmental and total knee replacement. J Bone Joint Surg Br. 1999;81(5):790–5.

126. Friesenbichler B, Item-Glatthorn JF, Wellauer V, von Knoch F, Casartelli NC, Maffiuletti NA. Short-term functional advantages after medial unicompartmental versus total knee arthroplasty. Knee. 2018;25(4):638–43.

127. Dunbar MJ, Richardson G, Robertsson O. I can't get no satisfaction after my total knee replacement: rhymes and reasons. Bone Joint J. 2013;95B(11):148–52.

128. Newman J, Pydisetty RV, Ackroyd C. Unicompartmental or total knee replacement: the 15-year results of a prospective randomized controlled trial. J Bone Joint Surg Br. 2009;91:52–7.

129. Sun PF, Jia YH. Mobile bearing UKA compared to fixed bearing TKA: a randomized prospective study. Knee. 2012;19(2):103–6.

130. Costa CR, Johnson AJ, Mont MA, Bonutti PM. Unicompartmental and total knee arthroplasty in the same patient. J Knee Surg. 2011;24(4):273–8.

131. Kulshrestha V, Datta B, Kumar S, Mittal G. Outcome of unicondylar knee arthroplasty vs total knee arthroplasty for early medial compartment arthritis: a randomized study. J Arthroplasty. 2017;32(5):1460–9.

132. Beard DJ, Davies LJ, Cook JA, MacLennan G, Price A, Kent S, Hudson J, Carr A, Leal J, Campbell H, Fitzpatrick R, Arden N, Murray D, Campbell MK, TOPKAT Study Group. The clinical and cost-effectiveness of total versus partial knee replacement in patients with medial compartment osteoarthritis (TOPKAT): 5-year outcomes of a randomised controlled trial. Lancet. 2019;394(10200):746–56.

133. Knifsund J, Niinimaki T, Nurmi H, Toom A, Keemu H, Laaksonen I, Seppänen M, Liukas A, Pamilo K, Vahlberg T, Äärimaa V, Mäkelä KT. Functional results of total-knee arthroplasty versus medial uni-compartmental arthroplasty: two-year results of a

randomised, assessor-blinded multicentre trial. BMJ Open. 2021;11(6):e046731.

134. Repicci JA. Total knee or uni? Benefits and limitations of the unicondylar knee prosthesis. Orthopedics. 2003;26(274):277.

135. Pandit H, Hamilton TW, Jenkins C, Mellon SJ, Dodd CAF, Murray DW. The clinical outcome of minimally invasive phase 3 Oxford unicompartmental knee arthroplasty: a 15 year follow-up of 1000 UKAs. Bone Joint J. 2015;97-B:1493–500.

136. Faour-Martín O, Valverde-García JA, Martín-Ferrero MA, Vega-Castrillo A, de la Red Gallego MA, Suárez de Puga CC, Amigo-Liñares L. Oxford phase 3 unicondylar knee arthroplasty through a minimally invasive approach: long-term results. Int Orthop. 2013;37(5):833–8.

137. Emerson RH, Alnachoukati O, Barrington J, Ennin K. The results of Oxford unicompartmental knee arthroplasty in the United States: a mean ten-year survival analysis. Bone Joint J. 2016;98-B:34–40.

138. Kim KT, Lee S, Kim JH, Hong SW, Jung WS, Shin WS. The survivorship and clinical results of minimally invasive unicompartmental knee arthroplasty at 10- year follow-up. Clin Orthop Surg. 2015;7:199.

139. Lisowski LA, Meijer LI, van den Bekerom MP, Pilot P, Lisowski AE. Ten- to 15-year results of the Oxford phase III mobile unicompartmental knee arthroplasty: a prospective study from a non-designer group. Bone Joint J. 2016;98 B(10 Suppl B):41–7.

140. Foran JR, Brown NM, Della Valle CJ, Berger RA, Galante JO. Long-term survivorship and failure modes of unicompartmental knee arthroplasty. Clin Orthop Relat Res. 2013;471(1):102–8.

141. Rothwell Chairman A; Supervisor Peter Devane Orthopaedic Surgeon Simon Young Orthopaedic Surgeon Dawson Muir Orthopaedic Surgeon, Andrew Oakley R, Griffin H, Pettett A; Hobbs Registry Coordinator T. Rothwell Registry supervisor Toni Hobbs Registry Coordinator Chris Frampton statistician James Taylor Hip A, Dawson Muir K: the New Zealand Joint Registry. Seventeen year report: January 1999 to December 2015. 1999. www.nzoa.org.nz/nz-joint-registry. Accessed 28 Sept 2021.

142. Norwegian Arthroplasty Register annual report 2016. 2016. http://nrlweb.ihelse.net. Accessed 28 Sept 2021.

143. Amin AK, Patton JT, Cook RE, Gaston M, Brenkel IJ. Unicompartmental or total knee arthroplasty?: results from a matched study. Clin Orthop Relat Res. 2006;451:101–6.

144. Lum ZC, Lombardi AV, Hurst JM, Morris MJ, Adams JB, Berend KR. Early outcomes of twin-peg mobile-bearing unicompartmental knee arthroplasty compared with primary total knee arthroplasty. Bone Joint J. 2016;98-B(Suppl B):28–33.

145. Horikawa A, Miyakoshi N, Shimada Y, Kodama H. Comparison of clinical outcomes between total knee arthroplasty and unicompartmental knee arthroplasty for osteoarthritis of the knee: a retrospective analysis of preoperative and postoperative results. J Orthop Surg Res. 2015;10:168.

146. Di Martino A, Bordini B, Barile F, Ancarani C, Digennaro V, Faldini C. Unicompartmental knee arthroplasty has higher revisions than total knee arthroplasty at long term follow-up: a registry study on 6453 prostheses. Knee Surg Sports Traumatol Arthrosc. 2021;29(10):3323–9.

147. Niinimäki T, Eskelinen A, Mäkelä K, Ohtonen P, Puhto A-P, Remes V. Unicompartmental knee arthroplasty survivorship is lower than TKA survivorship: a 27 year Finnish registry study. Clin Orthop Relat Res. 2014;472:1496–501.

148. Curtin B, Malkani A, Lau E, Kurtz S, Ong K. Revision after total knee arthroplasty and unicompartmental knee arthroplasty in the Medicare population. J Arthroplasty. 2012;27:1480–6.

149. Willis-Owen CA, Brust K, Alsop H, Miraldo M, Cobb JP. Unicondylar knee arthroplasty in the UK National Health Service: an analysis of candidacy, outcome and cost efficacy. Knee. 2009;16:473–8.

150. Goodfellow JW, O'Connor JJ, Murray DW. A critique of revision rate as an outcome measure: reinterpretation of knee joint registry data. J Bone Joint Surg Br. 2010;92(12):1628–31.

151. Chawla H, van der List JP, Christ AB, Sobrero MR, Zuiderbaan HA, Pearle AD. Annual revision rates of partial versus total knee arthroplasty: a comparative meta-analysis. Knee. 2017;24(2):179–90.

152. Deshmukh RV, Scott RD. Unicompartmental knee arthroplasty: long-term results. Clin Orthop Relat Res. 2001;392:272–8.

153. Pandit H, Gulati A, Jenkins C, Barker K, Price AJ, Dodd CA, Murray DW. Unicompartmental knee replacement for patients with partial thickness cartilage loss in the affected compartment. Knee. 2011;18(3):168–71.

154. Niinimäki TT, Murray DW, Partanen J, Pajala A, Leppilahti JI. Unicompartmental knee arthroplasties implanted for osteoarthritis with partial loss of joint space have high re-operation rates. Knee. 2011;18:432–5.

155. Zhang Q, Zhang Q, Guo W, Liu Z, Cheng L, Yue D, Zhang N. The learning curve for minimally invasive Oxford phase 3 unicompartmental knee arthroplasty: cumulative summation test for learning curve (LC-CUSUM). J Orthop Surg Res. 2014;9:81.

156. Lewold S, Robertsson O, Knutson K, Lidgren L. Revision of unicompartmental knee arthroplasty: outcome in 1,135 cases from the Swedish knee arthroplasty study. Acta Orthop Scand. 1998;69:469–74.

157. van der List JP, Zuiderbaan HA, Pearle AD. Why do medial unicompartmental knee arthroplasties fail today? J Arthroplasty. 2016;31:1016–21.

158. Citak M, Dersch K, Kamath AF, Haasper C, Gehrke T, Kendoff D. Common causes of failed unicompartmental knee arthroplasty: a single-centre analysis

of four hundred and seventy one cases. Int Orthop. 2014;38(5):961–5.

159. Epinette JA, Brunschweiler B, Mertl P, Mole D, Cazenave A, French Society for Hip and Knee. Unicompartmental knee arthroplasty modes of failure: wear is not the main reason for failure: a multicentre study of 418 failed knees. Orthop Traumatol Surg Res. 2012;98(6 Suppl):S124–30.

160. Khamaisy S, Zuiderbaan HA, van der List JP, Nam D, Pearle AD. Medial unicompartmental knee arthroplasty improves congruence and restores joint space width of the lateral compartment. Knee. 2016;23(3):501–5.

161. Park CN, Zuiderbaan HA, Chang A, Khamaisy S, Pearle AD, Ranawat AS. Role of magnetic resonance imaging in the diagnosis of the painful unicompartmental knee arthroplasty. Knee. 2015;22(4): 341–6.

162. Cross M, Yi P, Moric M. Revising an HTO or UKA to TKA: is it more like a primary TKA or a revision TKA? J Arthroplasty. 2014;229:31.

163. Wynn Jones H, Chan W, Harrison T, Smith TO, Masonda P, Walton NP. Revision of medial Oxford unicompartmental knee replacement to a total knee replacement: similar to a primary? Knee. 2012;19(4):339–43.

164. Chou DT, Swamy GN, Lewis JR, Badhe NP. Revision of failed unicompartmental knee replacement to total knee replacement. Knee. 2012;19(4):356–9.

165. Pearse AJ, Hooper GJ, Rothwell A, Frampton C. Survival and functional outcome after revision of a unicompartmental to a total knee replacement: the New Zealand National Joint Registry. J Bone Joint Surg Br. 2010;92(4):508–12.

166. Hang JR, Stanford TE, Graves SE, Davidson DC, de Steiger RN, Miller LN. Outcome of revision of unicompartmental knee replacement. Acta Orthop. 2010;81(1):95–8.

167. Sierra RJ, Kassel CA, Wetters NG, Berend KR, Della Valle CJ, Lombardi AV. Revision of unicompartmen-

tal arthroplasty to total knee arthroplasty: not always a slam dunk! J Arthroplasty. 2013;28:128–32.

168. Ghomrawi HM, Eggman AA, Pearle AD. Effect of age on cost-effectiveness of unicompartmental knee arthroplasty compared with total knee arthroplasty in the U.S. J Bone Joint Surg Am. 2015;97(5):396–402.

169. Shankar S, Tetreault MW, Jegier BJ, Andersson GB, Della Valle CJ. A cost comparison of unicompartmental and total knee arthroplasty. Knee. 2016;23(6):1016–9.

170. Goodfellow JW, Kershaw CJ, Benson MK, O'Connor JJ. The Oxford knee for unicompartmental osteoarthritis. The first 103 cases. J Bone Joint Surg Br. 1988;70(5):692–701.

171. Gulati A, Chau R, Pandit HG, Gray H, Price AJ, Dodd CA, Murray DW. The incidence of physiological radiolucency following Oxford unicompartmental knee replacement and its relationship to outcome. J Bone Joint Surg Br. 2009;91(7):896–902.

172. Witjes S, Gouttebarge V, Kuijer PP, van Geenen RC, Poolman RW, Kerkhoffs GM. Return to sports and physical activity after total and unicondylar knee arthroplasty: a systematic review and meta-analysis. Sports Med. 2016;46(2):269–92.

173. Walton NP, Jahromi I, Lewis PL, Dobson PJ, Angel KR, Campbell DG. Patient-perceived outcomes and return to sport and work: TKA versus mini-incision unicompartmental knee arthroplasty. J Knee Surg. 2006;19(2):112–6.

174. Jacofsky DJ, Allen M. Robotics in arthroplasty: a comprehensive review. J Arthroplasty. 2016;31:2353–63.

175. Liddle AD, Pandit H, O'Brien S, Doran E, Penny ID, Hooper GJ, Burn PJ, Dodd CA, Beverland DE, Maxwell AR, Murray DW. Cementless fixation in Oxford unicompartmental knee replacement: a multicentre study of 1000 knees. Bone Joint J. 2013;95-B(2):181–7.

Bi-compartmental and Bi-unicondylar Knee Arthroplasty

11

Amy Garner and Justin Cobb

Abbreviations

ACL	Anterior cruciate ligament
BCA-L	Bi-compartmental knee arthroplasty (medial)
BCA-M	Bi-compartmental knee arthroplasty (lateral)
Bi-UKA	Bi-unicondylar knee arthroplasty
CPKA	Combined partial knee arthroplasty
EQ-5D	EuroQol-5D index of quality of life
OKS	Oxford knee score
PFA	Patellofemoral joint arthroplasty
PFJ	Patellofemoral joint
PKA	Partial knee arthroplasty
TCA	Tricompartmental knee arthroplasty
TKA	Total knee arthroplasty
UKA	Uni-compartmental knee arthroplasty

Introduction

Gonarthrosis commonly occurs as a consequence of excessive varus load. This form of gonarthrosis commonly starts anteromedially, but may not present until some patellofemoral wear has devel-

A. Garner · J. Cobb (✉)
Advanced Musculoskeletal Research and Treatment, Imperial College London, London, UK
e-mail: a.garner@imperial.ac.uk; j.cobb@imperial.ac.uk

oped [1]. In a recent systematic review, we reported that wear precipitated by medial meniscal failure is the most common pattern of presentation accounting for 27% of all cases, while wear affecting both the medial and patellofemoral joints is the second most common at 23% (Fig. 11.1) [2]. Tri-compartmental damage is only seen in 17% of cases. Altogether, a third of knees present with two compartments affected in this study. Other authors have put the figure higher: 59% of those presenting with gonarthrosis [3] in one study had arthritis in two compartments, while 40% of patients over 50 years old with knee pain had radiographic evidence of combined medial compartment and PFJ wear. It is thus fair to conclude that the majority of patients undergoing total knee arthroplasty (TKA) have at least one healthy compartment excised.

In modern TKA practice, the Anterior Cruciate Ligament (ACL) is found to be present in up to 78% of cases [4, 5]. The fundamental role of the ACL in knee stability and functional gait is well described [6], yet most contemporary TKA systems necessitate its resection, while bi-cruciate retaining TKA designs have yet to demonstrate favourable outcomes [7].

Dissatisfaction rates of up to 20% are commonly reported after TKA [8], while TKA pose increased peri-operative risk [9] and limited function when in the absence of a native

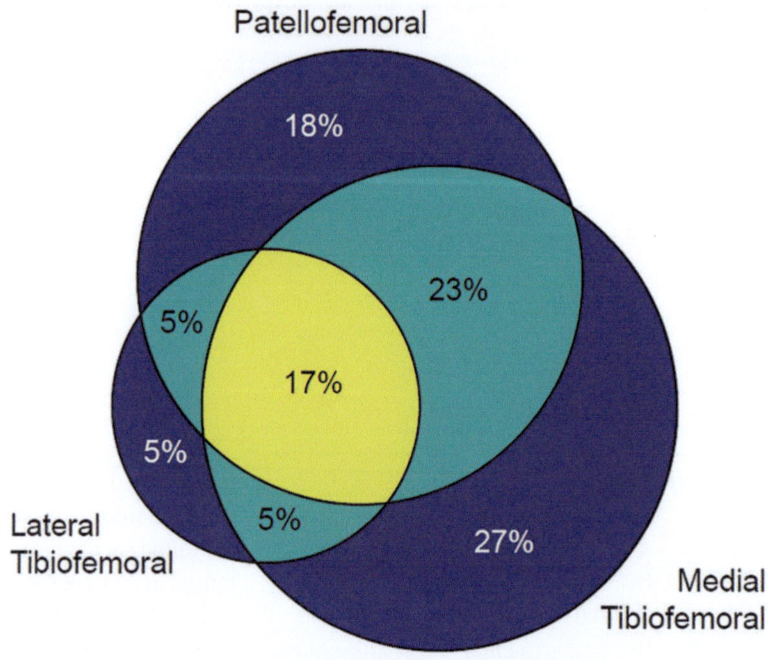

Fig. 11.1 Incidence of arthrosis by compartments of the knee. (From Stoddard et al. 2020 with permission)

ACL. However, TKA remains the most common treatment for multi-compartment arthrosis [10].

Combined Partial Knee Arthroplasty (CPKA), the implantation of multiple Partial Knee Arthroplasties (PKA) within the same knee to address multi-compartment disease, preserves the healthy remaining compartment; periarticular tissues including the meniscus if a tibiofemoral compartment is spared and, most importantly, functional cruciate ligaments. CPKA are an alternative to TKA and may be performed as a single procedure, or staged, in the event of native compartment degeneration following successful single PKA [11]. Four combinations of CPKA are described (Fig. 11.2): Bicompartmental Arthroplasty (BCA) refers to the combination of a Patellofemoral Arthroplasty (PFA) with either medial (BCA-M) or lateral (BCA-L) Unicompartmental Knee Arthroplasty (UKA), whilst Bi-Unicondylar Arthroplasty (Bi-UKA) describes ipsilateral medial and lateral UKA. Tricompartmental Arthroplasty (TCA) describes rare situation of all three PKAs used in combination, most typically in the staged setting. CPKA is not a new idea. Charnley's 'Load Angle Inlay' knee, the original Gunston Knee, the Cartier Knee; the Marmor Modular Knee; and Oxford partial knee systems all initially followed in a bi-unicondylar configuration. More recently, some reports of favourable outcomes following

compartmental arthroplasty have been reported in Europe [12, 13] and the USA [14].

In the 'staged' setting, conversion of PKA to CPKA for native compartment degeneration is potentially advantageous in that the second operation most likely carries the low-operative risk profile [9], operating times and hospital lengths of stay as that of a primary PKA. When PKA are revised to TKA, bone loss can cause significant problems with stability, and require metaphyseal augments and stems. Preserving a well-fixed, well-functioning PKA and, instead, tailoring the surgery to the exact disease pattern of the patient, may avoid revision to TKA altogether, though subsequent degeneration of the remaining native compartment remains a possibility. If second surgery in PKA involves conversion to a standard primary TKA, this is a relatively straightforward process, especially if a kinematic technique is employed [15]. The cost-benefit of the compartmental approach is, as yet, unknown. The cost of two implants, and, in the staged setting, two procedures and two short hospital stays is, potentially, offset against the shorter overall operating times, reduced peri-operative risk and the burden of, for example, longer hospital stays requiring more blood products, expensive revision implants, higher risks of peri-operative infections, serious medical complications and the

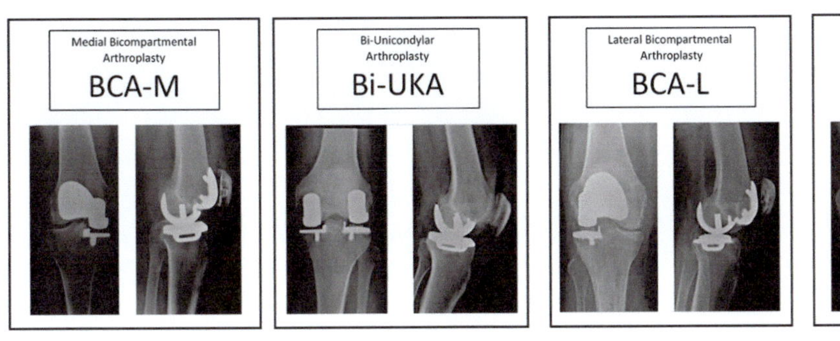

Fig. 11.2 Classification of combined partial knee arthroplasty (CPKA). (From Garner et al. 2019 with permission)

additional rehabilitation needs of the patient, who, if young, may never return to work. This echoes the cost-savings reported in the TOPKAT randomised trial, which compared primary PKA to primary TKA, owing to the additional non-revision costs incurred [16].

Case One

A 64-year-old male with a 3-year history of antero-medial right knee pain; pain on stair climbing; difficulty standing up from a chair; night pain; occasional giving way, and a new requirement for walking aids, is keen to return to playing tennis. A moderate effusion is found on examination, along with a correctable varus deformity, range of motion was 5–130°. The knee was stable, Anterior Drawer and Lachman Test were negative. The medial meniscus was extruded, but valgus stress did not result in extrusion of the lateral meniscus.

Varus alignment with significant medial joint space loss, osteophytes and subchondral sclerosis are observed on the pre-operative radiographs (Fig. 11.3). There tibia is medially translated on the femur. The lateral facet of the patellofemoral joint has severe arthrosis. The lateral compartment is well preserved. On the lateral view, the ACL appears to be functional, no evidence of anterior translation of the tibia on the femur is observed.

Management options include non-operative therapies, a compartmental approach or primary TKA. The patient prioritised an anticipated higher post-operative function, and accepted the risk of further surgery in the future, should the lateral compartment subsequently fail, and, on balance, with informed consent, opted for the bone, meniscus and ACL preserving BCA-M. In the operating theatre, the patient was positioned supine to optimise ease of PFA implantation, despite making the UKA-M more technically challenging than the standard 'dangle' setup. The knee joint was approached through a midline incision and medial parapatellar arthrotomy. Inspection of the lateral compartment confirmed little to no wear, and anterior-posterior movement of the tibia on the femur was appropriately restrained by a functional ACL. The medial compartment was prepared to accept a mobile-bearing UKA-M, undertaken first so as to correct the alignment. With trial implants left in situ, the patellar-femoral joint was prepared for an onlay trochlear component and a distalised and medialised patellar button. All components were implanted simultaneously, once all bony cuts had been performed. A 64-min tourniquet time was recorded (19 min longer than the surgeon average for UKA-M, of 45 min). The patient was discharged within 48 h of surgery and recovered without peri-operative complication. Full and active participation in tennis was achieved within 4 months of surgery. His 6 month post-operative Oxford Knee Score was 44, rising to 47 at 12 months. Six years post-surgery his OKS continues at 47.

Post-operative radiographs (Fig. 11.4) depict an onlay PFA and a cementless mobile-bearing UKA-M in situ. The varus deformity and tibial translation have been corrected, while the lateral compartment is preserved. The ACL appears functional. On examination, the knee is stable in all planes, the patella button tracks adequately

Fig. 11.3 Pre-operative radiographs case one

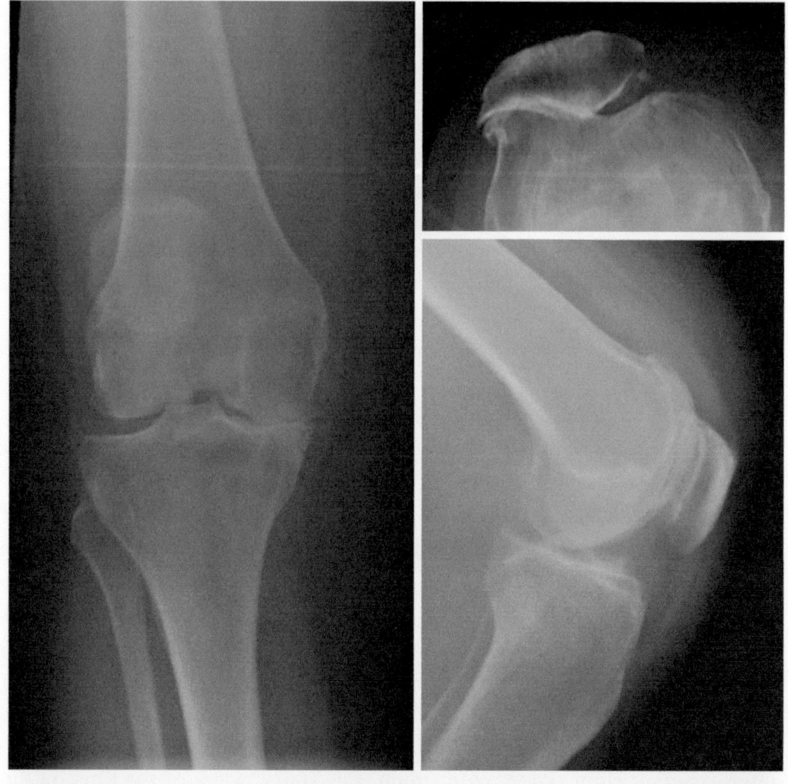

Fig. 11.4 Post-operative radiographs case one with BCA-M in situ

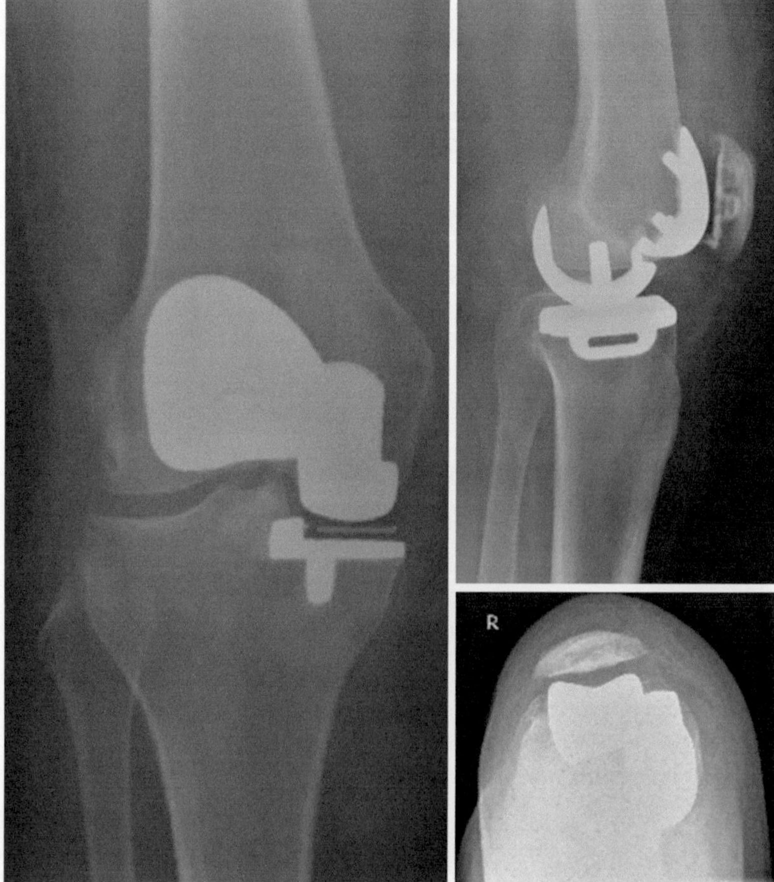

over the resurfaced trochlea and the lateral meniscus remains normal.

Case Two

A 54-year-old male reports lateral knee pain, with difficulty walking on slopes. For many years, he has been a keen hill walker but now reports knee swelling, requiring regular anti-inflammatory medications, even to walk short distances. Examining him, he has a good range of motion, but the lateral meniscus is felt to extrude. The knee was stable, Lachman test was negative, no medial meniscal extrusion was felt when a varus stress was applied.

Weight-bearing radiographs (Fig. 11.5) demonstrate a valgus deformity of the right knee, with Ahlback grade IV loss laterally, and some medial opening. Severe degeneration of the lateral PFJ is observed on the lateral radiograph, no evidence of anterior translation of the tibia on the femur is seen, suggesting that the ACL is functional.

Since high post-operative function was considered a priority, the patient elected to undergo single-stage BCA-L. The patient was set up on the operating table as per case one, but a lateral parapatellar arthrotomy was employed to opti-

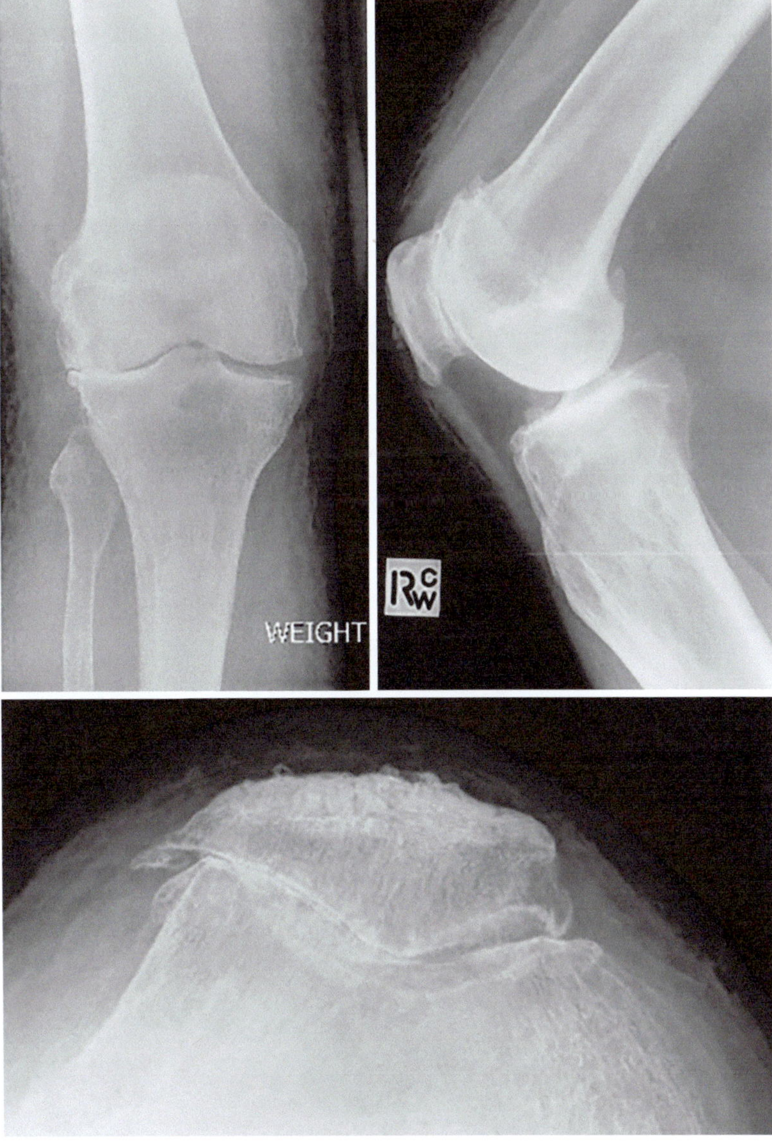

Fig. 11.5 Pre-operative radiographs case two

mise access to the lateral compartment. Additional care is required to sublux the patella medially and facilitate adequate exposure, including extension of the arthrotomy into the quadriceps tendon, as necessary. On inspection of the joint, the medial compartment was well-preserved. The ACL was functional and intact. For the BCA-L, particular care is taken to ensure the patella has a smooth transition between the components of the PFA, the UKA and the femoral condylar cartilage to optimise accurate patellar tracking. In this case, a mobile-bearing UKA-L design was used; however, our contemporary practise is to use a fixed bearing on the lateral side to avoid the risk of bearing dislocation. The patient spend 36 h in hospital, experienced no peri-operative complications, did not require a blood transfusion and returned to hill walking within 6 months. At 12 months post-surgery, his

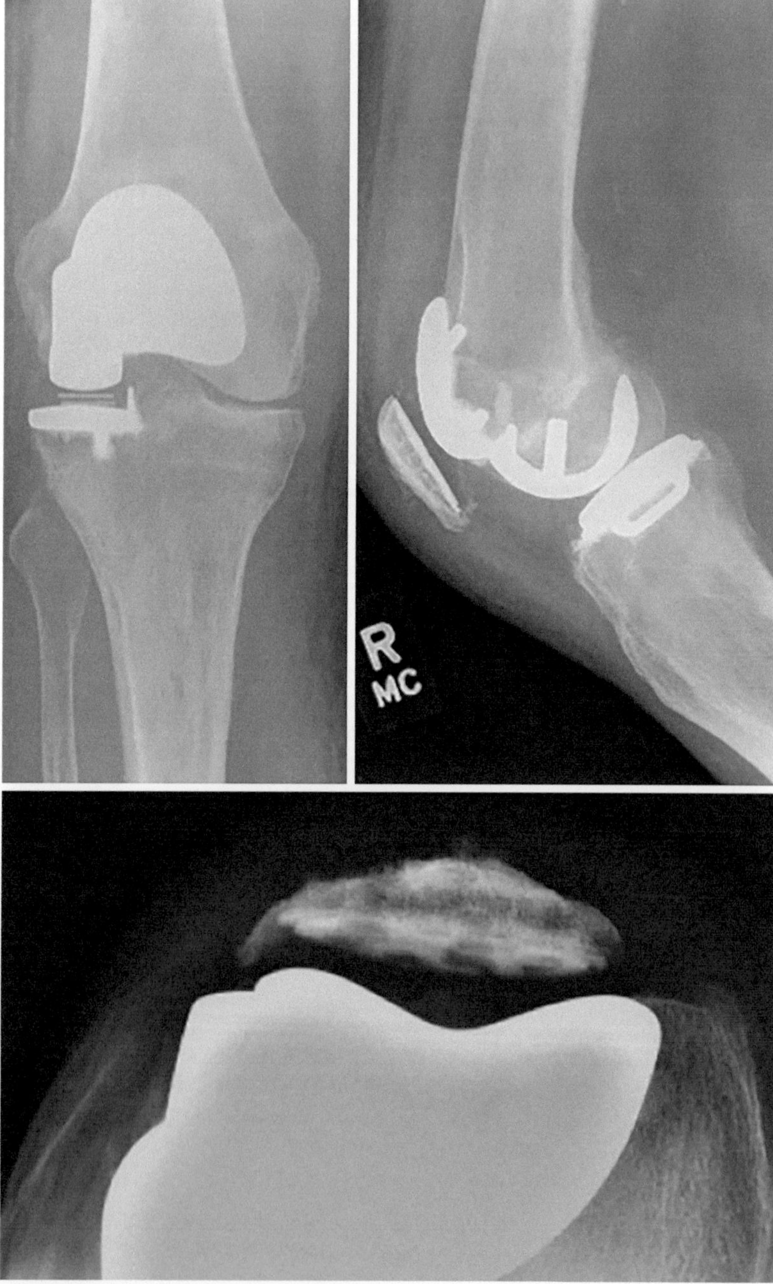

Fig. 11.6 Post-operative radiographs case two demonstrating a BCA-L in situ

Oxford Knee Score was 44, EQ-5D 0.95/1. Post-operative radiographs (Fig. 11.6) confirm that the medial compartment is preserved and valgus alignment corrected.

Case Three

Following a UKA-M 14 years ago, an 82-year-old lady presents with knee pain, requiring a walking stick. She can stand from a chair with the use of one-arm rest only. She uses the stairs without particular difficulty but reports a sense of "instability" and impending collapse. Her Diabetes Mellitus Type II is controlled with insulin; 2 years ago, she had three cardiac stents implanted; she had a transient ischaemic attack 5 years ago with no residual neurological deficit. Her hypertension is controlled on dual therapy. To examine her, she has a moderate effusion; 0–120 range of movement, correctable valgus deformity of <10°, the UKA-M appears stable and functional, though some anterior-posterior laxity is palpable. Pre-operative radiographs (Fig. 11.7) demonstrate failure of the lateral compartment in the presence of a well-fixed UKA-M and a relatively well-preserved patellofemoral joint. The status of the ACL is unclear.

In the absence of surgical intervention, progression of lateral compartment OA in patients with medial arthrosis is rare [17, 18]. Progression of lateral OA after UKA-M is a commonly reported mode of failure, prompting revision to TKA [19]. However, multiple 15–20-year follow-up studies place the revision rate as between 2.3 and 2.6% [20–22]. Our own group reported no instances of polyethylene dislocations in 64 UKA-M knees [23].

All surgical options for this lady carry considerable risk, given her age and comorbidities. The most commonly performed operation would be to remove the well-fixed, adequately functioning UKA-M, sacrifice the ACL and patellofemoral compartment and revise to a TKA. An alternative would be to pre-

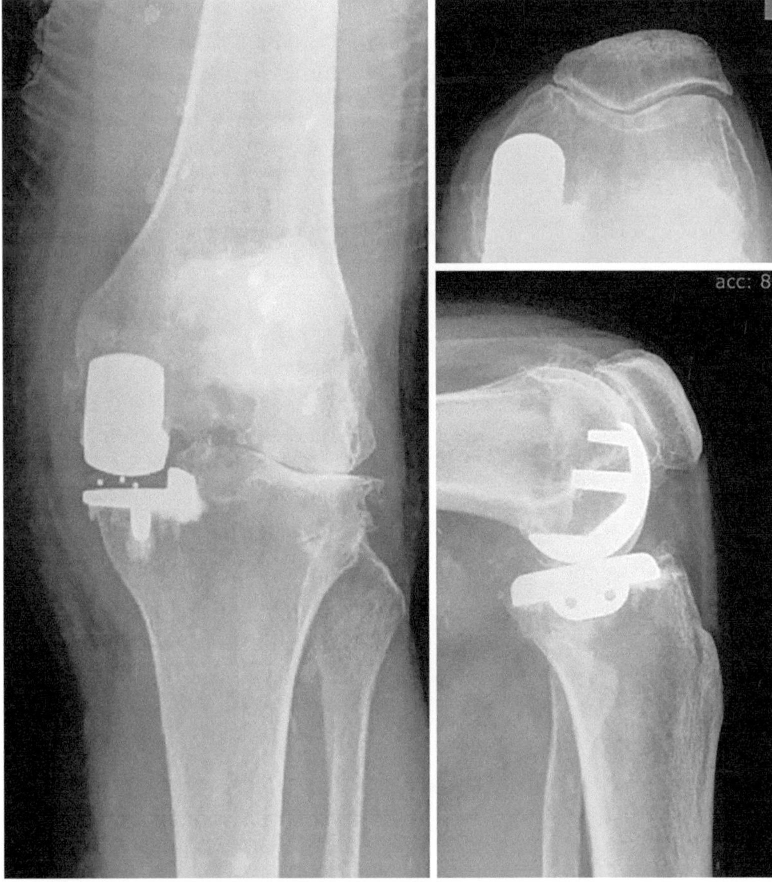

Fig. 11.7 Pre-operative radiographs case three demonstrating a UKA-M in situ

serve the UKA-M, and 'convert' to a Bi-UKA through the addition of a UKA-L, a so-called 'staged Bi-UKA' [24]. Some reports of the outcomes of stage Bi-UKA in this situation are favourable [24]. Revision to TKA carries significant peri-operative risk: a large surgical exposure is required, the risk of bone loss during implant removal may necessitate the requirement for stems and metaphyseal augments or cones. The peri-operative risk of stroke, myocardial infarction or death is considerable [9]. Although conversion to Bi-UKA would be regarded by joint registries as a 'revision' of the medial UKA, it is possible to perform it as though it were a primary procedure, with a small incision; lateral parapatellar arthrotomy through virgin tissue, small implants, short tourniquet times and likely earlier hospital discharge. The National Institute for Health and Clinical Excellence (NICE) recently reported that these additional procedures may be considered 'minor' revisions, and should be distinguished from 'major' revisions of TKA procedures [25]. Such a philosophy encourages a conservative, targeted and joint preserving compartmental approach to the management of gonarthrosis.

During the process of informed consent, the patient and surgeon discussed the need for formal inspection of the compartments prior to the final decision to proceed with staged Bi-UKA. Specifically, should the PFJ be significantly worn or the ACL completely dysfunctional at the time of surgery, there would be a low threshold for conversion to TKA.

The patient was positioned with the leg 'dangling' on a gutter support. When the primary incision is midline, this is the preferred approach through the skin; however, if the previous UKA-M incision were considerably medial to the mid-line, a parallel lateral incision would be made, with no less than a 6 cm skin bridge between the wounds. Once beneath the skin, a lateral parapatellar arthrotomy is made. On inspection, the ACL was functional, although degenerate. In elderly, low-demand patients, the absence of a functional ACL is not an absolute contraindication, since the joint is inherently stiff and anterior-posterior instability is less problematic than in younger, fitter patients. The UKA-M was well-fixed, with minimal evidence of polyethylene wear so was preserved. In high-functioning patients, the polyethylene is often exchanged if signs of wear are evident, though this adds considerably to the technical challenge

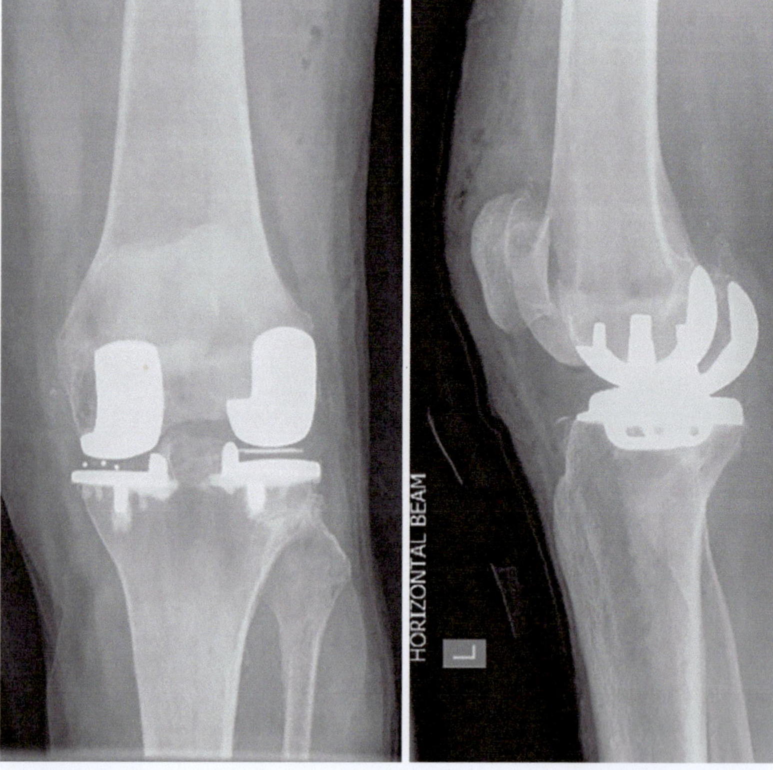

Fig. 11.8 Post-operative radiographs demonstrate conversion to bi-UKA through the addition of a lateral UKA

of the operation and may necessitate an additional medial parapatellar arthrotomy. The tourniquet time was 48 min. The patient was mobilised the following day and, after adequate post-operative radiographs (Fig. 11.8), physiotherapy support and acceptable blood results, the patient was discharged to her own home on the second post-operative day, with no reported perioperative complications.

Function Post-CPKA

There is some evidence that BCA is associated with superior performance in strenuous activities such as stair climbing and jogging, compared to TKA [26], in part due to restored isokinetic quadriceps function [27, 28]. BCA is consistently reported to result in high function, independent chair rising and reciprocal stair ascent [29, 30]. Gait patterns and kinematics associated with BCA are similar to those of healthy controls [29, 31]. Several studies report that compared to those with a TKA, BCA patients have higher levels of comfort and satisfaction following surgery [32, 33], with 85% of patients reporting excellent or good pain outcomes up to 12 years following surgery [34]. Intra-operative blood loss rarely results in the need for transfusion [13] and greater post-operative range of movement has been reported, compared to matched groups undergoing TKA [35].

In case one, the femur has been addressed through two, unlinked components, with one advantage being that each component can be orientated according to the specific anatomy of the compartment [19, 33]. An alternative is to use a monolithic femoral component, though early examples including the Journey-Deuce (Smith and Nephew Inc., Memphis, TN, US) performed very poorly, with high rates of early revision as a consequence of malalignment, poor durability, sizing difficulties, anterior knee pain, implant fracture, limited range of movement and tibial fractures, were all recorded as causes for early failure [27]. One short-term study reported a 12% revision rate, with 25% of patients complaining of anterior knee pain [36]. Of 25 Journey Deuce in a different study, three were revised—one for

patella instability and two for fractured tibial trays [37]. These, and other reports suggesting tibial subsidence, contributed to recall of the Journey-Deuce prosthesis in 2010.

Contemporary monolithic designs include custom-built models, utilising assistive technologies including 3D-printed patient-specific instrumentation, navigation and robotics in an effort to decrease the technical demands of the procedure and improve the accuracy and predictability of the alignment outcomes [38, 39]. It remains unclear whether this may lead to a resurgence in interest in linked components. Modular CPKA allows the surgeon more freedom, enabling subtle adjustments according to the femoral geometry, with promising results, but a well-described, steep learning curve [35, 36, 40–42] which may potentially be flattened with robotic assistance [43]. At 17 years, aseptic loosening of the PFA implant was the main cause of failure in 20/27 revised BCA-M—poor-quality polyethylene may have been a contributing factor to this high-revision rate [44]. Experience from BCA failure, however, provided evidence that conversion to TKA was typically straightforward, and primary TKA implants could often be utilised [12, 42, 45, 46]. Second generation, onlay, cemented patello-femoral components are associated with improved clinical and biochemical outcomes compared to their earlier counterparts [47–49], while unlinked CPKA components enable more accurate alignment [47]. Single-staged Bi-UKA has been associated with shorter hospital stays than TKA [12].

In a study by Biazzo et al., 19 patients undergoing single-stage Bi-UKA were compared to a matched cohort undergoing computer-assisted TKA. The results showed superior outcome of the Bi-UKA in terms of function and stiffness on the WOMAC indexes, and equivalent KSS and WOMAC Arthritis Index (pain score) [13].

Objectively, ACL retention and utilisation of a CPKA approach enables more normal gait [50]. While UKA returns knees to a near normal gait, patients with TKA are substantially less mobile, with shorter strides and lower cadence [51]. In a study comparing patients following BCA-M (n = 14) with age and sex matched healthy con-

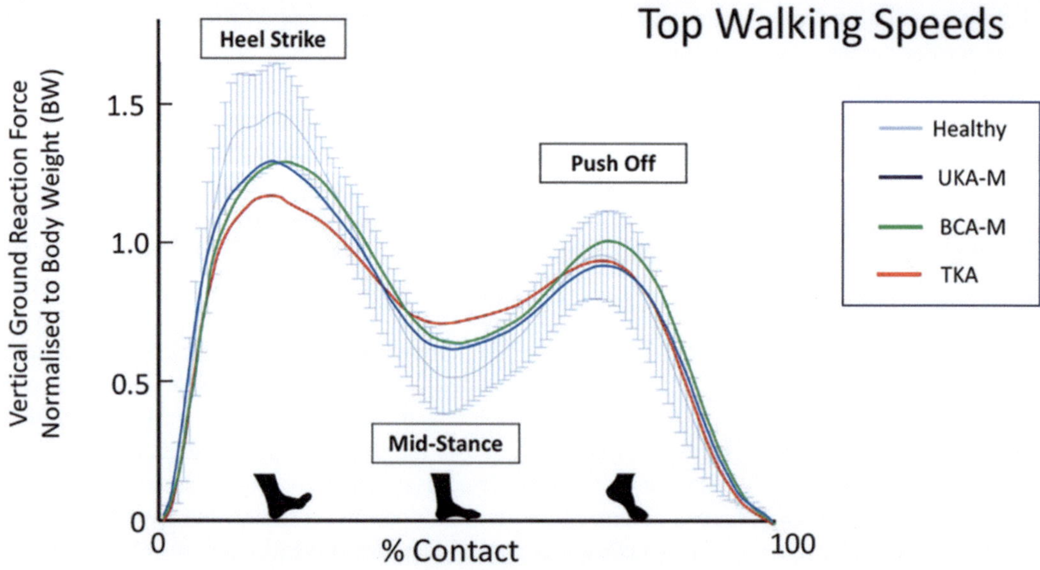

Fig. 11.9 Gait analysis of UKA, BCA-M, and TKA compared with healthy controls

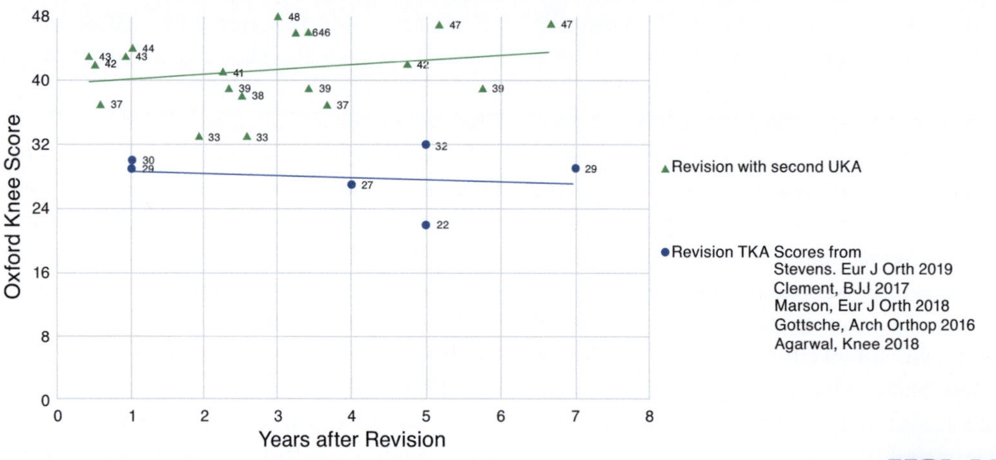

Fig. 11.10 Oxford Knee Scores of patients following addition of a second UKA compared with contemporary results of revision TKA

trols, UKA-M patients ($n = 18$) and those with a TKA ($n = 15$), BCA-M gait closely resembled that of UKA-M, 18% faster than TKA (BCA-M 6.5 km/h, UKA-M 6.4 km/h, TKA 5.5 km/h $p = 0.003$) with advantages seen, particularly in terms of heel-strike, maximum weight accep-tance and mid-stance forces, longer step and stride lengths and more normal cadence (Fig. 11.9). Early data regarding the medium-term patient reported outcomes following CPKA appear to show an advantage over widely pub-lished literature values for TKA (Fig. 11.10).

Summary

CPKA is a conservative alternative to TKA with an increasing body of evidence to support its use [33]. It may be appropriate for young, high-demand patients looking for excellent post-operative function, despite a potentially higher revision rate, though the exact figures are unknown. Further, it may be a safer alternative for high-risk patients facing revision of a PKA to TKA as a consequence of single native compartment failure. The conservative nature of UKA results in more active patients, who stay healthier for longer. To those with two-compartment disease, primary compartmental arthroplasty offers the potential benefits of PKA in the treatment of more widespread disease. Further, the compartmental approach to revision of PKA in the presence of single native-compartment degeneration following successful PKA presents an interesting alternative to revision to TKA.

References

1. Keyes GW, Carr AJ, Miller RK, Goodfellow JW. The radiographic classification of medial gonarthrosis. Correlation with operation methods in 200 knees. Acta Orthop Scand. 1992;63(5):497–501.
2. Stoddart JC, Dandridge O, Garner A, Cobb J, van Arkel RJ. The compartmental distribution of knee osteoarthritis—a systematic review and meta-analysis. Osteoarthr Cartil. 2020;29(4).445–55. Epub 2020/11/27.
3. Ledingham J, Regan M, Jones A, Doherty M. Radiographic patterns and associations of osteoarthritis of the knee in patients referred to hospital. Ann Rheum Dis. 1993;52(7):520–6. Epub 1993/07/01.
4. Johnson AJ, Howell SM, Costa CR, Mont MA. The ACL in the arthritic knee: how often is it present and can preoperative tests predict its presence? Clin Orthop Relat Res. 2013;471(1):181–8.
5. Scott CEH, Powell-Bowns MFR, MacDonald DJ, Simpson PM, Wade FA. Revision of unicompartmental to total knee arthroplasty: does the unicompartmental implant (metal-backed vs all-polyethylene) impact the total knee arthroplasty? J Arthroplast. 2018;33(7):2203–9. Epub 2018/03/12.
6. Duthon VB, Barea C, Abrassart S, Fasel JH, Fritschy D, Menetrey J. Anatomy of the anterior cruciate ligament. Knee Surg Sports Traumatol Arthrosc. 2006;14(3):204–13. Epub 2005/10/20.
7. Baumann F. Bicruciate-retaining total knee arthroplasty compared to cruciate-sacrificing TKA: what are the advantages and disadvantages? Expert Rev Med Devices. 2018;15(9):615–7. Epub 2018/08/23.
8. Bourne RB, Chesworth BM, Davis AM, Mahomed NN, Charron KD. Patient satisfaction after total knee arthroplasty: who is satisfied and who is not? Clin Orthop Relat Res. 2010;468(1):57–63. Epub 2009/10/22.
9. Liddle AD, Judge A, Pandit H, Murray DW. Adverse outcomes after total and unicompartmental knee replacement in 101,330 matched patients: a study of data from the National Joint Registry for England and Wales. Lancet (London, England). 2014;384(9952):1437–45. Epub 2014/07/12.
10. Cobb J. Osteoarthritis of the knee. Precise diagnosis and treatment. BMJ. 2009;339:b3747. Epub 2009/09/16.
11. Garner A, van Arkel RJ, Cobb J. Classification of combined partial knee arthroplasty. Bone Joint J. 2019;101-B(8):922–8.
12. Confalonieri N, Manzotti A, Cerveri P, De Momi E. Bi-unicompartmental versus total knee arthroplasty: a matched paired study with early clinical results. Arch Orthop Trauma Surg. 2009;129(9):1157–63. Epub 2008/08/13.
13. Biazzo A, Silvestrini F, Manzotti A, Confalonieri N. Bicompartmental (uni plus patellofemoral) versus total knee arthroplasty: a match-paired study. Musculoskelet Surg. 2018;103(1):63–8. Epub 2018/04/15.
14. Kamath AF, Levack A, John T, Thomas BS, Lonner JH. Minimum two-year outcomes of modular bicompartmental knee arthroplasty. J Arthroplast. 2014;29(1):75–9.
15. Toliopoulos P, LeBlanc MA, Hutt J, Lavigne M, Desmeules F, Vendittoli PA. Anatomic versus mechanically aligned Total knee arthroplasty for unicompartmental knee arthroplasty revision. Open Orthop J. 2016;10:357–63. Epub 2016/08/27.
16. Beard DJ, Davies LJ, Cook JA, MacLennan G, Price A, Kent S, et al. The clinical and cost-effectiveness of total versus partial knee replacement in patients with medial compartment osteoarthritis (TOPKAT): 5-year outcomes of a randomised controlled trial. Lancet. 2019;394(10200):746–56. Epub 2019/07/17.
17. Neogi T, Felson D, Niu J, Nevitt M, Lewis CE, Aliabadi P, et al. Association between radiographic features of knee osteoarthritis and pain: results from two cohort studies. BMJ. 2009;339:b2844. Epub 2009/08/25.
18. Felson DT, Nevitt MC, Yang M, Clancy M, Niu J, Torner JC, et al. A new approach yields high rates of radiographic progression in knee osteoarthritis. J Rheumatol. 2008;35(10):2047–54. Epub 2008/09/17.
19. Romagnoli S, Marullo M, Massaro M, Rustemi E, D'Amario F, Corbella M. Bi-unicompartmental and combined uni plus patellofemoral replacement: indications and surgical technique. Joints. 2015;3(1):42–8. Epub 2015/07/08.

20. Pandit H, Jenkins C, Gill HS, Barker K, Dodd CA, Murray DW. Minimally invasive Oxford phase 3 unicompartmental knee replacement: results of 1000 cases. J Bone Joint Surg. 2011;93(2):198–204. Epub 2011/02/02.

21. Goodfellow J, O'Connor J, Pandit H, Dodd CA, Murray D. Unicompartmental arthroplasty with the Oxford knee. 2nd ed. Goodfellow Publishers Limited; 2016. p. 288.

22. Price AJ, Svard U. A second decade lifetable survival analysis of the Oxford unicompartmental knee arthroplasty. Clin Orthop Relat Res. 2011;469(1):174–9. Epub 2010/08/14.

23. Altuntas AO, Alsop H, Cobb JP. Early results of a domed tibia, mobile bearing lateral unicompartmental knee arthroplasty from an independent Centre. Knee. 2013;20(6):466–70. Epub 2013/01/01.

24. Pandit H, Mancuso F, Jenkins C, Jackson WFM, Price AJ, Dodd CAF, et al. Lateral unicompartmental knee replacement for the treatment of arthritis progression after medial unicompartmental replacement. Knee Surg Sports Traumatol Arthrosc. 2017;25(3):669–74. Epub 2016/03/28.

25. Joint replacement (primary): hip, knee and shoulder NICE guideline [NG157]. 2020.

26. Thienpont E, Price A. Bicompartmental knee arthroplasty of the patellofemoral and medial compartments. Knee Surg Sports Traumatol Arthrosc. 2013;21(11):2523–31. Epub 2012/11/28.

27. Palumbo BT, Henderson ER, Edwards PK, Burris RB, Gutierrez S, Raterman SJ. Initial experience of the journey-deuce bicompartmental knee prosthesis: a review of 36 cases. J Arthroplast. 2011;26(6 Suppl):40–5. Epub 2011/05/10.

28. Garner A, Dandridge O, Amis AA, Cobb JP, Arkel RJ. The extensor efficiency of unicompartmental, bicompartmental, and total knee arthroplasty. Bone Joint Res. 2021;10(1):1–9.

29. Wang H, Dugan E, Frame J, Rolston L. Gait analysis after bi-compartmental knee replacement. Clin Biomech (Bristol, Avon). 2009;24(9):751–4. Epub 2009/08/22.

30. Argenson JN, Parratte S, Bertani A, Aubaniac JM, Lombardi AV Jr, Berend KR, et al. The new arthritic patient and arthroplasty treatment options. J Bone Joint Surg Am. 2009;91(Suppl 5):43–8. Epub 2009/08/08.

31. Leffler J, Scheys L, Plante-Bordeneuve T, Callewaert B, Labey L, Bellemans J, et al. Joint kinematics following bi-compartmental knee replacement during daily life motor tasks. Gait Posture. 2012;36(3):454–60. Epub 2012/07/04.

32. Parratte S, Ollivier M, Opsomer G, Lunebourg A, Argenson JN, Thienpont E. Is knee function better with contemporary modular bicompartmental arthroplasty compared to total knee arthroplasty? Short-term outcomes of a prospective matched study including 68 cases. Orthop Traumatol Surg Res. 2015;101(5):547–52. Epub 2015/06/07.

33. Heyse TJ, Khefacha A, Cartier P. UKA in combination with PFR at average 12-year follow-up. Arch Orthop Trauma Surg. 2010;130(10):1227–30. Epub 2009/11/06.

34. Cartier P, Sanouiller JL, Grelsamer R. Patellofemoral arthroplasty. 2-12-year follow-up study. J Arthroplast. 1990;5(1):49–55. Epub 1990/03/01.

35. Tan SM, Dutton AQ, Bea KC, Kumar VP. Bicompartmental versus total knee arthroplasty for medial and patellofemoral osteoarthritis. J Orthop Surg (Hong Kong). 2013;21(3):281–4. Epub 2013/12/25.

36. Rolston L, Bresch J, Engh G, Franz A, Kreuzer S, Nadaud M, et al. Bicompartmental knee arthroplasty: a bone-sparing, ligament-sparing, and minimally invasive alternative for active patients. Orthopedics. 2007;30(8 Suppl):70–3. Epub 2007/09/11.

37. Engh GA. A bi-compartmental solution: what the deuce? Orthopedics. 2007;30(9):770–1. Epub 2007/09/29.

38. Steinert AF, Beckmann J, Holzapfel BM, Rudert M, Arnholdt J. Bicompartmental individualized knee replacement: use of patient-specific implants and instruments (iDuo). Operat Orthopad Traumatol. 2017;29(1):51–8. Epub 2017/02/02.

39. Beckmann J, Steinert AF, Huber B, Rudert M, Köck FX, Buhs M, et al. Customised bi-compartmental knee arthroplasty shows encouraging 3-year results: findings of a prospective, multicenter study. Knee Surg Sports Traumatol Arthrosc. 2020;28(6):1742–9. Epub 2019/06/30.

40. Argenson JN, Chevrol-Benkeddache Y, Aubaniac JM. Modern unicompartmental knee arthroplasty with cement: a three to ten-year follow-up study. J Bone Joint Surg Am. 2002;84-a(12):2235–9. Epub 2002/12/11.

41. Wunschel M, Lo J, Dilger T, Wulker N, Muller O. Influence of bi- and tri-compartmental knee arthroplasty on the kinematics of the knee joint. BMC Musculoskelet Disord. 2011;12:29. Epub 2011/01/29.

42. Zanasi S. Innovations in total knee replacement: new trends in operative treatment and changes in peri-operative management. Eur Orthop Traumatol. 2011;2(1–2):21–31. Epub 2011/09/06.

43. Banger MS, Johnston WD, Razii N, Doonan J, Rowe PJ, Jones BG, et al. Robotic arm-assisted bi-unicompartmental knee arthroplasty maintains natural knee joint anatomy compared with total knee arthroplasty: a prospective randomized controlled trial. Bone Joint J. 2020;102-B(11):1511–8.

44. Parratte S, Pauly V, Aubaniac JM, Argenson JN. Survival of bicompartmental knee arthroplasty at 5 to 23 years. Clin Orthop Relat Res. 2010;468(1):64–72. Epub 2009/08/12.

45. Lonner JH. Modular bicompartmental knee arthroplasty with robotic arm assistance. Am J Orthop

(Belle Mead NJ). 2009;38(2 Suppl):28–31. Epub 2009/04/08.

46. Pradhan NR, Gambhir A, Porter ML. Survivorship analysis of 3234 primary knee arthroplasties implanted over a 26-year period: a study of eight different implant designs. Knee. 2006;13(1):7–11. Epub 2005/08/30.

47. Shah SM, Dutton AQ, Liang S, Dasde S. Bicompartmental versus total knee arthroplasty for medio-patellofemoral osteoarthritis: a comparison of early clinical and functional outcomes. J Knee Surg. 2013;26(6):411–6. Epub 2013/04/12.

48. Pritchett JW. Anterior cruciate-retaining total knee arthroplasty. J Arthroplast. 1996;11(2):194–7. Epub 1996/02/01.

49. Andriacchi TP, Galante JO, Fermier RW. The influence of total knee-replacement design on walking and stair-climbing. J Bone Joint Surg Am. 1982;64(9):1328–35. Epub 1982/12/01.

50. Wiik AV, Manning V, Strachan RK, Amis AA, Cobb JP. Unicompartmental knee arthroplasty enables near normal gait at higher speeds, unlike total knee arthroplasty. J Arthroplast. 2013;28(9 Suppl):176–8.

51. Jones GG, Kotti M, Wiik AV, Collins R, Brevadt MJ, Strachan RK, et al. Gait comparison of unicompartmental and total knee arthroplasties with healthy controls. Bone Joint J. 2016;98-B(10 Supple B):16–21.

Osteotomies for Knee Arthritis

Wiemi A. Douoguih, Blake M. Bodendorfer, and Henry Tout Shu

Introduction

Symptomatic unicompartmental osteoarthritis (UCOA) is a substantial orthopaedic problem representing one-third of patients with knee osteoarthritis (OA) [1]. Total knee arthroplasty is the treatment of choice for multicompartmental OA in older, less active patients, but less invasive treatment strategies may be beneficial for active patients with UCOA under the age of 60. One less invasive option, osteotomy about the knee, aims to transfer stress away from the involved compartment to healthy areas of the knee unaffected by disease, thereby decreasing pain and increasing function. Favorable results have been reported in biomechanical and clinical studies for isolated lateral tibiofemoral OA, isolated medial tibiofemoral OA, and patellofemoral OA [2–15]. Osteotomies preserve intra-articular structures and do not involve intra-articular implants, which allows for unrestricted loading and activity postoperatively. Osteotomies thus can provide functional advantages over arthroplasty options for younger, more active populations [16].

Proximal Tibial Osteotomy for Medial Compartment OA

Background

High tibial osteotomy (HTO) for the treatment of varus medial compartment knee OA was first described by Jackson and Waugh in 1960 [17]. Coventry popularized the lateral closing wedge HTO (LCWHTO) in 1965, [18] and in 1987 Hernigou described a medial opening wedge HTO [19] (MOWHTO). Since then, numerous studies have shown the benefits of these techniques in improving pain and function for patients with varus medial compartment arthrosis of the knee [20–24]. Resurgent interest in the use of HTO as an alternative to total knee arthroplasty (TKA) has been driven largely by inferior results demonstrated in TKA patients under the age of 60 [25] and those engaged in higher demand physical activities [26, 27]. Improved surgical technology and better understanding of indications for HTO have also supported increased use of HTO. One recent study showed a 5-year

W. A. Douoguih (✉)
MedStar Georgetown University Medical Center, Washington, DC, USA

B. M. Bodendorfer
Midwest Orthopaedics at Rush, Chicago, IL, USA

MedStar Georgetown University Hospital, Washington, DC, USA

Omaha Sports Doctor, Omaha Sports Doctor, NE, Omaha, USA
e-mail: Blake.bodendorfer@rushortho.com

H. T. Shu
Department of Orthopaedic Surgery, The Johns Hopkins University, School of Medicine, Baltimore, MD, USA
e-mail: hshu5@jhmi.edu

increase in HTO, unicompartmental knee arthroplasty (UKA), and TKA of 210%, 138% and 18%, respectively, with the largest increase in patients 55–64 years old undergoing HTO or unicompartmental knee arthroplasty (UKA) [28].

Patients undergoing HTO for medial arthritis have the option of opening wedge, closing wedge, or dome osteotomy. Although HTO has been shown to be a durable and highly successful procedure for younger, highly active patients with isolated medial compartment arthrosis, there is no consensus in comparison studies as to whether MOWHTO or LCWHTO is better [29, 30]. Overall, 10-year survival rates for HTO to treat UCOA varus malalignment have been reported to range between 65 and 95% [4, 10, 12–14].

Two Surgical Considerations

The ideal candidate for HTO is an active patient with medial UCOA with isolated medial symptoms, deformity <15° varus, >90° ROM, and <20° flexion contracture, and age <60 years. We consider the procedure for patients up to age 65 who want to maintain an active lifestyle if their bone quality is satisfactory and they are motivated. A trial with a valgus unloader is useful to assess the response, particularly in a patient who also has patellofemoral disease. If the valgus unloader eliminates pain and improves function, the patient is likely to have a successful result with HTO regardless of whether he or she has patellofemoral disease [31]. We recommend UKA if the patient has minimal mechanical axis deformity but persistent medial pain while wearing the brace.

Understanding the natural history of knee OA is critical to optimize the patient's outcome. Varus malalignment in patients with medial compartment OA has been shown to cause a fourfold increase in the risk of progression of disease within 18 months of diagnosis (Fig. 12.1). Additionally, the severity of varus significantly correlates with progression, as does an absolute

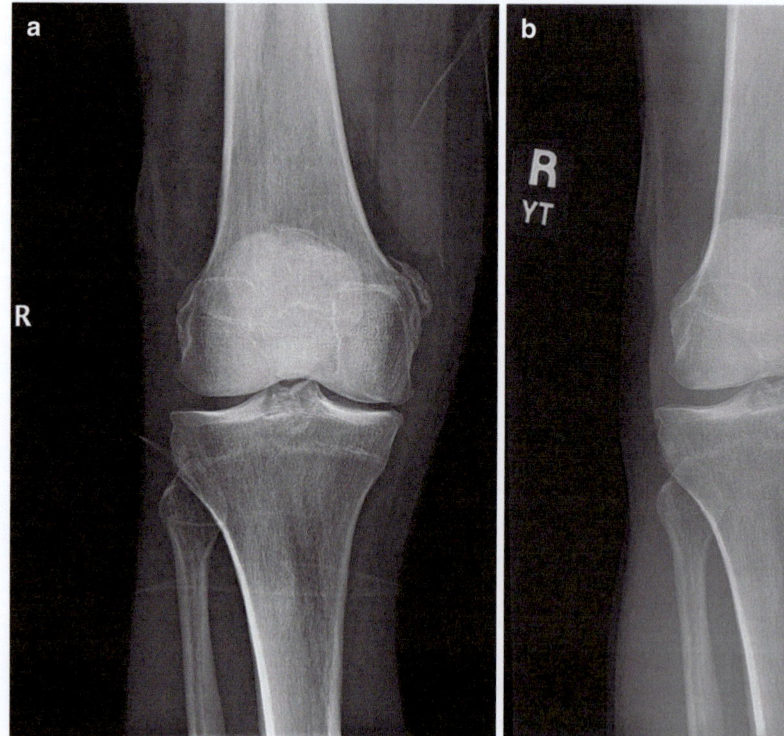

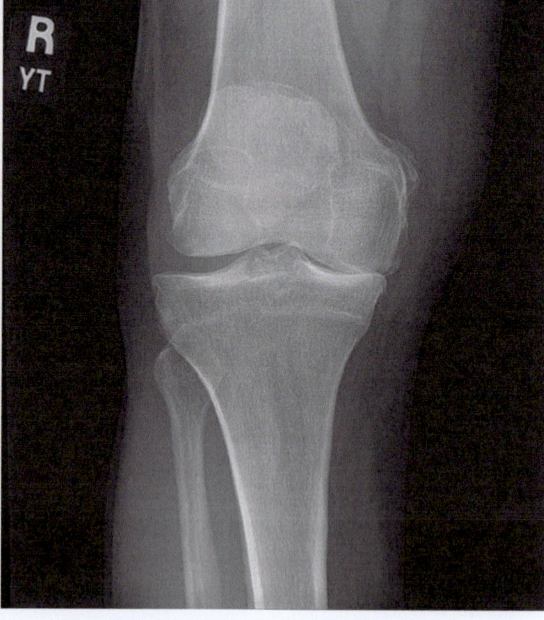

Fig. 12.1 Standing anteroposterior radiographs of 55-year-old patient with UCOA who developed increasing knee pain. The patient had substantial improvement with the use of a valgus unloader brace in the 3 months prior to visit in April 2019. HTO was recommended, but the patient was unable to undergo surgery because of insurance restrictions. (**a**) Right knee in April 2019 shows moderate medial compartment joint space narrowing. (**b**) Same knee in July 2019 shows progression of arthrosis with complete loss of the medial joint space

varus mechanical axis of >5° [32]. Because of the risk of progression and poorer results with higher grade arthrosis, we consider HTO after a 6-week trial with a valgus unloader and physical therapy. For lower grade arthrosis and lesser mechanical axis deformity, a longer nonoperative approach is warranted including physical therapy, valgus unloader bracing, NSAIDS, and injections for up to 6 months. Although biomechanical and computer-simulated data have helped inform clinicians about the effects of different angular corrections on joint kinematics [2, 15], the degree of angular correction needed to unload the joint to obtain optimal clinical results remains a controversial topic. Coventry et al. [33] found that when valgus angulation was 8° or more or if the patient's weight was less than 1.32 times the ideal weight, the probability of survival at 5 years was at least 90% and at 10 years was at least 65%, compared to 38% and 19%, respectively, when valgus angulation was less than 8° or if patient weight was more than 1.32 times the ideal weight. Those investigators concluded that there is considerable risk of failure if the alignment is not overcorrected to at least 8° of valgus angulation and if the patient is substantially overweight. These findings were in contrast to Hernigou et al. [19] who found that overcorrection >6° portended a poorer result. The best results were obtained in 20 knees with hip-knee-ankle angle of 183–186°. All five knees with an angle of more than 186° had progressive degenerative changes in the lateral compartment. Deterioration occurred at an average of 7 years after the osteotomy and was always associated with recurrence of pain.

Preoperative Planning

All patients who present with medial knee pain should undergo thorough history and physical examination to assess patient activity level, comorbidities, and character, location, and duration of pain. Patients typically present with isolated medial joint line pain and increased pain with high-impact activity. On physical exam, any limited ROM and ligamentous instability should be assessed because both can be contraindications for HTO. Additionally, body mass index (BMI), smoking status, and rheumatological issues need to be considered. Care should be taken to rule out any signs of infection or neoplastic disease.

Patients with signs and symptoms of UCOA undergo standing anteroposterior (AP), flexed lateral, sunrise, and posteroanterior (PA) 45° standing X-rays. For patients who have been deemed appropriate candidates for HTO, full-length bilateral standing lower extremity films are obtained to calculate the mechanical axis and assess extent of malalignment. The intersection of the biomechanical axis of the femur and tibia are drawn to the desired point of correction on the tibial plateau (Fig. 12.2a). Alternatively, femoral and tibial malalignment can be identified by calculating the lateral distal femoral angle (LDTA) and medial proximal tibial angle (MPTA) as described by Paley et al. [34]. We seek to restore a neutral mechanical axis (50%) in patients with Kellgren Lawrence grades II and III degenerative changes and 3–5° of overcorrection (62% lateral) in patients with grade IV degenerative changes. Avoidance of excessive overcorrection is critical because overcorrection has been shown to adversely affect joint kinematics and may lead to lateral tibiofemoral joint degeneration [15, 32].

Surgery

Although both closing and opening wedge HTO techniques have shown comparable long-term results, [4, 10, 12] opening wedge techniques allow for more flexibility in adjusting tibial slope and coronal plane angular correction. Modern plate constructs provide excellent fixation to mitigate issues around loss of correction and hardware failure. The medial approach virtually eliminates problems associated with the lateral approach particularly with regards to risk of peroneal nerve injury [35]. For these reasons, we prefer an opening wedge technique.

Medial Opening Wedge Technique

A diagnostic arthroscopy is performed first to address loose bodies, degenerative meniscal tears, and any inflamed synovium. Arthroscopy also serves to confirm the extent of the medial

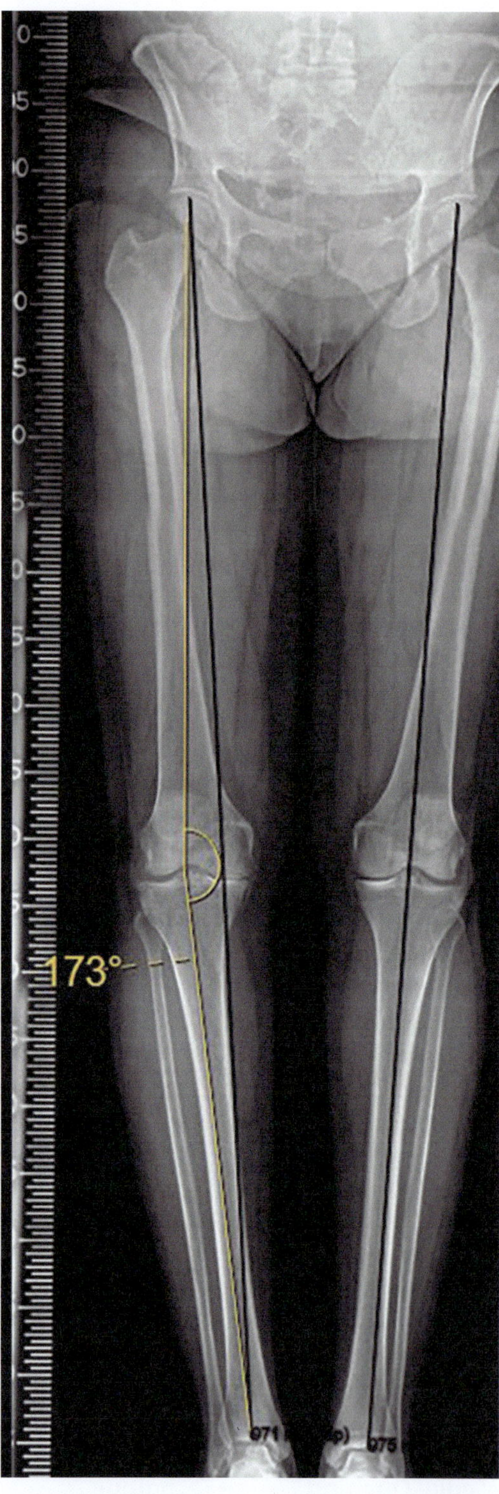

Fig. 12.2 Image shows 7° varus mechanical axis in standing full length weightbearing alignment radiograph

compartment disease and any unexpected lateral tibiofemoral degenerative changes that could confound results. Once arthroscopy is complete, a longitudinal incision is made at the midpoint between the tibial tubercle and the posteromedial border of the tibia. The incision extends from the medial joint line distally for a length of 5–10 cm, depending on the type of plating system used. The tibial tubercle is identified, and two guide pins are placed under fluoroscopic guidance from the medial cortex at the level of the tibial tubercle, 3.5 cm distal to the joint line, directed proximally and laterally towards the fibular head. These pins are drilled to within 1 cm of the lateral tibial cortex as a guide to assist in leaving the lateral cortex intact. The tibial tubercle is identified and a retro-tubercular cut is made in the coronal plane. This biplanar cut separates the extensor mechanism from the body of the horizontal HTO and has been shown to increase stability of the HTO construct [36]. A retractor is placed deep into the medial collateral ligament (MCL) around the posteromedial tibia to protect the popliteal vessels. The osteotomy is then made with a saw over the guide pins anteriorly and centrally. The posterior cortex is cut with an osteotome, taking care not to penetrate too far posteriorly. Once the osteotomy is complete, wedges are used anteriorly and posteriorly to open the osteotomy site to the desired angular correction. A medial locking plate is then placed and secured with screws proximal and distal to the osteotomy site (Fig. 12.3).

Lateral Closing Wedge Technique

A longitudinal incision or transverse incision can be made. Careful dissection down to the fibular head is performed, identifying, and protecting the peroneal nerve. The fibular head is then resected through the same incision as is used for the osteotomy. This gives access to the lateral tibial plateau, removes the tibiofibular joint and ligaments, and allows for reattachment of the biceps tendon and fibular collateral ligament to the neck of the fibula under physiologi-

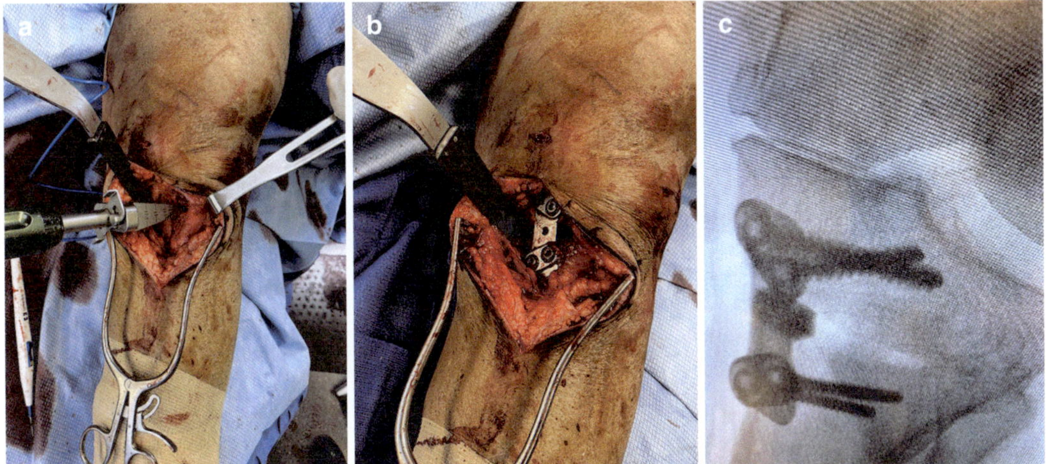

Fig. 12.3 (**a**) Photograph shows wedges inserted to gradually open osteotomy site to desired angular correction in preparation for placement of plate. (**b**) Photograph shows 7.5°, four-hole locking plate; fixation maintaining desired correction. (**c**) Intra-operative fluoroscopic image confirming proper plate placement and intact lateral tibial hinge

cal tension. In this way, the peroneal nerve is visualized and injury to it can be avoided. Removing the fibular head also allows for clear visualization of the osteotomy site and avoids impact on the proximal tibial fragment as the wedge is closed.

The osteotomy passes through the tibia between the joint and the tibial tubercle. A proximal guide pin is placed from lateral to medial, parallel to the tibial plateau and 1.5–2 cm distal to the joint line. This proximal pin is drilled to within 1 cm of the medial tibial cortex. A second guide pin is placed distally, angled towards the medial tip of the proximal pin. Placement of the distal pin is based on preoperative calculations to achieve the desired correction.

Historically, the size of the wedge to be removed would be measured by transposing the measurements from a print radiograph to the tibia and by accurately measuring the base of the wedge. Electronical radiographs have measuring tools that allow for easy calculation of requisite angular correction based on standing weightbearing full-length lower extremity films. In general, a 1-mm wedge correlates with 1° of correction. Fixation is achieved with two staples or a plate and screws.

Current Concepts and Techniques

Although most studies show excellent pain relief and return of function for properly selected patients undergoing lateral closing wedge techniques, these techniques have been associated with an incidence of peroneal nerve injury and concerns about lateral ligamentous instability and damage to musculotendinous structures about the knee [37]. A novel LCWHTO technique [38, 39] preserves the lateral ligamentous complex by selectively removing only the anterior aspect of the fibular head. Resection of the anterior aspect of the proximal part of the fibular head allows for excellent exposure of the proximal tibia. A calibrated slotted wedge resection guide is used to perform the osteotomy proximal to the tuberosity under fluoroscopic guidance to achieve the desired correction. Fixation of the osteotomy site is achieved with two-step staples (Fig. 12.4).

Because overcorrection has been associated with inferior outcomes, it is useful to understand measures that could help mitigate this risk. A concept that has received recent attention is the joint line convergence angle (JLCA), defined as the angle between the tangent to the subchondral

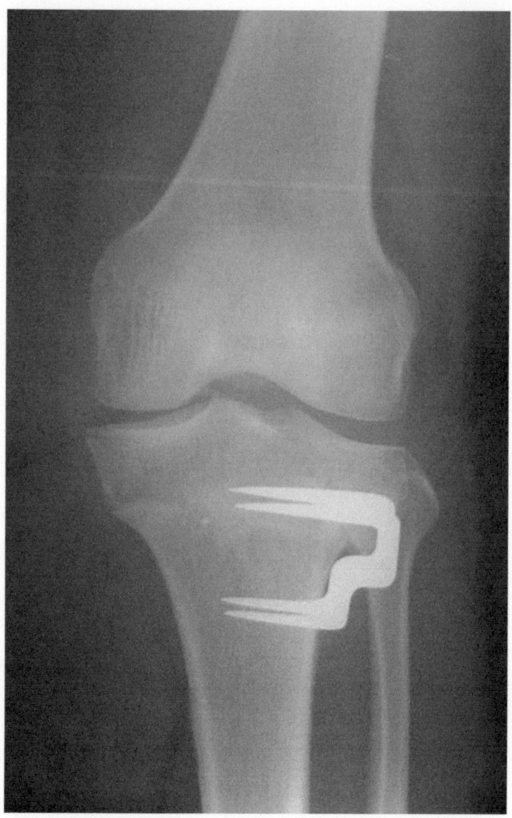

Fig. 12.4 Photograph shows lateral closing wedge osteotomy fixed with two-step staples. (Reprinted with permission from Brouwer et al. Osteotomy for medial compartment arthritis of the knee using a closing wedge or an opening wedge controlled by a Puddu plate: a one-year randomized, controlled study. 2006;88-B:1454–1459)

plates of the femoral condyle and the tibial plateau. This angle has been suggested as a tool to identify the contribution of ligamentous laxity to malalignment [40]. Not taking the JLCA into account may lead to inadvertent overcorrection. JLCA >4° has been correlated with a significantly higher risk of overcorrection [40].

Postoperative Rehabilitation

We favor an early weightbearing (WB) protocol. In a prospective randomized controlled trial of MOWHTO, Schroter et al. found better results with restricted WB for 11 days versus 6 weeks, demonstrating superior Lysholm and Lequesne outcome scales postoperatively at 6 months [41].

The first 2 weeks we have the patient toe-touch weightbear and then weightbear as tolerated and wean crutches over the next 4 weeks. Physical therapy begins at 2 weeks, and a strengthening program begins at 6 weeks if the patient is pain free. Treadmill jogging can be started at 3 months if desired with return to heavy activity between 6 and 9 months.

Distal Femoral Osteotomy

Background

Varus-producing distal femoral osteotomy (DFO) has been used as an effective treatment for treatment of lateral compartment osteoarthrosis with valgus malalignment. In 1973, Coventry [31] reported that distal femoral varus osteotomy (DFO) was superior to HTO if the valgus deformity exceeded 12° and the joint line was inclined greater than 10°. Other early studies corroborated these results [42, 43]. Valgus malalignment with attendant lateral UCOA is less common than varus medial compartment disease [44]. As a result, there is a relative paucity of literature surrounding osteotomies for the treatment of lateral compartment UCOA with valgus malalignment. These limitations notwithstanding, DFO has shown consistently good results for the treatment of lateral UCOA with valgus malalignment. A recent systematic review of 20 studies comparing LOWDFO versus MCWDFO reported no differences in outcomes between the two techniques [5]. Overall, studies have reported between 71 and 83% good or excellent outcomes for DFO [11, 22, 42], with 10-year survival rates ranging between 64 and 87% [3, 8, 9, 11]. It should be noted that outcomes after conversion from DFO to TKA are favorable, but tend to be worse than primary TKA, [8] likely in part because DFO may make subsequent TKA technically more demanding. DFO can be combined with other joint preservation procedures such as osteoarticular allograft and meniscal transplant [45, 46]. As with HTO, complications have been reported with DFO for valgus malalignment with UCOA including hardware-related pain and nonunion [47].

Surgical Considerations

In patients with UCOA and valgus malalignment, there is a nearly fivefold increase in the odds of lateral OA progression [32]. Severity of valgus has also been shown to correlate with greater subsequent lateral joint space loss. Alignment of more than 5° valgus is associated with significantly greater functional deterioration during the 18 months after diagnosis compared with alignment of 5° or less, after adjusting for age, sex, body mass index, and pain [32]. For patients who have previously sustained lateral meniscal injuries or who have undergone partial or subtotal lateral meniscectomies, the weightbearing load to the lateral compartment can change substantially, shifting the load-bearing and shock absorption to the chondral surface. Unfortunately, this can lead to progressive valgus and rapid articular cartilage degeneration [32]. An additional consideration that can be overlooked is the effect of genu valgum on patellofemoral tracking. DFO can reduce the Q angle and medialize the tibial tubercle, unloading the patellofemoral compartment laterally. This may improve patellar tracking, anterior knee pain, and instability in select patients [11, 48].

DFO is indicated in physiologically young and active patients with unicompartmental moderate to severe (Kellgren-Lawrence grades III or IV) lateral knee OA with valgus malalignment that have not responded to management with medication, injections, physical therapy, and activity modification [43, 49]. In patients with >5° valgus deformity associated with lateral compartment OA, early surgical intervention may be warranted to avoid deformity and arthritis progression. In contrast to the inherent activity restrictions after unicompartmental knee arthroplasty, DFO can allow patients to return to unrestricted high-impact activities.

Absolute contraindications of DFO include symptomatic medial or tricompartmental OA, medial meniscus deficiency, severe valgus deformity with tibial subluxation >1 cm, knee flexion contracture >15°, and gross knee instability [49]. There is no optimal cut-off for degrees of valgus deformity, but DFO may be contraindicated in patients with greater than 20° of valgus [50].

Nonetheless, successful outcomes have been reported with DFO in patients with up to 27° of valgus [11]. Relative contraindications include severe patellofemoral OA, high BMI, rheumatologic OA, age >65 years, severe lateral compartment bone loss, and history of septic knee arthritis [49].

Preoperative Assessment and Planning

Evaluation of a patient with symptomatic valgus deformity begins with a thorough history and physical exam and radiologic examination. Appropriate candidates for DFO exhibit isolated lateral joint line pain with activity. Considerations regarding patient size and comorbidities are the same as for patients with isolated medial-sided disease. Patients who have improved pain and function with a lateral unloading brace may benefit from a DFO because the brace simulates the effect of a DFO. Because progression of lateral UCOA has been shown to occur in the presence of significant valgus deformity [32], DFO should be considered as an early intervention in physiologically young, active patients who respond to bracing.

Once a patient decides to proceed with DFO, preoperative planning begins with quantification of the degree of valgus deformity. AP full-length standing radiographs are obtained where the mechanical axis of the lower extremity is determined by drawing a line from the center of the femoral head to the tibial plafond. Valgus deformity is present if the mechanical axis passes through the lateral compartment of the knee. The normal mechanical axis deviation (MAD) is typically 10 mm medial to the center of the knee joint, which is in the region of the medial tibial spine [34]. As with varus unicompartmental disease, femoral and tibial malalignment can be further identified by calculating the LDTA and medial proximal tibial angle (MPTA). The degree of correction (alpha or a) is then identified by calculating the angle between the femoral mechanical axis and the tibial mechanical axis (Fig. 12.5). The femoral mechanical axis is identified by drawing a

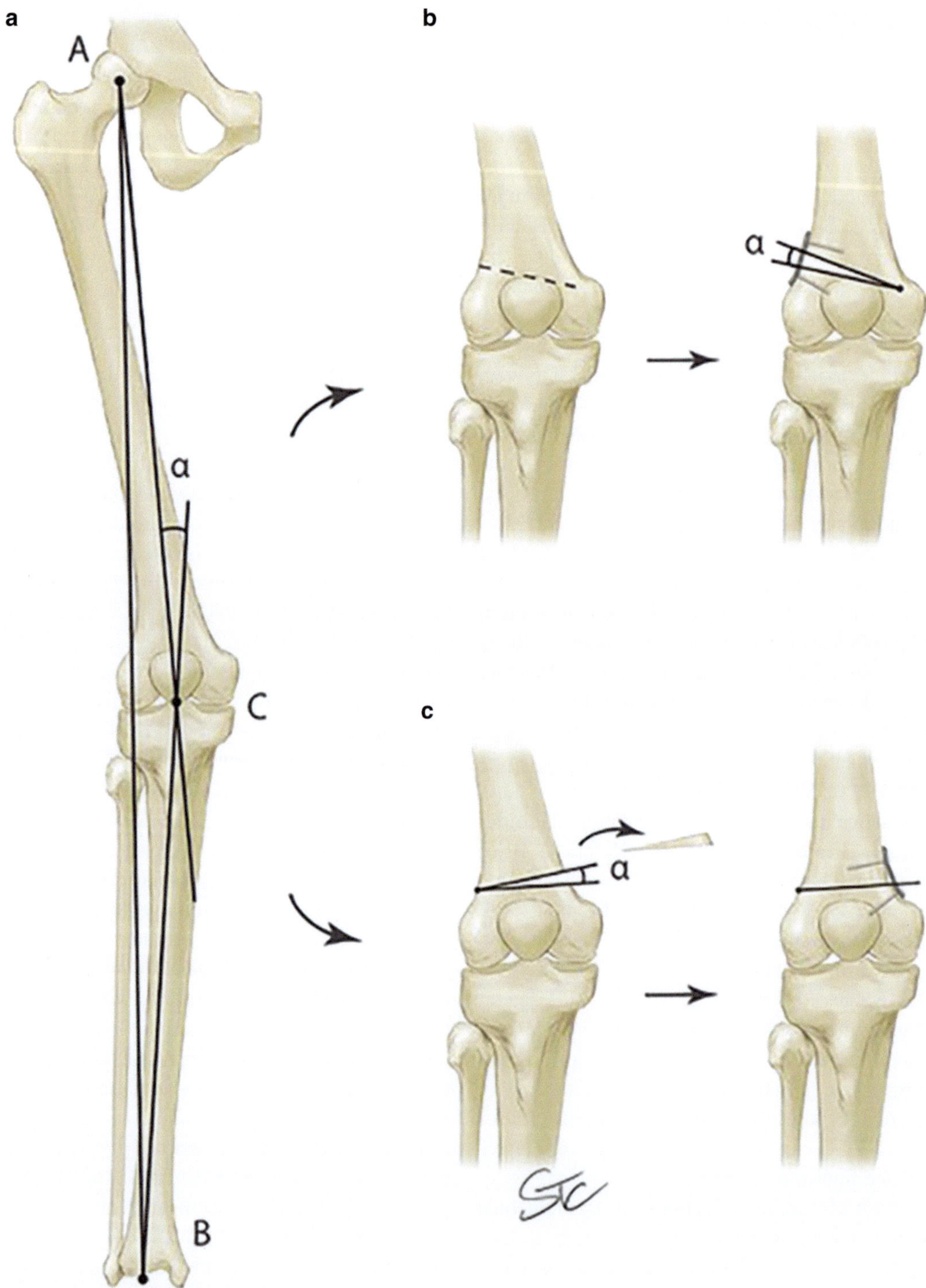

Fig. 12.5 Illustration shows preoperative planning for distal femoral varus osteotomy. The mechanical axis is determined by drawing a line from the center of the femoral head to the center of the ankle joint (line A–B). The point of correction (C) is chosen and marked on the tibial plateau. Two additional lines are drawn, one extending from the center of the femoral head through the desired point of correction on the tibial plateau and one extending from the center of the talus through the point of correction. The angle of correction (α) is the angle at which these two lines intersect. This angle may be used for the lateral opening wedge (**b**) or medial closing wedge (**c**) distal femoral osteotomy. (Reprinted with permission of Missouri Orthopaedic Institute, University of Missouri Health Care, Columbia, MO)

line from the center of the femoral head to center of the knee. The tibial mechanical axis is identified by drawing a line from the tibial plafond to the center of the knee. In treating UC lateral knee OA, correction is typically performed 50–62.5% of the way into the medial compartment.

Preoperative magnetic resonance imaging (MRI) may be useful in identifying ligamentous, meniscal, or chondral defects, especially in the medial and patellofemoral compartments. However, arthroscopy remains the gold standard in evaluating chondral and meniscal lesions. Recently, Salem et al. have demonstrated the value in staging arthroscopy prior to chondral restoration procedures and meniscal allograft transplant, with a change in treatment made in 47% of cases in which staging arthroscopy was utilized [51]. Thus, staging arthroscopy prior to DFO may be useful in identifying any necessary concomitant chondral restoration procedures and meniscal procedures that should be performed. In patients with previous knee arthroscopic surgeries, previous arthroscopic images should be reviewed to rule out medial and patellofemoral OA changes, meniscal deficiency, and identify progression of knee OA.

Current Concepts and Techniques

With the advent of modern implants and bone grafting, lateral opening wedge DFO has become the preferred technique versus DFO with a medial closing wedge. Lateral opening wedge DFO provides some key advantages, including a more straightforward surgical approach, more predictable and accurate deformity correction, and a single cut osteotomy [49]. Despite these advantages, there are some important potential complications associated with lateral opening wedge DFO. Painful hardware is a common problem postoperatively. As a result, when obtaining informed consent, the surgeon should note that plate removal may be required in as many as 47–86% of patients undergoing DFO after healing has occurred [52]. Additionally, although nonunion has been reported in patients undergoing lateral opening wedge DFO, when bone graft is utilized lateral opening wedge DFO has demonstrated to similar nonunion rates to medial closing wedge DFO techniques [5]. Medial closing wedge DFO may still be used in cases with a limb length discrepancy requiring shortening of the operative limb, in cases where the angle of correction exceeds 17.5°, and in cases where there are risk factors for delayed bone healing or nonunion [49].

Historically, medial closing wedge DFO has been performed with 90° angled blade plates or staples. Current fixation techniques for medial closing wedge DFO involve stainless steel or titanium pre-contoured locking plates. Similarly, lateral opening wedge DFO is typically performed with a lateral locking plate, such as the TomoFix (DePuy Synthes, Warsaw, IN, USA) or ContourLock (Arthrex, Naples, FL, USA) plates. Recently, the use of carbon-fiber-reinforced (CFR) polymer locking plates have been reported in DFO due to their radiolucency and higher load to failure than titanium implants [53]. However, CFR polymer plates were associated with significantly greater time to union, osteotomy displacement, and overall complication rate when compared to a titanium plate [53]. Recently, attention has been turned to the potential of DFO in treating patella instability associated with genu valgum because DFO medializes the tibial tubercle with respect to the trochlear groove [48, 54, 55]. Thus, DFO may be especially beneficial in patients with lateral OA and patellofemoral syndrome.

Medial Closing Wedge DFO Technique

The patient is positioned supine with the knee in full extension. A longitudinal anteromedial incision is made from 8–10 cm above the patella down to the middle third of the patella. Dissection is carried down through the vastus medialis oblique (VMO) fascia and through the intermuscular septum. To optimize exposure for plate positioning, the proximal third of the medial patellofemoral ligament can be incised at the insertion of the VMO to mobilize it from the patella. A blunt, curved rasp is used to elevate the posterior soft tissues from the femoral cortex. Care should be taken to work as close to the femoral cortex as possible to prevent neurovascular injury. A wide, blunt

Hohmann retractor can then be placed behind the femoral shaft to protect the neurovasculature. Another Hohmann retractor can be used to expose the anteromedial aspect of the femur.

The osteotomy site is identified with the use of two Kirschner wires (K-wires) both proximal and distal to the osteotomy site. The first two K-wires are placed anteriorly and posteriorly to mark the distal cut of the osteotomy. Care should be taken to ensure that the K-wires are placed parallel to each other to prevent any flexion or extension deformity. The next two K-wires are then placed proximally in a similar manner to mark the proximal osteotomy site, with the distance between the two sets of K-wires equal to the desired width of the wedge. The distal osteotomy cut is performed with an oscillating saw to a depth of about 5–10 mm from the lateral cortex to ensure that the lateral hinge is intact. Once the proximal cut is made, the wedge should be easily removed. If there is any difficulty in removing the wedge, the anterior and posterior portions may not be fully cut. Carefully inspect the osteotomy site if this occurs. A Freer elevator should be used to ensure that the anterior and posterior cortices are fully cut. If not, the surgeon can complete the cut with osteotomes as needed. After the wedge is removed, the osteotomy should be gently closed by applying lateral leg pressure while stabilizing the knee joint. If there is resistance with closing the osteotomy, a Freer elevator again can be used to ensure that the anterior and posterior cortices are fully cut, and K-wires may be used to gently perforate the lateral cortex to prevent fracture while closing. Complete closure can also be assessed by fluoroscopy. Once the osteotomy is closed, the femoral plate is typically fixed with 4.5-mm unicortical locking screws. The medial patellofemoral ligament and VMO are then reattached to the patella and the soft tissue is closed in layers.

Lateral Opening Wedge DFO Technique

The patient is positioned supine with the knee in full extension. Two approaches can be used to access the distal femur. If a concomitant intrarticular procedure is performed, the lateral parapa-tellar approach can be extended proximally to access the distal femur. The extraarticular lateral DFO approach begins with a longitudinal incision of 12–15 cm about 2 cm anterior to the iliotibial band. The incision should be started distally about 2 cm distal to the lateral femoral epicondyle and should extend proximally. Dissection is carried down to the iliotibial band, which is subsequently split, and the intermuscular septum is identified. The intermuscular septum is then divided at the metaphyseal-diaphyseal junction and the vastus lateralis is elevated off the femur and retracted anteriorly. A retractor is placed posteriorly to protect the neurovasculature.

The osteotomy site is marked with two K-wires placed parallel to each other and perpendicular to the femoral shaft to avoid flexion or extension deformity. With fluoroscopic guidance, the K-wires should be started 3–4 cm superior to the lateral epicondyle and run medially and inferiorly towards the medial epicondyle, with care not to disrupt the patellofemoral articulation during guide-pin placement. An oscillating saw is then used to perform the osteotomy, with the medial cortex left intact to act as a hinge. Once the osteotomy is complete, it can be opened to the desired amount of correction with a laminar spreader, osteotomes, or specialized, calibrated wedges or spreaders. The medial cortex can be gently perforated with a drill bit or K-wire to allow for more opening to decrease the risk of fracture. Once the desired amount of correction (50–62.5% medial, width of the tibial plateau) is obtained, the osteotomy is held by a locking plate and 6.5-mm unicortical cancellous screws distally and by 4.5-mm cortical screws proximally. Bone allograft, autograft, or commercially manufactured bone graft substitutes can be used to fill the osteotomy site to aid osteogenesis and reduce the risk of nonunion, especially in cases with >10° angular correction. Fluoroscopy is used to confirm the final construct, and the soft tissue is closed in layers with care to repair the intermuscular septum.

Postoperative Care

Immediate range of motion exercises should be implemented unless concomitant procedures prevent it. Deep venous thrombosis prophylaxis should be strongly considered during the first 6 postoperative weeks. Patients are made foot flat weightbearing for the first 2 weeks after surgery with LOWDFO and weightbearing as tolerated with MCWDFO. From 2 to 6 weeks, all patients are weightbearing as tolerated with crutches in a hinged brace gradually unlocked to accommodate comfortable ROM. Low-impact and light duty activities can resume at 3 months after surgery, and high-impact activities such as sport or heavy labor work can start at approximately 6–9 months, depending on the patient's progress with return to sport criteria.

Tibial Tubercle Osteotomy

Background

The patellofemoral joint is maintained through a complex relationship between the patella soft-tissue attachments and the trochlear morphology. Trauma can directly lead to degenerative damage by acute damage to the osteochondral tissue of the patellofemoral articulation or indirectly as a result of damage to soft-tissue restraints, which can lead to repetitive microtrauma and consequent wear of the articular cartilage surfaces. Some of the greatest contact forces in the body are experienced across the patellofemoral joint, with 385 N during walking, 2400 N while ascending or descending stairs, and 6000 N while landing a jump [23].

With careful patient selection and consideration of both the nature of patellofemoral OA and the awareness of any concomitant instability, TTO generally yields excellent short-term results and pain relief [56]. Satisfactory outcomes were reported to be as high as 94% [6], with return to sport as high as 83% overall, 60% at the same level [7].

Surgical Considerations

The first-line treatment for patellofemoral arthrosis is nonoperative, including anti-inflammatories, activity modification, and therapy. Therapy should emphasize quadriceps strengthening and closed chain short-arc quadriceps exercises. Intra-articular injections may also be used for symptomatic relief. For patients that fail an extensive trial of nonoperative treatment, realignment procedures are considered. Patients with diffuse patellofemoral DJD are not good candidates for TTO. The Fulkerson osteotomy or variations of anteromedialization (AMZ) procedures should be considered for lateral and distal pole lesions and patients with an abnormally high Q angle or TT-TG distance. However, AMZ is contraindicated with superomedial arthrosis and in skeletally immature patients.

Preoperative Assessment and Planning

A thorough history and examination is performed. Patients will typically report diffuse pain in the peripatellar or retropatellar region, and this is typically insidious and vague in nature. Pain may be aggravated by ascending or descending stairs, prolonged sitting with the knee bent or kneeling. Palpable crepitus may be evident throughout knee range of motion, and pain may be present with compression of the patella with range of motion or resisted knee extension. Attention should be paid to any signs of associated instability.

Standard radiographic examination includes anteroposterior, lateral, and sunrise knee radiographs, which may demonstrate obvious chondrosis, shallow sulcus, patella alta or baja, or lateral patellar tilt. Patellar height can be determined by methods including the Insall-Salvati, Blackburne-Peele, Caton-Deschamps, and plateau patella angle or their modifications Trochlear dysplasia may also be graded in severity by the Dejour classification [21]. CT can be performed for assessment of patellofemoral alignment, trochlear geometry, calculation of the TT-TG distance, and torsion of the lower extremity. TT-TG distance is measured between two perpendicular lines from the posterior cortex to the tibial tubercle and the trochlear groove, with more than 20 mm considered abnormal, MRI can serve as a proxy for CT in calculating the TT-TG interval. However, MRI tends to underestimate the TT-TG interval when compared with the CT and this must be taken into account. There is a role for staging arthroscopy if there is any doubt regarding interpretation of concomitant pathologies and is advocated in some instances as obligatory, such as with Fulkerson or AMZ procedures when superomedial arthrosis would potentially contraindicate the realignment procedure done in isolation.

Surgical Technique

Most contemporary techniques are adaptations of the Fulkerson AMZ osteotomy. However, the type of osteotomy is ultimately dictated by the nature of the patellofemoral OA and the presence or absence of instability [57].

TTO Surgical Technique

For anteromedialization of the tibial tubercle, we make an 8- to 10-cm longitudinal incision just lateral to midline to avoid the incision lying directly over the tibial tubercle and allow for optimal visualization of the lateral tibial cortex when performing the osteotomy. We use a 2.5-mm drill bit to mark out the ostetomy site from proximal to distal medially and laterally. The osteotomy is made from medial to lateral angling posterolaterally 40–45°. The cut should taper from proximal to distal with maximal thickness of 4 cm proximally, thinning out distally and preserving a periosteal hinge at the distal apex. With the tibial tubercle now freed, desired medial correction is performed manually and the osteotomy is held in place provisionally by placing a 0.064-in. K-wire just medial to the medially translated tibial tubercle. Fixation of the osteotomy can then be achieved with two to three bicortical 3.5-mm screws or 4.5-mm countersunk screws (Fig. 12.6). While plate and screw constructs can be considered, this is often unnecessary and hardware irritation with potential skin breakdown can be a significant problem [58]. Patients are placed in a hinged brace postoperatively locked in extension until there is clinical and radiographic evidence that the osteotomy has healed. Crutches are used during the first 6 weeks. PT begins at

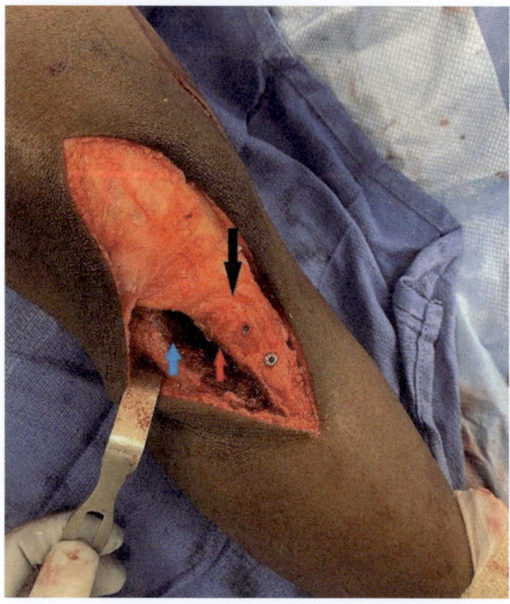

Fig. 12.6 Photograph shows tibial tubercle (anteromedialization) osteotomy performed in conjunction with medial patellofemoral ligament reconstruction for lateral patellar instability, lateral patellofemoral arthritis, and abnormal TT-TG interval (25 mm). Black arrow, osteotomized TT. Red arrow, lateral border of the osteotomized TT. Blue arrow, lateral border of the native tibia. Medialization of 1.5 cm resulted in 1 cm anteriorization with osteotomy. Osteotomy fixed with two 3.5-mm bicortical screws

week 2 emphasizing early active-assisted range of motion (AAROM) in flexion and passive extension in non-painful arcs, targeting 90° by 6 weeks. Unrestricted weightbearing can be initiated once radiographic and clinical healing have been established, typically by 6 weeks. Full return to high-level activity is anticipated by 6–9 months postoperatively.

Summary

Osteoarthritis of the knee is a growing problem with incidence continuing to increase steadily in parallel with an aging population worldwide. Symptomatic unicompartmental knee osteoarthritis has received increasing attention because increased prevalence in young active patient populations is driving demand for less invasive treatment strategies. The preservation of intra-articular structures and avoidance of implants with osteotomies about the knee allow for unrestricted loading and activity postoperatively. Greater functional benefit has been found with osteotomy versus arthroplasty in younger, more active populations. With advancements in surgical technology and materials and improved understanding of rehabilitation principles, osteotomies about the knee are an excellent treatment option for select patients with UCOA.

References

1. Ledingham J, Regan M, Jones A, Doherty M. Radiographic patterns and associations of osteoarthritis of the knee in patients referred to hospital. Ann Rheum Dis. 1993;52(7):520–6. https://doi.org/10.1136/ard.52.7.520.
2. Agneskirchner JD, Hurschler C, Wrann CD, Lobenhoffer P. The effects of valgus medial opening wedge high tibial osteotomy on articular cartilage pressure of the knee: a biomechanical study. Arthroscopy. 2007;23(8):852–61. https://doi.org/10.1016/j.arthro.2007.05.018.
3. Backstein D, Morag G, Hanna S, Safir O, Gross A. Long-term follow-up of distal femoral varus osteotomy of the knee. J Arthroplast. 2007;22(4 Suppl 1):2–6. https://doi.org/10.1016/j.arth.2007.01.026.
4. Gstottner M, Pedross F, Liebensteiner M, Bach C. Long-term outcome after high tibial osteotomy. Arch Orthop Trauma Surg. 2008;128(1):111–5. https://doi.org/10.1007/s00402-007-0438-0.
5. Kim YC, Yang JH, Kim HJ, Tawonsawatruk T, Chang YS, Lee JS, et al. Distal femoral varus osteotomy for valgus arthritis of the knees: systematic review of open versus closed wedge osteotomy. Knee Surg Relat Res. 2018;30(1):3–16. https://doi.org/10.5792/ksrr.16.064.
6. Klinge SA, Fulkerson JP. Fifteen-year minimum follow-up of anteromedial tibial tubercle transfer for lateral and/or distal patellofemoral arthrosis. Arthroscopy. 2019;35(7):2146–51. https://doi.org/10.1016/j.arthro.2019.02.030.
7. Liu JN, Wu HH, Garcia GH, Kalbian IL, Strickland SM, Shubin Stein BE. Return to sports after tibial tubercle osteotomy for patellofemoral pain and osteoarthritis. Arthroscopy. 2018;34(4):1022–9. https://doi.org/10.1016/j.arthro.2017.09.021.
8. Nelson CL, Saleh KJ, Kassim RA, Windsor R, Haas S, Laskin R, et al. Total knee arthroplasty after varus osteotomy of the distal part of the femur. J Bone Joint Surg Am. 2003;85(6):1062–5. https://doi.org/10.2106/00004623-200306000-00012.
9. Saithna A, Kundra R, Getgood A, Spalding T. Opening wedge distal femoral varus osteotomy for lateral compartment osteoarthritis in the valgus knee. Knee. 2014;21(1):172–5. https://doi.org/10.1016/j.knee.2013.08.014.
10. Sprenger TR, Doerzbacher JF. Tibial osteotomy for the treatment of varus gonarthrosis. Survival and failure analysis to twenty-two years. J Bone Joint Surg Am. 2003;85(3):469–74.
11. Wang JW, Hsu CC. Distal femoral varus osteotomy for osteoarthritis of the knee. Surgical technique. J Bone Joint Surg Am. 2006;88(Suppl 1 Pt 1):100–8. https://doi.org/10.2106/JBJS.E.00827.
12. Yasuda K, Majima T, Tsuchida T, Kaneda K. A ten- to 15-year follow-up observation of high tibial osteotomy in medial compartment osteoarthrosis. Clin Orthop Relat Res. 1992;282:186–95.
13. Floerkemeier S, Staubli AE, Schroeter S, Goldhahn S, Lobenhoffer P. Outcome after high tibial open-wedge osteotomy: a retrospective evaluation of 533 patients. Knee Surg Sports Traumatol Arthrosc. 2013;21(1):170–80. https://doi.org/10.1007/s00167-012-2087-2.
14. Hantes ME, Natsaridis P, Koutalos AA, Ono Y, Doxariotis N, Malizos KN. Satisfactory functional and radiological outcomes can be expected in young patients under 45 years old after open wedge high tibial osteotomy in a long-term follow-up. Knee Surg Sports Traumatol Arthrosc. 2018;26(11):3199–205. https://doi.org/10.1007/s00167-017-4816-z.
15. Kuriyama S, Watanabe M, Nakamura S, Nishitani K, Sekiguchi K, Tanaka Y, et al. Classical target coronal alignment in high tibial osteotomy demonstrates validity in terms of knee kinematics and kinetics in a computer model. Knee Surg Sports Traumatol Arthrosc. 2020;28(5):1568–78. https://doi.org/10.1007/s00167-019-05575-3.
16. Jacquet C, Gulagaci F, Schmidt A, Pendse A, Parratte S, Argenson JN, et al. Opening wedge high tibial osteotomy allows better outcomes than unicompartmental knee arthroplasty in patients expecting to return to impact sports. Knee Surg Sports Traumatol Arthrosc. 2020;28(12):3849–57. https://doi.org/10.1007/s00167-020-05857-1.
17. Jackson JP, Waugh W. Tibial osteotomy for osteoarthritis of the knee. Proc R Soc Med. 1960;53(10):888.
18. Coventry MB. Osteotomy of the upper portion of the tibia for degenerative arthritis of the knee. A preliminary report. J Bone Joint Surg Am. 1965;47:984–90.
19. Hernigou P, Medevielle D, Debeyre J, Goutallier D. Proximal tibial osteotomy for osteoarthritis with varus deformity. A ten to thirteen-year follow-up study. J Bone Joint Surg Am. 1987;69(3):332–54.
20. Atkinson HD, Bailey CA, Anand S, Johal P, Oakeshott RD. Tibial tubercle advancement osteotomy with bone allograft for patellofemoral arthritis: a retrospective cohort study of 50 knees. Arch Orthop Trauma Surg. 2012;132(4):437–45. https://doi.org/10.1007/s00402-011-1433-z.
21. Dejour H, Walch G, Nove-Josserand L, Guier C. Factors of patellar instability: an anatomic radiographic study. Knee Surg Sports Traumatol Arthrosc. 1994;2(1):19–26.

22. Edgerton BC, Mariani EM, Morrey BF. Distal femoral varus osteotomy for painful genu valgum. A five-to-11-year follow-up study. Clin Orthop Relat Res. 1993;288:263–9.

23. Feller JA, Amis AA, Andrish JT, Arendt EA, Erasmus PJ, Powers CM. Surgical biomechanics of the patellofemoral joint. Arthroscopy. 2007;23(5):542–53. https://doi.org/10.1016/j.arthro.2007.03.006.

24. Finkelstein JA, Gross AE, Davis A. Varus osteotomy of the distal part of the femur. A survivorship analysis. J Bone Joint Surg Am. 1996;78(9):1348–52. https://doi.org/10.2106/00004623-199609000-00008.

25. Vessely MB, Whaley AL, Harmsen WS, Schleck CD, Berry DJ. The Chitranjan Ranawat award: long-term survivorship and failure modes of 1000 cemented condylar total knee arthroplasties. Clin Orthop Relat Res. 2006;452:28–34. https://doi.org/10.1097/01.blo.0000229356.81749.11.

26. Argenson JN, Boisgard S, Parratte S, Descamps S, Bercovy M, Bonnevialle P, et al. Survival analysis of total knee arthroplasty at a minimum 10 years' follow-up: a multicenter French nationwide study including 846 cases. Orthop Traumatol Surg Res. 2013;99(4):385–90. https://doi.org/10.1016/j.otsr.2013.03.014.

27. Lutzner C, Kirschner S, Lutzner J. Patient activity after TKA depends on patient-specific parameters. Clin Orthop Relat Res. 2014;472(12):3933–40. https://doi.org/10.1007/s11999-014-3813-5.

28. Koh IJ, Kim MW, Kim JH, Han SY, In Y. Trends in high tibial osteotomy and knee arthroplasty utilizations and demographics in Korea from 2009 to 2013. J Arthroplast. 2015;30(6):939–44. https://doi.org/10.1016/j.arth.2015.01.002.

29. Smith TO, Sexton D, Mitchell P, Hing CB. Opening- or closing-wedged high tibial osteotomy: a meta-analysis of clinical and radiological outcomes. Knee. 2011;18(6):361–8. https://doi.org/10.1016/j.knee.2010.10.001.

30. Kim JH, Kim HJ, Lee DH. Survival of opening versus closing wedge high tibial osteotomy: a meta-analysis. Sci Rep. 2017;7(1):7296. https://doi.org/10.1038/s41598-017-07856-8.

31. Coventry MB. Osteotomy about the knee for degenerative and rheumatoid arthritis. J Bone Joint Surg Am. 1973;55(1):23–48.

32. Sharma L, Song J, Felson DT, Cahue S, Shamiyeh E, Dunlop DD. The role of knee alignment in disease progression and functional decline in knee osteoarthritis. JAMA. 2001;286(2):188–95. https://doi.org/10.1001/jama.286.2.188.

33. Coventry MB, Ilstrup DM, Wallrichs SL. Proximal tibial osteotomy. A critical long-term study of eighty-seven cases. J Bone Joint Surg Am. 1993;75(2):196–201. https://doi.org/10.2106/00004623-199302000-00006.

34. Paley D, Herzenberg JE, Tetsworth K, McKie J, Bhave A. Deformity planning for frontal and sagittal plane corrective osteotomies. Orthop Clin North Am. 1994;25(3):425–65.

35. Agarwala S, Sobti A, Naik S, Chaudhari S. Comparison of closing-wedge and opening-wedge high tibial osteotomies for medial compartment osteoarthritis of knee in Asian population: mid-term follow-up. J Clin Orthop Trauma. 2016;7(4):272–5. https://doi.org/10.1016/j.jcot.2016.06.012.

36. Pape D, Lorbach O, Schmitz C, Busch LC, Van Giffen N, Seil R, et al. Effect of a biplanar osteotomy on primary stability following high tibial osteotomy: a biomechanical cadaver study. Knee Surg Sports Traumatol Arthrosc. 2010;18(2):204–11. https://doi.org/10.1007/s00167-009-0929-3.

37. Coventry MB. Upper tibial osteotomy for osteoarthritis. J Bone Joint Surg Am. 1985;67(7):1136–40.

38. van Raaij TM, Brouwer RW. Proximal tibial valgus osteotomy: lateral closing wedge. JBJS Essent Surg Tech. 2015;5(4):e26. https://doi.org/10.2106/JBJS.ST.N.00104.

39. Brouwer RW, Bierma-Zeinstra SM, van Raaij TM, Verhaar JA. Osteotomy for medial compartment arthritis of the knee using a closing wedge or an opening wedge controlled by a Puddu plate. A one-year randomised, controlled study. J Bone Joint Surg Br. 2006;88(11):1454–9. https://doi.org/10.1302/0301-620X.88B11.17743.

40. Park JG, Kim JM, Lee BS, Lee SM, Kwon OJ, Bin SI. Increased preoperative medial and lateral laxity is a predictor of overcorrection in open wedge high tibial osteotomy. Knee Surg Sports Traumatol Arthrosc. 2020;28(10):3164–72. https://doi.org/10.1007/s00167-019-05805-8.

41. Schroter S, Ateschrang A, Lowe W, Nakayama H, Stockle U, Ihle C. Early full weight-bearing versus 6-week partial weight-bearing after open wedge high tibial osteotomy leads to earlier improvement of the clinical results: a prospective, randomised evaluation. Knee Surg Sports Traumatol Arthrosc. 2017;25(1):325–32. https://doi.org/10.1007/s00167-015-3592-x.

42. Healy WL, Anglen JO, Wasilewski SA, Krackow KA. Distal femoral varus osteotomy. J Bone Joint Surg Am. 1988;70(1):102–9.

43. McDermott AG, Finklestein JA, Farine I, Boynton EL, MacIntosh DL, Gross A. Distal femoral varus osteotomy for valgus deformity of the knee. J Bone Joint Surg Am. 1988;70(1):110–6.

44. Cooke TD, Li J, Scudamore RA. Radiographic assessment of bony contributions to knee deformity. Orthop Clin North Am. 1994;25(3):387–93.

45. Drexler M, Gross A, Dwyer T, Safir O, Backstein D, Chaudhry H, et al. Distal femoral varus osteotomy combined with tibial plateau fresh osteochondral allograft for post-traumatic osteoarthritis of the knee. Knee Surg Sports Traumatol Arthrosc. 2015;23(5):1317–23. https://doi.org/10.1007/s00167-013-2828-x.

46. Liu JN, Agarwalla A, Garcia GH, Christian DR, Gowd AK, Yanke AB, et al. Return to sport and work after high tibial osteotomy with concomitant medial meniscal

allograft transplant. Arthroscopy. 2019;35(11):3090–6. https://doi.org/10.1016/j.arthro.2019.05.053.

47. Jacobi M, Wahl P, Bouaicha S, Jakob RP, Gautier E. Distal femoral varus osteotomy: problems associated with the lateral open-wedge technique. Arch Orthop Trauma Surg. 2011;131(6):725–8. https://doi.org/10.1007/s00402-010-1193-1.

48. Flury A, Jud L, Hoch A, Camenzind RS, Fucentese SF. Linear influence of distal femur osteotomy on the Q-angle: one degree of varization alters the Q-angle by one degree. Knee Surg Sports Traumatol Arthrosc. 2020;29:540. https://doi.org/10.1007/s00167-020-05970-1.

49. Sherman SL, Thompson SF, Clohisy JCF. Distal femoral varus osteotomy for the management of valgus deformity of the knee. J Am Acad Orthop Surg. 2018;26(9):313–24. https://doi.org/10.5435/JAAOS-D-16-00179.

50. Rosso F, Margheritini F. Distal femoral osteotomy. Curr Rev Musculoskelet Med. 2014;7(4):302–11. https://doi.org/10.1007/s12178-014-9233-z.

51. Salem HS, Chaudhry ZS, Lucenti L, Tucker BS, Freedman KB. The importance of staging arthroscopy for chondral defects of the knee. J Knee Surg. 2020;35:145. https://doi.org/10.1055/s-0040-1713126.

52. Shivji FS, Foster A, Risebury MJ, Wilson AJ, Yasen SK. Ten-year survival rate of 89% after distal femoral osteotomy surgery for lateral compartment osteoarthritis of the knee. Knee Surg Sports Traumatol Arthrosc. 2020;29:594. https://doi.org/10.1007/s00167-020-05988-5.

53. Fragomen AT, McCoy TH Jr, Fragomen FR. A preliminary comparison suggests poor performance of carbon fiber reinforced versus titanium plates in distal femoral osteotomy. HSS J. 2018;14(3):258–65. https://doi.org/10.1007/s11420-017-9587-z.

54. Frings J, Krause M, Akoto R, Wohlmuth P, Frosch KH. Combined distal femoral osteotomy (DFO) in genu valgum leads to reliable patellar stabilization and an improvement in knee function. Knee Surg Sports Traumatol Arthrosc. 2018;26(12):3572–81. https://doi.org/10.1007/s00167-018-5000-9.

55. Swarup I, Elattar O, Rozbruch SR. Patellar instability treated with distal femoral osteotomy. Knee. 2017;24(3):608–14. https://doi.org/10.1016/j.knee.2017.02.004.

56. Saltzman BM, Rao A, Erickson BJ, Cvetanovich GL, Levy D, Bach BR Jr, et al. A systematic review of 21 tibial tubercle osteotomy studies and more than 1000 knees: indications, clinical outcomes, complications, and reoperations. Am J Orthop (Belle Mead NJ). 2017;46(6):E396–407.

57. Hall MJ, Mandalia VI. Tibial tubercle osteotomy for patello-femoral joint disorders. Knee Surg Sports Traumatol Arthrosc. 2016;24(3):855–61. https://doi.org/10.1007/s00167-014-3388-4.

58. Stevens JM, Barton SB, Alexander M, Eldridge JD, Clark D. Plate and screw fixation of arthroscopically assisted tibial tuberosity osteotomy: technique and results. Eur J Orthop Surg Traumatol. 2020;30(1):139–45. https://doi.org/10.1007/s00590-019-02536-x.

Planning Bone and Soft-Tissue Management During Revision Knee Reconstruction

13

Paolo Salari, Michele d'Amato, and Andrea Baldini

Introduction

Total Knee Arthroplasty, the second most common joint replacement procedure, is a cost effective and successful operation. However, the literature reports up to 30% of failures and dissatisfaction that often result in implant revision [1]. Moreover, registry data has highlighted an increasing number of TKAs in a younger and higher-demand population, suggesting a potential rise in future of RTKAs [2]. Outcomes after primary TKA are reasonably predictable and reproducible. Otherwise, RTKA is a technically demanding procedure and is usually associated with worse results than after primary arthroplasty, due to a multitude of factors including the complexity of the procedure associated with bone and soft-tissue problems. As a result of these technical demands, higher complication rate, and a lengthier hospital stay and period of convalescence, the cost of RTKA is approximately double that of a primary procedure.

Over the last decade, failure mechanisms of a TKA have changed due to improvements in the surgical technique and implants performance. The most frequently reported mechanisms of failure in primary TKA have varied but consistently include Periprosthetic Joint Infection (PJI), loosening, instability and stiffness [3]. In 2006, Mulhall et al. [4] classified TKA failure mechanisms in early (<2 years) and late (>2 years). Early revisions (31% of patients) were primarily due to infection (25%); 69% of patients were revised after 2 years for mechanical instability (29%), polyethylene wear (25%) and component loosening (41%). In recent literature [5], pain, instability, and stiffness are more likely to be reported as causes of failure after TKA. Surgeons should approach knee revision surgery only after an accurate planning of implant type and fixation to avoid pitfalls.

Preoperative Evaluation

Clinical Evaluation

Understanding the cause of implant failure is the key to success in the subsequent revision. Several studies showed that revising a TKA for pain symptoms, without identifying the reason for failure, inevitably leads to not succeed [6]. Figuring out why a huge bone or soft-tissue defect occurred is essential to not make the same mistake again. Become essential to collect an accurate clinical history of the patient, evaluating parameters such as age, gender, occupation and patients' expectations from surgery. Comorbidities, such as diabetes, vasculopathies, coagulopathies, obesity, mental state, smoking

P. Salari · M. d'Amato · A. Baldini (✉)
Institute for Complex Arthroplasty and Revisions at Istituto Fiorentino di Cura e Assistenza,
Florence, Italy

© The Author(s), under exclusive license to Springer Nature Switzerland AG 2023
A. J. Deshmukh et al. (eds.), *Surgical Management of Knee Arthritis*,
https://doi.org/10.1007/978-3-031-47929-8_13

and drugs, must also be carefully evaluated. Any type of infection affecting other body's districts or close to the joint must be excluded. It is also necessary to evaluate pre-existing neuromuscular pathologies, such as Parkinson's or neurological paralysis, which, due to the intrinsic instability of the joint, would lead to high stress on the implant in the long term [7]. The physical examination starts observing patient walking straight for few meters. It allows to observe how the joint reacts to the weight-bearing stress in a dynamic condition and to seek for pathological conditions of the nearby articulation like hips and ankles, that could influence the outcome of our surgery. A patient with a dynamic thrust sign may indicate excessive laxity of the lateral compartment structures or a varus alignment of the implant [8]. Instead, a patient walking with the knee in hyperextension may indicate an excessive residual laxity of the TKA in extension, a lesion of the posterior capsule, or a chronic insufficiency of the extensor mechanism with a subsequent stretching of the posterior capsule (Fig. 13.1). The trigger of the recurvatum deformity should be carefully evaluated to choose the right reconstructive technique and implant. Hyperextension caused by chronically stretched posterior capsule need an anti-recurvatum implant and cannot be corrected overfilling the extension space [9]. Patients' ambulation can be also affected by a varus or valgus deformity of the affected knee. Deformities of the contralateral limb should be considered during the correction planning.

Limping for a leg length discrepancy must be closely analyzed to uncover the origin excluding any flexion joints contracture [10]. Knee stability examination is completed with the patient in supine position. Varus and valgus stress is applied at different range of flexion, usually at 0°, 15° and 90°. Is important to notice that collaterals ligaments act as main stabilizers only after 15° of flexion, the posterior capsule is the main varus-valgus constraint from 0 to 15° and a positive stress in complete extension is a sign of posterior structures insufficiency. Antero-posterior stability is checked with an anterior and posterior drawer test [11]. Skin examination is another fundamental step. Knee is inspected to determine the number and the position of previous scar incisions, the mobility of the skin from the subcutaneous fascia and the presence of sinus tracts. Multiple surgical scars and adhesions to deeper layers is a risk for skin necrosis. Surgeons should figure out the most appropriate surgical approach considering all the soft-tissue complications could happen in a pluri-operated knee. In complex situations, plastic surgical consultation is recommended [12] for the design of the most suitable skin approach and for muscle flap procedures (Fig. 13.2). The range of motion evaluation (ROM), the last step of the clinical evaluation, is the most important to plan the right surgical gestures in the operating room.

Active and passive ROM have to be carefully assessed, it is necessary to distinguish an extension problem due to stiffness or a lag. Extension

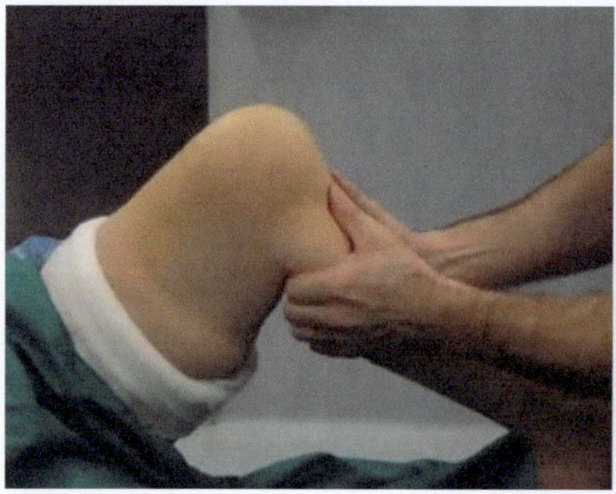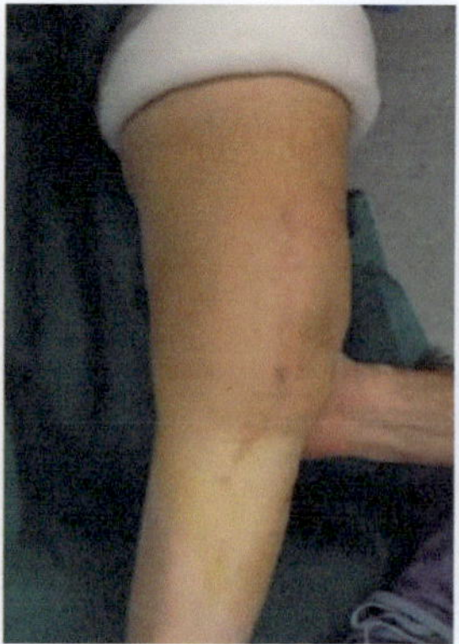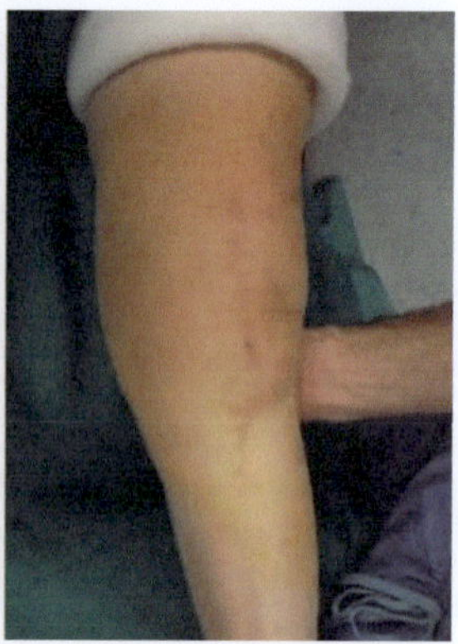

Fig. 13.1 The images show a patient with posterior capsule insufficiency and severe varus-valgus instability

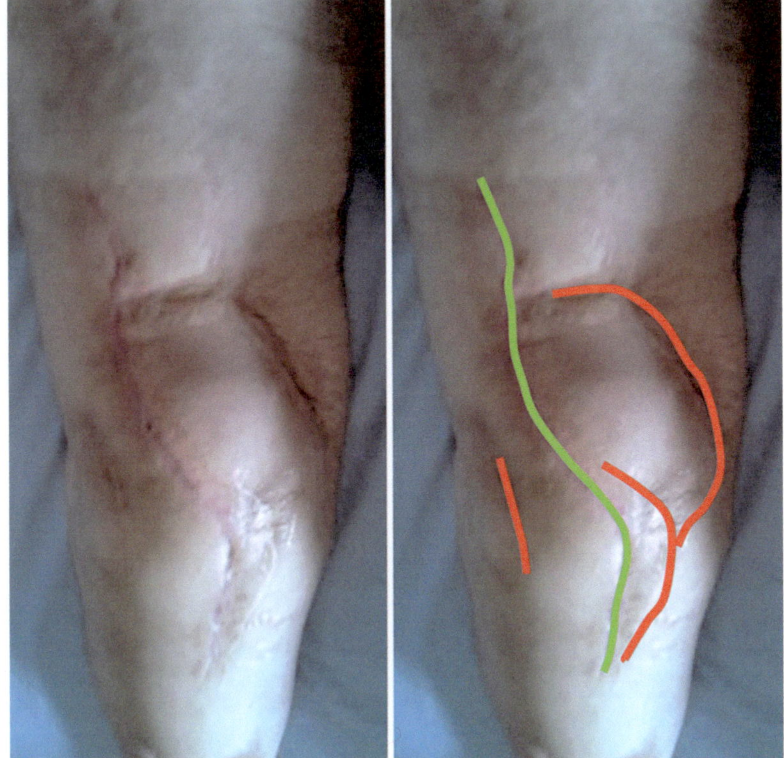

Fig. 13.2 When dealing with multiple scars, the most lateral one has the lower change to cause skin necrosis

lag is defined as a discrepancy between the active and passive extension of the knee. Lag is related to a disruption of the extensor apparatus, which can occur at various levels: quadriceps, patella, or patellar tendon [13]. Generally, to understand where the lesion is located, the clinical examination is sufficient: the area affected by the injury has a depression and is often painful at palpation. The lateral x-ray view could help us in the diagnosis: a lesion on the quadriceps tendon will show a remarkably low patella, instead a lesion of the patellar tendon will show a very high patella (Fig. 13.3).

It is important to make an accurate diagnosis to plan the right treatment. An acute lesion can be treated with a side-to-side suture and with autologous tissue augmentation. On the other side, chronic extensor mechanism discontinuity or lesions involving a resurfaced patella may necessitate a complete extensor mechanism allograft reconstruction. This requires the availability in the operating room of the specific allograft.

Unstable knees usually present an abnormal ROM that does not correlate with pain symptoms. In the other hand, stiff joints have a restricted motion in flexion and/or extension [14]. A flexion contracture has to be differentiated from an extension lag where the passive extension is always possible.

The key to success in an arthrofibrotic knee is to create a sort of iatrogenic "instability". All the adhesions and the scar tissue should be removed, the extensor mechanism should be stretched with a progressive intraoperative mobilization and the quadriceps elevated from the anterior femoral cortex. In severe flexion contractures, the posterior capsule become rigid and is usually sacrificed. Even a partial or sub-total detachment of collateral ligament could be performed to gain access to the joint. Despite these wide-releasing maneuvers, a stiff knee does rarely evolve into a condition of instability and a semi-constrained implant is usually enough [15]. In presence of a restricted flexion ROM, a liner impingement for

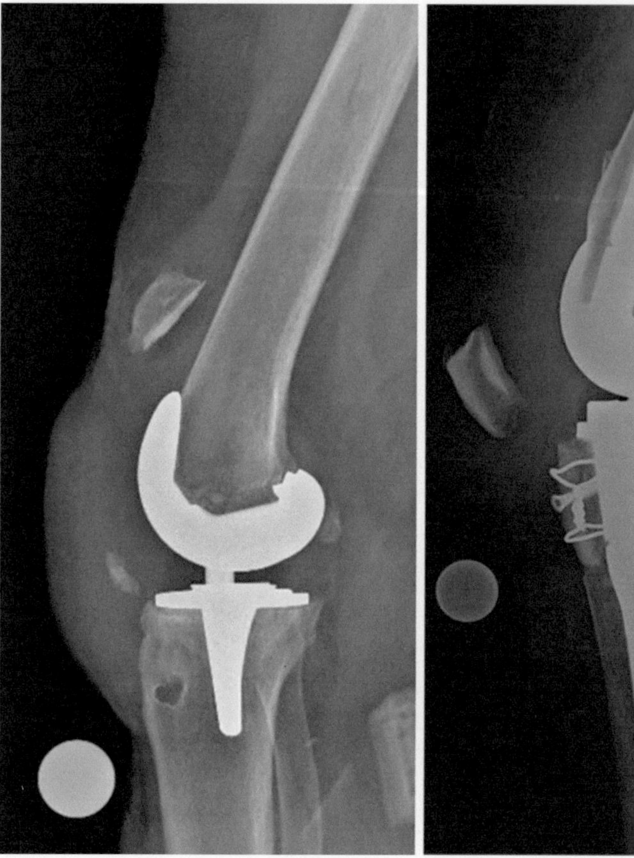

Fig. 13.3 Lateral view X-ray of patient with patellar tendon lesion on the left, and with quadriceps tendon lesion on the right

patella baja or an extensor mechanism clunk should be always excluded during physical examination. Obtaining complete patients records is mandatory before approaching every revision. Information about implant type and size and other surgical details or clinical data about the perioperative and post-operative period are useful to understand the failure mechanism and plan the correct reconstruction strategy. To optimize the surgical flow, this information should be shared promptly with all the operating team.

Radiographic Evaluation

The standard radiographic evaluation of a failed TKA includes standing antero-posterior and lateral images and a full weight bearing long leg view. If components loosening is suspected, knee X-rays tangential to the bone-implant interface should be performed using a fluoroscopic guide [16]. An axial 45° Merchant patellar view may be useful in case of patellar problems.

Properly performed radiographs play perhaps the most crucial role in the preoperative planning of a TKA revision. The necessary images are latero-lateral (LL), and long leg full weight bearing.

Knee rotation and correct projection in all radiographs are important to respect. For example, in long-leg and in AP X-ray, the patella must always be centered in the middle of the femoral condyles and the fibular head should only for one-third by tibia. In the LL X-ray, the posterior condyles of the femur must always be well overlapped. A rotational or oblique X-ray could mislead the measurements, a limb internally or externally rotated by only 3° can affect the measurement of the mechanical axis by even 5–6°. To obtain the correct projections, it is recommended to check the position of the limb under fluoroscopy, taking only then the final X-ray [17].

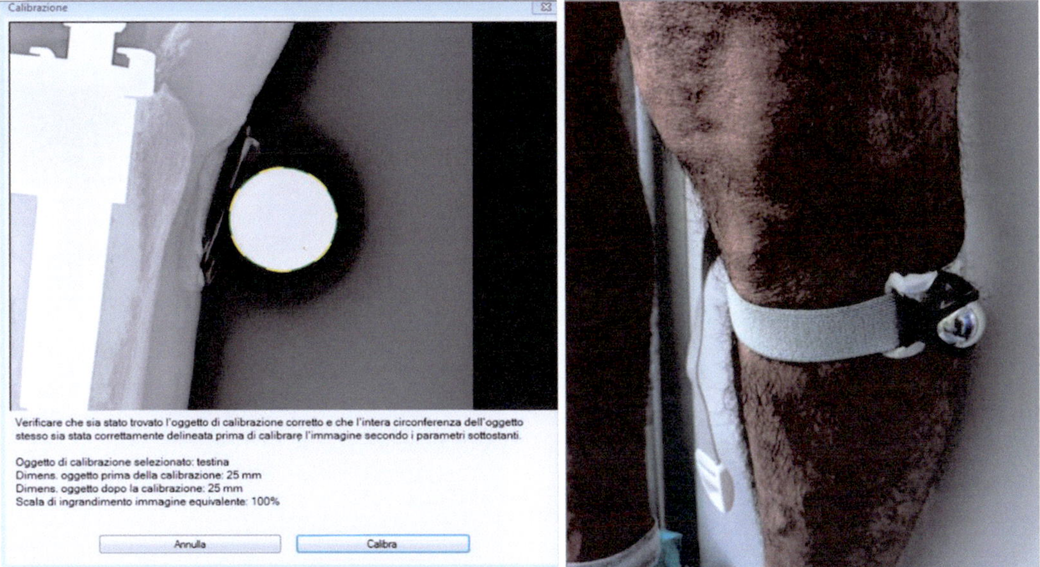

Fig. 13.4 Calibration marker used to avoid magnification issues during templating

It is also of fundamental importance to use a radiopaque spherical marker of known size during imaging execution to check the magnification (Fig. 13.4). Kniesel et al. [18] have shown that in TKA, there is a high correlation between the implanted and planned sizes only when a reference marker is used on the X-rays. Using a digital PACS and a templating software, the calibration can be automatic, otherwise a mathematical ratio has to be performed. Templating on calibrated images is important for an accurate planning in very large or very small-sized patients, because sometimes it may be necessary to have on-the-shelf extra-small or extra-large size implants, or even custom-made implants, situation that surgeons should be prepared to afford intraoperatively. Nuclear medicine scans should be performed only in strictly selected cases when diagnosis of failure is highly probable and cannot be diagnosed with standard methods [19]. Magnetic resonance imaging with metal artefacts reduction sequences is used in case of soft-tissue and bone-marrow issues [20]. Computer tomography (CT) scans with metal artefacts reduction protocols or dual-energy CT may be useful to detect micro-loosening and components malrotation or for a better preoperative estimation of the bone loss [21].

Planning Fixation and Bone-Defects Management

One of the greatest challenges in revision TKA is to overcome the bone loss and to find an adequate support for implant fixation. The removal of prosthetic implant, osteolysis for aseptic loosening, or stress shielding and debridement or resection for infection are common causes of bone deficiencies in a revision scenario [22]. There are various classification systems of bone defects mainly based on type, severity, and location of the defects useful to provide a valid algorithm of treatment. The Anderson Orthopedic Research Institute (AORI) bone defect classification is the most widely accepted because of its simplicity [23]. According to it, bone defects are classified into three types for tibia (T1, T2, T3) and femur (F1, F2, F3) separately. To establish the correct amount of bone defect, weight-bearing X-rays are usually sufficient. It is highly recommended understanding the precise extension and position of the defect preoperatively, but the effective bone loss must be confirmed or modified intra-operatively after implant removal. The Type 1 defect has preoperative radiographs negative for component migration and osteolysis, a normal joint line level is demonstrated by the patellar height and the distance of the prosthesis from epicondyles and fibular head. The Type 2 bone defect is characterized by osteolysis or significant proximal migration of the femoral component or a subsidence of the tibial plateau typically in varus. The subtype 2A can involve either condyle. There is a unilateral collapse of the cancellous bone of the involved condyle and the bone of the opposite condyle is near intact and at the level of the right joint line. The defect in a Type 2B is identical to the 2A defect except that it involves both condyles. The damaged metaphyseal bone requires reconstruction of both condyles. The damage may extend to the level of the fibular head or near epicondyles but should not include extensive destruction of bone beyond this level. The metaphysis of the tibia is reduced but still present. Type 3 femoral defects have extensive structural bone loss, involving a major portion of one or both condyles and metaphysis. The preoperative radiographs of F3 defects demonstrate osteolysis and/or severe component migration to the level of the epicondyles. Preoperative radiographs of a T3 defect reveal either severe tibial component migration and instability or destruction of a major segment of the proximal tibial metaphysis. Bone loss is severe, so that the patellar tendon insertion or collateral ligament attachment on one or both sides is often compromised. A high patella may be present as sign of extensor mechanism failure. Obtaining a solid primary fixation of implants into host bone is the primary goal in a revision TKA scenario. It is essential to allow early post-operative mobilization and rehabilitation and to guarantee the longevity of the construct. Morgan-Jones et al. [24] identified three anatomical zones in which fixation for a revision TKA implant should be achieved: zone 1, the joint surface or epiphysis; zone 2, the metaphysis; and zone 3, the diaphysis (Fig. 13.5). In literature, there is still no agreement and shared decision in this regard. The authors suggest that a solid and durable fixation should be obtained in two of the three zones at least. In addition, presence of sclerotic bone must be anticipated to plan a non-cemented fixation methods at this level as

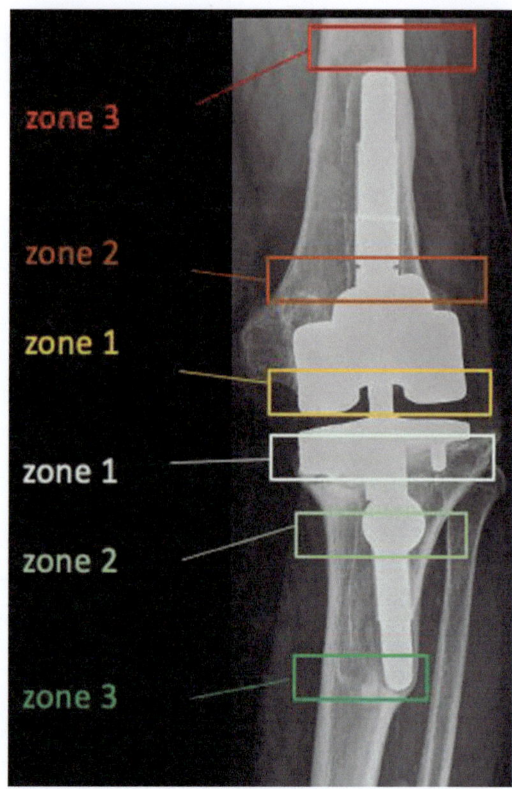

Fig. 13.5 Morgan-Jones zonal classification

there are no longer trabeculae available for cement penetration (Fig. 13.6).

In most of the cases, zone 1 is partially or completely compromised by the process of implant failure and removal. The zone should be cleared from cement debris, avascular bone, and fibrous membrane to improve fixation. If the defect in this zone is uncontained, the authors suggest obtaining solid fixation in zones 2 and 3 and to fill the defect in zone 1 with cement or metal augments. Instead, when the defect is not massive, the epiphysis must be regularized with aligned cuts, and the bone fixation or augmentation can be performed by cement, bone graft or metal augment [25]. Cement is not a biological scaffold and may cause thermal necrosis of the surrounding bone and blood supply to the bone, which is a cause for long-term loosening of the prostheses; in case of sclerotic bone, the quality of cementing technique is poor. For all these rea-

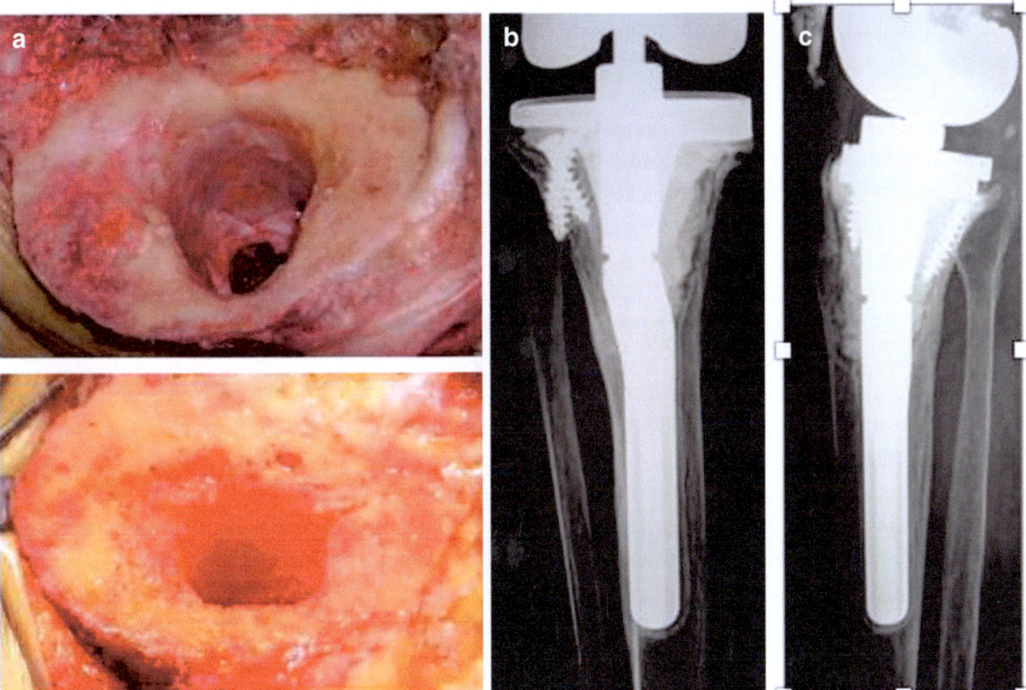

Fig. 13.6 How appear sclerotic (**a**) and cancellous bone (**b**) intraoperatively. In (**c**) is shown an early loosening of tibia where cemented technique was used in sclerotic bone, without interdigitation into trabecular bone

sons, it is recommended only for small contained defects with a healthy medullary bone. For tibial or femoral defects from 5 to 10 mm in height, the cement can be augmented with a titanium screw [26]. The screw should be inserted to a depth that its head does not reach the prosthetic surface or go beyond the cortical bone. It is a reliable, reproducible, easily performed, inexpensive technique and results in 30% less displacement of the prosthesis than cement alone. Impacted, morselized bone grafts is preferred to restore the bone stock, especially in younger patients with contained bone defects. The main disadvantage of the technique is that to ensure a solid fixation, the graft has to be integrated into the host bone with a long-term process [27]. If this is the preferred option, the authors suggest obtaining a solid fixation in zones 2 and 3. Impaction bone grafting is not recommended for repairing cortical or uncontained defects because the cortical rim is important to ensure stability until integration. Moreover,

in cases of infection, the use of prosthetic augments and antibiotic bone cement is a safer option. Metal augments in titanium or porous metal are available in different sizes and shapes for both femoral and tibial defects. They are frequently used to restore appropriate alignment for a varus/valgus deformity with a medial/lateral tibial defect, to reconstruct the appropriate condylar offset of the femur or to restore proper femoral component rotation and balance the flexion/extension gap. Metal augments are used especially in elderly, low-demand patients and appeared to be superior in terms of forces resisting deflections. Zone 2 has been recently considered as the most important zone for a long-term implant fixation, as it avoids stress-shielding phenomena correlated with a diaphyseal fixation alone. A closer fixation to the joint line provides better restoration of joint line and axial/rotational stability, even in the presence of cortical or cancellous bone defects and may be an alternative to long stems. An uncontained defect in this zone could be managed only with mega-prosthesis or structural allograft, but fortunately is a rare scenario. If part of zone 2 is still available, as for zone 1, it can be reconstructed with cement, bone graft or using sleeves and trabecular metal cones [28]. Trabecular metals have a structure similar to cancellous bone and is highly biocompatible and osteoconductive; they offer the advantages of an intra-operative press-fit stability for its high-frictional characteristics, allowing immediate weight-bearing. The porosity permits bone in growth in the mid-term and preserves in a long term the bone stock for the low modulus of elasticity. Trabecular metal cones are used to reconstruct large cavitary defects and, recreating the cortical rim, they can also manage cortical defects eliminating the need for extensive bone grafting. The authors suggest using trabecular metal cones in all situations where the bone in this zone is sclerotic or when the defect is so large that a cemented fixation would result in a cement mantle greater than 7 mm, with the subsequent risk of fracture (Fig. 13.7). Augments and cones of trabecular metal can be available in different sizes and shapes and can also be custom-made with 3D-printing technology. Zone 3 fixation remains

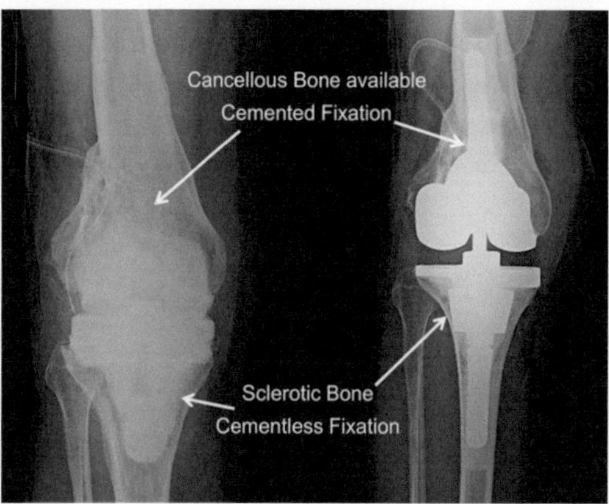

Fig. 13.7 An example of two different types of fixation in Zone 2 in the same joint. The metaphyseal bone of the femur is still available, so a cemented fixation is a valid solution. The metaphyseal bone of the tibia instead is no more available, with a big cavitary defect and with sclerotic bone interface. In this case, a cementless fixation with trabecular metal cone or sleeve is the best solution to achieve strong and long-lasting fixation

fundamental in revision TKA to protect the juxta-articular bone until the metaphyseal implant integration or in cases where zones 1 and 2 are completely absent. It is important to notice that a stem cannot be a substitute for optimal component fixation in a long-term follow-up; it plays only an adjunctive role in transferring the loads from the compromised metaphysis to the stronger diaphysis. The balance between overshielding and overloading the juxta-articular bone would provide zone 2 protection and avoid stress-shielding. Two methods of stem fixation are available: total cementation technique and hybrid technique with a cementless press-fit stem. The former technique is the most widely used. Based on the available literature, no superiority of any type of stem fixation has been found. Advantages of cemented stems include allowing for intraoperative adjustment in cases with osseous anatomical abnormalities, the ability to deliver antibiotics locally, a proven 10-year record of good results and the ability to gain satisfactory fixation in patients with large medullary canal diameter and severe osteopenia. Disadvantages with the use of cemented stems are centered on difficulty with removal, as substantial bone loss or fracture can occur. Cemented stems are preferred in patients with poor diaphyseal bone and large canal diameter; in patients whose canal geometry does not allow a reliable press-fit for uncemented stems and those with sclerotic or damaged metaphyseal bone (which results in inadequate fixation requiring extension of cementing into the diaphyseal canal). Cemented stem fixation allows the use of shorter stems, provides immediate fixation and, in infected revisions, allows the delivery of antibiotics. Advantages of cementless stems include ease use and removal in the early post-operative period, facilitation in gaining proper alignment when there are no extraarticular deformity or bowed diaphysis, and compatibility with most intramedullary-based revision instrumentation systems. Disadvantages of the use of cementless stems are the possible inferior immediate fixation, and distortion of proper condylar implant position in cases with anatomical deformities in either the metaphyseal or diaphyseal regions (Fig. 13.8). Cementless stems are indicated in

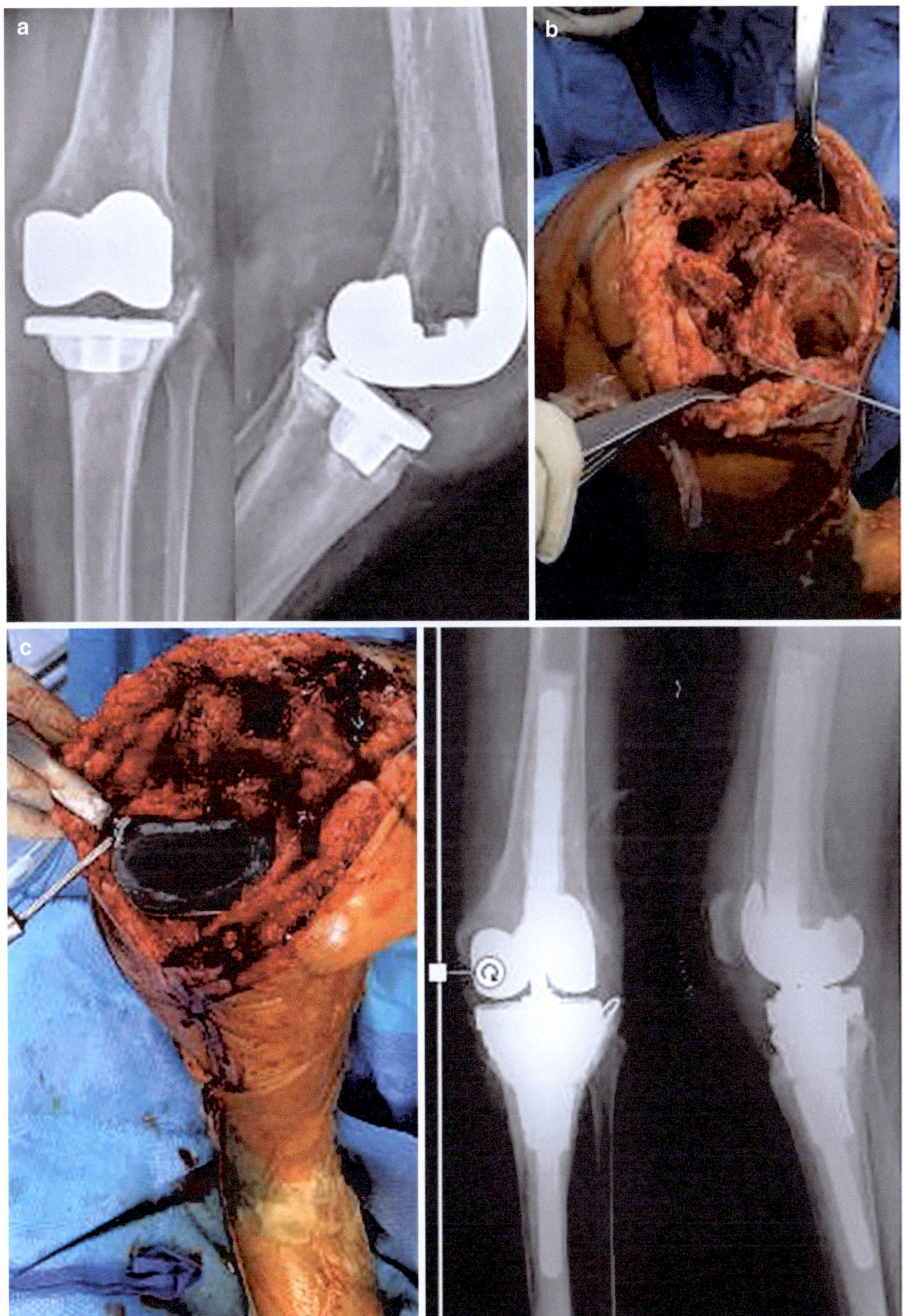

Fig. 13.8 The preoperative X-ray (**a** and **b**) and the intraoperative findings (**c**) show a deficient metaphysis on the tibia but an intact diaphysis. In this case, it is fundamental to obtain a strong fixation with a long cemented stem and with a diaphyseal trabecular metal cone, in order to transfer the load from the deficient and sclerotic metaphysis. In the metaphysis, a cone was placed with the purpose to fill the defect and to help the long-term stability of the implant with the bone ingrowth of lateral surface of the metaphysis

patients with good diaphyseal bone and favorable canal geometry allowing a press-fit engagement. Cementless stems are also preferred in the management of periprosthetic fracture and osteotomies. However, the optimal length and thickness of stems remain poorly defined for both cemented and uncemented designs [29].

The authors prefer, when possible, to use short cemented stem for fixation in the proximal part of zone 3. The reason for this choice is simple. In order to obtain a press-fit engagement with a cementless stem, it should reach the distant portion of the shaft which consequently "guides" most of the times the prosthesis in varus/valgus or in recurvatum/procurvatum. Using a short and thinner cemented stem, the position of the prosthesis is no more "guided" by the diaphysis but controlled by the surgeon and by the epiphyseal preparation. Moreover, stems without offset can be more easily accommodated into the inner diameter of cones.

Planning Soft-Tissue Management

Surgical Exposure

Previous surgical scars and the joint stiffness often result in a challenging joint exposure in revision knee surgery. It is important to review previous operative reports to assess the surgical approach used and the additional soft-tissue procedures performed. It is recommended to mark out scars around the joint before prepping and draping the limb. The use of the same previous skin incision is recommendable, in case of different surgical scars the lateral most is often used to prevent a devascularization of a large lateral skin flap. The vascular supply to the skin of the anterior knee is derived primarily from the medial side and in proximity of the joint line the vascularization is enhanced [30]. It is safe to ignore previous short skin incisions or to cross at a perpendicular angle transverse incision, such as those seen after high tibial osteotomies. Creation of skin flaps at acute angle of less than 60° at the intersection of the incisions is a risk for the blood supply. Skin vascularization is dependent to the

dermal plexus, which originates from perforators arterioles crossing the subcutaneous fascia. Undermining the skin to create large skin flaps especially in presence of a thin subcutaneous tissue could lead to a damage at the underlying plexus increasing the risk for skin necrosis. Short skin bridges of less than 6–7 cm between prior incisions and new one is not recommended. The workhorse approach to the knee is the medial para-patellar capsular incision for its extensile capabilities. Firstly, a sub-periosteal dissection of the medial structures of the proximal tibia with the release of the deep medial collateral ligament to the postero-medial capsule is advised. To gain adequate joint exposure intra-articular adhesions are released and wide resection of intra-articular pseudo-capsule is performed in the supra-patellar pouch, medial and lateral gutters. A lateral retinacular release and a lateral patellar facetectomy may be performed if difficulties with patellar mobility persist. It allows external rotation of the tibia, reduces tension on the extensor mechanism and exposes the proximal tibia. If additional medial release is needed, extend the subperiosteal dissection more distally on the medial tibia by elevating the superficial MCL. One or both collateral ligaments can be sacrificed, through epicondyles detachment, in stiff knees to improve the exposure. A partial release of the patellar ligament is avoided because of an increased incidence of later patellar ligament rupture. If exposure remains inadequate, extensile exposure options such as extended Tibial Tubercle Osteotomy (TTO) should be considered. With this maneuver, surgeons easily gain access to the lateral gutter, the most difficult-to-reach recess of the knee. Given the risk of post-operative extensor lag, a V-Y quadricepsplasty is not indicated. In extension contracted knees, where a flexion mobilization under anesthesia MUA is advisable, TTO should be performed after the maximum range of flexion is obtained. Performing the osteotomy before the MUA does not allow to effectively stretch the retracted quadriceps sarcomers. The patella can be everted at this point or merely subluxated laterally without eversion. We generally do not prefer everting the patella, as it may increase the risk of injury to the patellar tendon and is often unnecessary for adequate exposure [31]. The osteotomized tubercle can be fixed proximally in case of patella-liner impingement or medialized in case of chronic patellar dislocation and has to be at least 6–7 cm long and 2 cm thick [32]. Obtaining a good exposure is mandatory to start an efficient and safe implant removal phase to avoid major bone loss and periprosthetic fractures.

Constraint Choice

Instability, the third most common mode of failure in TKAs that occurs in 7.3–28.9% of the cases is defined as abnormal and excessive displacement of a knee prosthesis accompanied by clinical symptoms [33]. Obesity, rheumatoid arthritis, connective tissue diseases, severe osteoporosis and neuromuscular pathology are risk factors associated with post-operative instability. TKA instability is highly related with the preoperative limb deformity. Correction procedures, such as wide ligament releases, could lead to iatrogenic post-operative knee instability. Obesity has also been associated with the increased risk of instability because ligament injuries tend to occur for a more difficult surgical exposure and a thinner stretched ligament.

Different classifications have been proposed for instability following TKA, based on the type and the possible treatment strategy. Vince et al. [34] described four types of instability according to the direction of deforming force: (1) varus/valgus, (2) recurvatum, (3) A-P in flexion and (4) global types. Parratte and Pagnano [35] proposed three different types: (1) extension instability, (2) flexion instability and (3) genu recurvatum. Extension instability can be divided into symmetric and asymmetric. An excessive femoral and/or tibial bone resection may result in a symmetric extension instability. Asymmetric extension instability is frequently encountered in the clinical practice; it is mainly associated with insufficient correction of deformity for an improper soft-tissue release. Another common cause of asymmetric extension instability is iatrogenic injury to the collateral ligament during

surgery. It is important to notice the posterior capsule is tight in extension and to assess a real medio-lateral gap unbalance the joint should be flexed at 10–20°.

Flexion instability can be defined as the presence of the flexion gap larger than the extension gap. It is mostly due to an over-resection or a bone loss in revisions of the posterior femoral condyles and the consequent under-sizing of the femoral component. Therefore, sizing of the femoral component has to be based not only on the bone stock but also assessing flexion stability. Excessive internal or external rotation of the femoral component results in the creation of a trapezoidal flexion gap, thus surgeons should pay attention to the rotational alignment of the component in revision scenario.

Flexion instability can also occur for insufficiency of Posterior Cruciate Ligament (PCL) in patients with cruciate retaining implants. In these patients, the resultant inappropriate flexion gap could cause flexion instability and even a dislocation in severe cases that can be easily treated with an ultra-congruent insert or a posterior stabilized (PS) implant. Recurvatum following TKA is one of the most challenging deformities. It is caused by a damage or a laxity of the posterior capsule. It is a common finding in patients with an insufficiency of quadriceps muscle for neuro-muscular diseases and to a lesser degree in valgus knee especially in obese patients. Under-resection of the distal femur up to the use of specific implants is mandatory to prevent recurvatum in these patients.

As a result, the implant choice depends on the state of collateral ligaments and other peripheral stabilizers of the knee and is indirectly related to the severity of bone loss. Moreover, large exposures and releases often required in revision surgery or acquired bone loss could lead to more constrained implants. Surgical treatment modalities for instability include several different procedures, according to the patient's characteristics and type of instability, ranging from the exchange of polyethylene insert to complete revision TKA. Isolated polyethylene exchange is an attractive treatment with low morbidity in selected patients. This procedure can be performed only in case of proper alignment and stable fixation of both components. It is mainly used in cases of global instability, where the joint has a laxity in extension and flexion and the liner appears not thick enough: the TKA presents a mild recurvatum deformity and A-P instability at 90° of flexion. Secondly, liner exchange is a valuable option in case of posterior cruciate insufficiency in cruciate-retaining implants: in this case, an ultra-congruent polyethylene insert may be implanted if commercially available. Rarely this procedure is appropriate in varus/valgus ligamentous imbalance, stretching soft tissues on the tight compartment and stretching. Unfortunately, it is well known that the results of isolated polyethylene exchange are usually poor and unpredictable.

A partial or complete component revision is indicated when there is malalignment of the components or inadequate constraint options of the existing implant. The revision of femoral and tibial components allows realignment, correct flexion/extension gaps balancing, and restoration of the joint line. PS implants provide only A-P stability, but varus/valgus stability is not influenced: they are mainly used to substitute for the posterior cruciate ligament. Differently, a Condylar Constrained Knee system (CCK) can help stabilize the knee in a variety of planes: it provides A-P and varus/valgus stability, and it is used primarily as substitute of a deficient collateral ligaments. The height of the post helps prevent posterior dislocation and is generally taller than a posterior stabilized construct. Constraint differs between manufacturers regarding varus/ valgus and rotational freedom. Hinged implant is the most constrained type of TKA [36]. Its primary indications are severe distal femoral bone loss, recurvatum deformity, severe flexion gap instability which cannot be matched by the extension gap and totally disrupted medial and posteromedial structures with a positive valgus-stress test in full extension. This option should be considered even in case of isolated medial collateral ligament insufficiency in the elderly population. Hinged knee implants have limited usage among relatively young and active patients because they have been associated with increased risk of a sec-

ondary revision due to early loosening caused by excessive stress at the fixation interface. An "hyperfixation" consisting of an appropriate full cementation technique and a large use of osteointegrating cones and/or stems should be considered with these types of implants.

Conclusion

RTKAs have worse clinical and functional outcomes and a greater incidence of post-operative complications compared to primary arthroplasties. All this results in a worse implants survivorship. An accurate algorithm to diagnose the cause of failure and a precise reconstructive planning are mandatory in revision knee surgery. The underlying concept is that revising an implant without a clear diagnosis of failure inevitably leads to fail again.

References

1. Font-Rodriguez DE, Scuderi GR, Insall JN. Survivorship of cemented total knee arthroplasty. Clin Orthop Relat Res. 1997;345:79–86.
2. Kurtz S, Ong K, Lau E, Mowat F, Halpern M. Projections of primary and revision hip and knee arthroplasty in the United States from 2005 to 2030. J Bone Joint Surg Am. 2007;89(4):780–5.
3. Sierra RJ, Cooney WP 4th, Pagnano MW, Trousdale RT, Rand JA. Reoperations after 3200 revision TKAs: rates, etiology, and lessons learned. Clin Orthop Relat Res. 2004;425:200–6.
4. Mulhall KJ, Ghomrawi HM, Scully S, Callaghan JJ, Saleh KJ. Current etiologies and modes of failure in total knee arthroplasty revision. Clin Orthop Relat Res. 2006;446:45–50.
5. Suarez J, Griffin W, Springer B, Fehring T, Mason JB, Odum S. Why do revision knee arthroplasties fail? J Arthroplast. 2008;23(6 Suppl 1):99–103.
6. Petersen KK, Simonsen O, Laursen MB, Nielsen TA, Rasmussen S, Arendt-Nielsen L. Chronic postoperative pain after primary and revision total knee arthroplasty. Clin J Pain. 2015;31(1):1–6.
7. Hofmann S, Seitlinger G, Djahani O, Pietsch M. The painful knee after TKA: a diagnostic algorithm for failure analysis. Knee Surg Sports Traumatol Arthrosc. 2011;19(9):1442–52.
8. Baldini A, Castellani L, Traverso F, Balatri A, Balato G, Franceschini V. The difficult primary total knee arthroplasty: a review. Bone Joint J. 2015;97-B(10 Suppl A):30–9.

9. Meding JB, Keating EM, Ritter MA, Faris PM, Berend ME. Genu recurvatum in total knee replacement. Clin Orthop Relat Res. 2003;416:64–7.

10. aidya SV, Patel MR, Panghate AN, Rathod PA. Total knee arthroplasty: limb length discrepancy and functional outcome. Indian J Orthop. 2010;44(3):300–7. https://doi.org/10.4103/0019-5413.65159.

11. Rossi R, Dettoni F, Bruzzone M, Cottino U, D'Elicio DG, Bonasia DE. Clinical examination of the knee: know your tools for diagnosis of knee injuries. Sports Med Arthrosc Rehabil Ther Technol. 2011;3:25.

12. Colen DL, Carney MJ, Shubinets V, Lanni MA, Liu T, Levin LS, Lee GC, Kovach SJ. Soft-tissue reconstruction of the complicated knee arthroplasty: principles and predictors of salvage. Plast Reconstr Surg. 2018;141(4):1040–8.

13. Vyas P, Cui Q. Management options for extensor mechanism discontinuity in patients with total knee arthroplasty. Cureus. 2020;12(7):e9225.

14. Rodríguez-Merchán EC. The stiff total knee arthroplasty: causes, treatment modalities and results. EFORT Open Rev. 2019;4(10):602–10.

15. Vince KG. The stiff total knee arthroplasty: causes and cures. J Bone Joint Surg Br. 2012;94(11 Suppl A):103–11.

16. Kumar N, Yadav C, Raj R, Anand S. How to interpret postoperative X-rays after total knee arthroplasty. Orthop Surg. 2014;6(3):179–86.

17. Aderbacher G, Baier C, Benditz A, Wagner F, Greimel F, Grifka J, Keshmiri A. Presence of rotational errors in long leg radiographs after total knee arthroplasty and impact on measured lower limb and component alignment. Int Orthop. 2017;41(8):1553–60.

18. Kniesel B, Konstantinidis L, Hirschmüller A, Südkamp N, Helwig P. Digital templating in total knee and hip replacement: an analysis of planning accuracy. Int Orthop. 2014;38(4):733–9.

19. Pinski JM, Chen AF, Estok DM, Kavolus JJ. Nuclear medicine scans in total joint replacement. J Bone Joint Surg Am. 2021;103(4):359–72.

20. Schröder FF, Post CE, Wagenaar FBM, Verdonschot N. Huis In't veld RMHA. MRI as diagnostic modality for analyzing the problematic knee arthroplasty: a systematic review. J Magn Reson Imaging. 2020;51(2):446–58. https://doi.org/10.1002/jmri.26874. Epub 2019 Jul 22.

21. Saffi M, Spangehl MJ, Clarke HD, Young SW. Measuring tibial component rotation following total knee arthroplasty: what is the best method? J Arthroplast. 2019;34(7S):S355–60.

22. Sharkey PF, Hozack WJ, Rothman RH, et al. Insall award paper. Why are total knee arthroplasties failing today? Clin Orthop. 2002;404:7–13.

23. Engh GA, Ammeen D. Classification and preoperative radiographic evaluation: knee. Orthop Clin North Am. 1998;29:205–17.

24. Morgan-Jones R, Oussedik SI, Graichen H, Haddad FS. Zonal fixation in revision total knee arthroplasty. Bone Joint J. 2015;97-B(2):147–9.

25. Daines BK, Dennis DA. Management of bone defects in revision total kneearthroplasty. Instr Course Lect. 2013;62:341–8.

26. Ritter MA. Screw and cement fixation of large defects in total knee arthroplasty. JArthroplasty. 1986;1(2):125–9.

27. Clatworthy MG, Ballance J, Brick GW, Chandler HP, Gross AE. The use of structural allograft for uncontained defects in revision total knee arthroplasty. A minimum five-year review. J Bone Joint Surg Am. 2001;83(3):404–11.

28. Brown NM, Bell JA, Jung EK, Sporer SM, Paprosky WG, Levine BR. The use of trabecular metal cones in complex primary and revision total knee arthroplasty. J Arthroplast. 2015;30(9 Suppl):90–3. https://doi.org/10.1016/j.arth.2015.02.048.

29. Driesman AS, Macaulay W, Schwarzkopf R. Cemented versus cementless stems in revision total knee arthroplasty. J Knee Surg. 2019;32(8):704–9.

30. Haertsch PA. The blood supply to the skin of the leg: a post-mortem investigation. Br J Plast Surg. 1981;34:470–7.

31. Fehring TK, Odum S, Griffin WL, Mason JB. Patella inversion method for exposure in revision total knee arthroplasty. J Arthroplast. 2002;17(1):101–4.

32. Dolin MG. Osteotomy of the tibial tubercle in total knee replacement. J Bone Joint Surg Am. 1983;65:704–6.

33. Lombardi AV Jr, Berend KR. The role of implant constraint in revision TKA: striking the balance. Orthopedics. 2006;29:847–9.

34. Vince KG, Abdeen A, Sugimori T. The unstable total knee arthroplasty: causes and cures. J Arthroplast. 2006;21(4 Suppl 1):44–9.

35. Parratte S, Pagnano MW. Instability after total knee arthroplasty. Instr Course Lect. 2008;57:295–304.

36. Joshi N, Navarro-Quilis A. Is there a place for rotating-hinge arthroplasty in knee revision surgery for aseptic loosening? J Arthroplast. 2008;23:1204–11.

Periprosthetic Knee Infection: The Multidisciplinary Oxford Bone Infection Unit Experience

14

T. W. Hamilton, A. Vogt, A. J. Ramsden, M. Scarborough, and A. Alvand

Introduction

Knee periprosthetic joint infection (PJI) is the most common indication for early revision following arthroplasty [1]. Overall the incidence of PJI is between 1 and 2% following a primary arthroplasty, but significantly higher following revision procedures [2]. In addition to an increased number of arthroplasty surgeries (both primary and revision) being performed, the incidence of PJI has also been rising. As a consequence, the burden of PJI on healthcare providers and healthcare payers is increasing rapidly [3].

The Oxford Bone Infection Unit (BIU) is a specialist adult National Health Service (NHS) tertiary referral centre and regional hub for PJI that receives local, national and international referrals. We receive nearly 1000 osteoarticular referrals per year and are the highest volume centre for bone and joint infection management in the United Kingdom, including for knee PJI. In addition to non-arthroplasty infection work, over 500 revision arthroplasty surgeries are conducted each year at the Nuffield Orthopaedic Centre,

with 95% of these being revision hip and knee procedures [1].

The BIU consists of a 28 bedded inpatient ward at the Nuffield Orthopaedic Centre, Oxford. Referral to the BIU is by way of a standardised proforma which is triaged by a multi-disciplinary team. For the majority of cases, the initial review is in a multi-disciplinary outpatient clinic, but in some cases, an inpatient 72-h assessment is required. A minority of patients are admitted acutely through the emergency on-call system. Patients admitted are managed under the combined care of an orthopaedic surgeon and an infectious disease physician, as well as a plastic surgeon where appropriate.

The Multidisciplinary Team

The successful management of bone and joint infections is best achieved through the combination of complete and careful surgical debridement, primary wound closure and appropriate microbiological treatment.

There is increasingly compelling evidence that the optimal management of bone and joint infections can be improved through the involvement of a multidisciplinary team (MDT) [4]. This should include an orthopaedic surgeon, ideally with a specialist interest in bone and joint infections, a plastic surgeon, an infectious diseases physician or clinical microbiologist, a specialist

T. W. Hamilton · A. Vogt · A. J. Ramsden ·
M. Scarborough · A. Alvand (✉)
Bone Infection Unit, Nuffield Orthopaedic Centre,
Oxford University Hospitals NHS Foundation Trust,
Oxford, UK
e-mail: thomas.hamilton@ndorms.ox.ac.uk;
Alexander.Vogt@ouh.nhs.uk; Alex.Ramsden@ouh.
nhs.uk; Matthew.Scarborough@ouh.nhs.uk;
abtin.alvand@ndorms.ox.ac.uk

© The Author(s), under exclusive license to Springer Nature Switzerland AG 2023
A. J. Deshmukh et al. (eds.), *Surgical Management of Knee Arthritis*,
https://doi.org/10.1007/978-3-031-47929-8_14

musculoskeletal radiologist and experienced nursing and therapy staff. We strongly advocate face-to-face meetings of this group on a weekly basis if possible. The orthopaedic surgeon should feel confident in their ability to undertake the necessary debridement, facilitated where necessary by the plastic surgeons to achieve primary closure at the same operation. From an infection point of view, we would counsel against relying solely on telephone advice from the laboratory because direct patient contact frequently influences management pathways. In addition, there is a clear evidence that involvement of an experienced musculoskeletal infection specialist improves outcomes, with a recent study reporting a relative risk of treatment failure of 4.6 (95% confidence interval 2.3–8.9) if management is undertaken by the surgical team alone [5].

Diagnosis

Clinical Presentation

The diagnosis of bone and joint infection is based on several variables, the most important of which is the clinical presentation of the patient. Patients most commonly present with local signs and symptoms of infection and only rarely do they become systemically unwell. Patients with a draining sinus in particular are unlikely to develop signs of systemic sepsis, although the presence of an established sinus is almost pathognomonic of a deep infection. Various scoring systems and diagnostic criteria have been established for the diagnosis of PJI, incorporating a mixture of clinical signs, microbiological, biochemical and intra-operative findings [6–14].

Imaging

Radiological investigation of bone and joint infection is usually based upon plain radiographs and some form of cross-sectional imaging; the latter is used principally to define the extent of disease and in surgical planning. In our experience, bone scintigraphy is of very limited utility although we are increasingly finding PET-CT of

benefit where other diagnostic measures have proven inconclusive [15].

Blood Tests and Biopsies

Pre-operative laboratory investigations play a minor role in determining the presence or absence of PJI. In particular, the CRP (and ESR) is insufficiently sensitive or specific to provide useful standalone information and should not be used in isolation for the diagnosis or exclusion of infection. Similarly, the CRP has a limited role in monitoring treatment response during therapy, with much more useful information being derived from the patient's symptoms and examination findings [16]. We do not routinely rely on other systemic inflammatory markers or intra-operative biochemical tests, although these are continuously evaluated during ongoing research studies.

The use of pre-operative biopsy is generally reserved for specific circumstances such as when an exotic infection or neoplasia form part of the differential, or where the choice and use of local antibiotics is likely to be an important consideration during surgery, particularly if there is a high chance of antibiotic resistance. The problem with pre-operative biopsy is that it yields only a limited number of samples, is prone to sampling error and it poses additional infection risks to the patient. We take the view that, if the patient is to undergo surgical intervention, optimal sampling is best achieved under direct vision at the time of surgery. Biopsy can of course reasonably be used when no surgical intervention is planned and/or suppressive therapy is likely to be the mainstay of treatment.

Intra-operative Sampling

To maximise the chance of identifying the infecting organism, we strongly believe in a rigorous standardised sampling framework. The pathway includes a period of at least 2 weeks off antibiotics prior to surgery where possible. In the majority of cases, this poses very little risk to the patient, but antibiotics should not be withheld where they are considered necessary, for example, in cases of overt sepsis.

We advocate the omission of pre-operative prophylactic antibiotics until deep surgical samples have been obtained. Deep surgical samples should be taken as soon as possible after the skin incision and prior to significant manipulation of the surgical site. Each sample should be taken with a clean set of surgical instruments and each sample should be separately labelled as to its anatomical source. We recommend five deep samples be sent for microbiology and at least two for histopathology in all cases of suspected or possible infection. We have demonstrated that this is the optimum number of samples to obtain the greatest yield in terms of diagnostic accuracy [17]. Samples should include any grossly infected or abnormal looking tissue, pus, periprosthetic membrane, avascular bone and pannus. Provided that deep samples have been obtained early during surgery, and with a no-touch technique, the surgeon's gloves should be clean at the end of the sampling framework. If this is achieved, the surgical team can be reassured that the risk of intraoperative contamination of the samples has been minimised.

Interpretation of Laboratory Results

A microbiological diagnosis is most likely if at least two deep surgical samples yield a phenotypically indistinguishable microorganism on culture [17]. Generally speaking, if a low virulent organism such as coagulase negative staphylococcus is obtained from only one sample out of five, it is likely that this represents contamination. On the other hand, if multiple samples yield the same organism, this is almost certainly the pathogen involved in the deep infection. Of note, surface swabs are notoriously unreliable for diagnosis because discharging wounds or sinuses are often colonised by skin organisms, which don't necessarily reflect the deep pathogen. For this reason, we advise against submission of an excised ulcer or sinus tract for microbiological diagnosis, although such a specimen may be sent for histopathology to exclude neoplastic transformation in a chronic discharging wound.

The utility of sonication of implant components remains a subject of debate. Data from our unit suggest that there is an additive effect with sonication samples but that this does not replace the established framework for tissue sampling [18].

Using histopathological diagnosis of infection as the gold standard comparator, the above technique allows a microbiological diagnosis in approximately 80% of infected cases: the remainder are considered culture negative and are treated empirically (or according to previous microbiological isolates). It is critically important that clinicians do not interpret a negative culture as being sufficient evidence to exclude active infection.

Infectious Disease Management

Antibiotic Choice

Empiric Antibiotic Choice

The most important variable governing the choice of antibiotic is the susceptibility of the infecting organism. Optimisation of a microbiological diagnosis is, therefore, a priority. Additional variables to consider when choosing the most appropriate antibiotic include the pharmacokinetics, history of drug allergy or intolerance, potential drug interactions, cost and convenience.

Immediately after completion of surgical sampling, patients are usually given intravenous meropenem and vancomycin: this combination has previously been shown to provide the most effective empiric cover [19]. Post-operatively, the meropenem is normally discontinued after 48 h of incubation if no gram-negative organisms have been identified. The vancomycin continues pending final culture results.

Directed Antibiotic Treatment

Staphylococcal Infections

Provided that the susceptibility pattern supports it, we would normally treat staphylococcal infections with the combination of rifampicin and one other highly bioavailable oral agent. Rifampicin should never be used as a monotherapy due to the risk of emergence of resistance. Whilst some specialists would restrict adjunctive rifampicin therapy to metalwork-related infection, we generally use it more widely, most commonly combined with ciprofloxacin. Alternative rifampicin combinations frequently include doxycycline, clindamycin and co-trimoxazole. Where the susceptibility pattern is less favourable, it may be necessary to use other agents, such as linezolid or an intravenous antibiotic. In this context, adjunctive rifampicin therapy is less commonly invoked. If intravenous therapy is deemed necessary, ceftriaxone and teicoplanin are the most commonly used agents. Preference for these agents is partially based upon the convenience they afford through once daily dosing. In order to improve our antimicrobial stewardship, we are now increasingly making use of continuous infusions of flucloxacillin through Silastic pumps where susceptibilities allow.

Streptococci and Enterococci

Amoxicillin is the most commonly used oral agent in the treatment of streptococcal infection. Although it has some limitations and variation in oral bioavailability, there seems to be little evidence in favour of other agents. If the patient is unable to take amoxicillin, alternative oral agents may include clindamycin, doxycycline or linezolid.

Enteric Gram-Negative Infections

Once the microbiological diagnosis has been established, monotherapy with any of the following agents may be appropriate: amoxicillin, co-amoxiclav, ciprofloxacin, co-trimoxazole, cefalexin. Patient factors determining which agent to use include variables such as QT interval, comorbidities, drug intolerances and perceived risk of complications, such as C. difficile.

Pseudomonas

Given the strong preference on our unit for oral therapy where possible, ciprofloxacin is the main anti-pseudomonal agent used. The dose for pseudomonas is normally 750 mg twice daily (as compared to 500 mg bd for most other gram-negative organisms).

Culture Negative Infection

Culture negative infections are normally treated as for staphylococcal disease unless there is previous microbiology to guide choice of therapy, or histopathology suggesting a specific alternative diagnosis.

Dose of Antibiotic

Factors that influence the dose of therapy include the mechanism of action of the individual antibiotic (some agents rely on the maximal concentration achieved whilst others rely on the time available above the minimum inhibitory concentration), the half-life of individual agents (and therefore the dosing interval), the oral bioavailability, the bone penetration and the activity against sessile organisms in a biofilm.

For most agents, the most appropriate dose is established according to its pharmacokinetics. However, in some cases, the dose must be adjusted according, for example, to renal function, concomitant medications and patient weight. For a small number of agents, therapeutic drug monitoring can be used to limit the risk of toxicity whilst maintaining efficacy.

Route of Antibiotic Therapy

For many years, we believed that intravenous therapy was required for the optimal treatment of bone and joint infections. However, recent evidence suggests that there is no advantage of intravenous therapy and we now preferentially rely on carefully selected, highly bioavailable oral therapy where possible [20]. Oral therapy has the advantages of earlier hospital discharge, fewer complications related to intravascular access devices and considerable savings to the health economy. For patients in whom there is no oral option available, either because of the reported susceptibilities or because of patient factors such as drug intolerances, intravenous therapy is usually administered via a peripherally inserted central catheter (PICC) line in the community.

Local antibiotic therapy, implanted at the time of surgery, is increasingly used in orthopaedics. Whilst there is no compelling prospective evidence that this approach can be used effectively without concomitant systemic therapy, observational studies suggest that local therapy may provide significant benefit. The theoretical advantages of local therapy include the high local concentration of antibiotic at the sight of infection, the limited systemic exposure/toxicity, reduced selection pressure for resistance as compared to oral or IV antibiotics, confidence in treatment adherence and the utility of the local carrier compound as a dead space filler at the time of surgery.

Duration of Therapy

The duration of therapy in orthopaedic infection is poorly defined but, based on emerging evidence, is becoming shorter over time. Generally speaking, patients with retained metalwork after surgery (e.g., after DAIR [debridement, antibiotics and implant retention] or single stage revision) are treated for longer than patients without metalwork in situ. A retrospective review of hip and knee arthroplasty infection managed by DAIR at our centre showed that there was no advantage of extending therapy beyond 6 months [21]. A more recent prospective study suggests that, in staphylococcal infection of prosthetic hip joints managed by DAIR, 8 weeks of therapy was not inferior to 12 weeks of therapy. Unfortunately, the study was discontinued before sufficient data had been collected to inform optimal duration for prosthetic knee joint infection [22]. In the absence of prosthetic material, 6 weeks of therapy is probably non-inferior to 12 weeks of therapy: the most compelling evidence for this comes from a prospective study in pyogenic vertebral osteomyelitis [23].

In addition to the presence or absence of metal where, duration of therapy may be influenced by the adequacy of the surgical clearance of abnormal tissue. In some cases, prolonged or indefinite suppressive therapy is indicated where the risk of treatment failure is high and the options for further surgical intervention are limited. In general, patients undergoing knee DAIR or single stage revision for infected TKR receive 6 months of antibiotics, and those undergoing two stage revision surgery receive 6 weeks of antibiotics after their first stage.

Surgical Management

Surgical treatment of PJI remains the gold standard. Whilst long-term antibiotic suppression is used in select patients, this is often not tolerated and there are concerns about the development of resistance in the longer term. The type of surgical management needs to be tailored to the patient and their pathology in the context of the patient's wishes about their care.

Surgical management has two goals:

- Identify the causative agent
- Eradicate the infection

Surgical Strategy

Every case is discussed in the MDT in order to agree surgical strategy based on host factors, infecting organism factors and prior history. Surgical options, listed in order from the least to most invasive, include:

- Debridement, Antibiotics and Implant Retention (DAIR) (Fig. 14.1)
- Single Stage Revision (Fig. 14.2)
- Two Stage Revision (Fig. 14.3)
- Arthrodesis (Fig. 14.4)
- Amputation (Fig. 14.5)

As the surgical options become more invasive, there is, at the population level, a higher chance of infection eradication. However, with increasing level of invasiveness comes lower functional outcomes, as well as increased morbidity and cost [24].

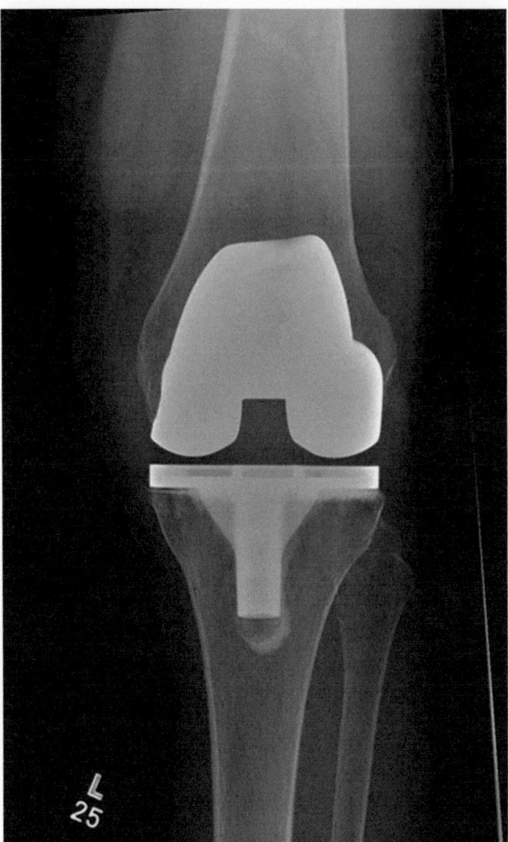

Fig. 14.1 DAIR: A 73-year-old patient presents 4 weeks after a primary total knee arthroplasty with a clinically infected knee and aspirate which cultured *Staphylococcus Aureus*. DAIR with exchange of modular components was undertaken with antibiotics for 6 months from the date of DAIR

Whilst in some cases more invasive surgical management is required to eradicate the infective organism, with appropriate case selection and antimicrobial therapy, we believe that the outcomes of less invasive surgery can deliver similar eradication rates, together with better functional outcomes and lower morbidity. Therefore, where appropriate, our preference is to offer single stage revision surgery where possible. We must stress, however, that this is an MDT decision that is discussed in detail with the patient prior to surgery, as well as being based on recent evidence-based guidelines [25].

Debridement, Antibiotics and Implant Retention

DAIR is considered where it is felt that there is a window of opportunity to intervene surgically prior to the establishment of a mature biofilm. It is frequently used in acute infection, either early postoperative or late haematogenous cases, as the success of DAIR decreases with chronicity [26]. There is controversy around the time frame for which DAIR is indicated but the chance of treatment failure is significantly reduced if DAIR is performed early in the course of an infection. However, important factors that should be considered prior to proceeding with DAIR include the history, host and infecting organism. Absolute contraindications to DAIR are loose, unstable or poorly functioning components. Relative contraindications to DAIR are the presence of a draining sinus and/or the immunocompromised patients. Whilst the absence of a pre-operative microbiological diagnosis is not a contraindication to DAIR, if the organism is known to be difficult to treat (e.g., fungi or multi-drug resistant bacteria), we would usually opt for an alternative surgical strategy.

DAIR should be performed by an experienced surgical team using an open approach. During DAIR, modular components should be removed and exchanged to reduce the bioburden and to allow access to all parts of well-fixed implants. A more detailed description of the DAIR technique has previously been published by our group [27]. The primary role for arthroscopic surgery is to stabilise the septic patient who is in extremis, in which case, the definitive surgical procedure should be performed shortly thereafter.

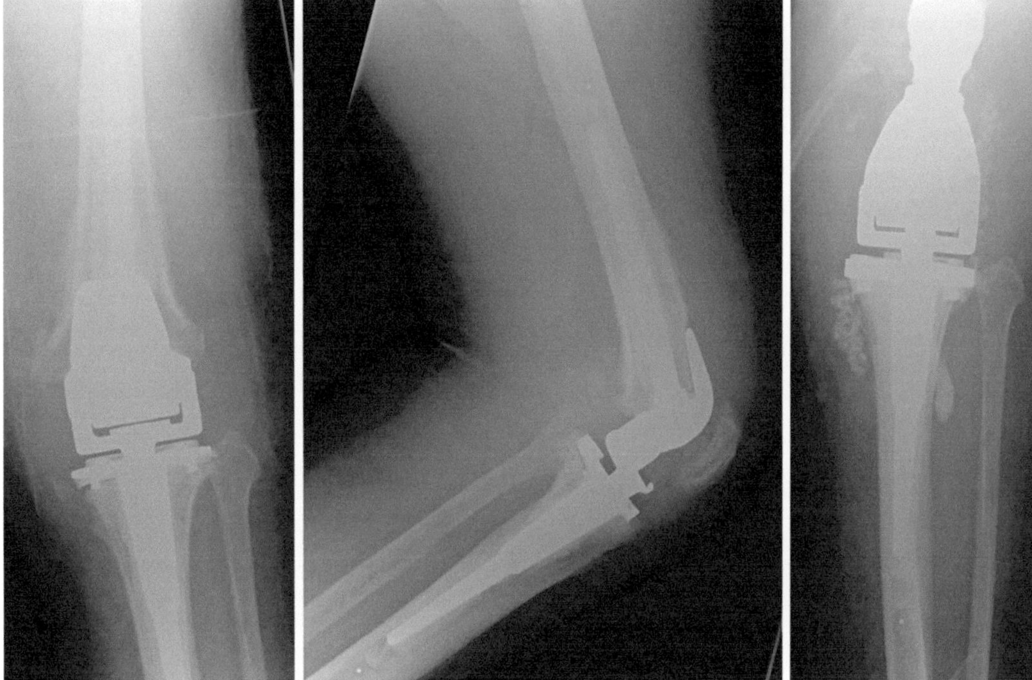

Fig. 14.2 Single Stage Revision: A 69-year-old patient presented with an infected, loose, knee arthroplasty. *Staphylococcus Aureus* was isolated from pre-operative ultrasound-guided biopsy. A single stage revision distal femoral replacement was performed with antibiotics for 6 months from the date of surgery

Single Stage Revision

Single stage revision is the most common treatment for PJI in Europe [28]. It involves removal of all implants (including the patella button), sampling, debridement, irrigation and then re-implantation of a new definitive prosthesis in a clean surgical bed during the same operation. Relative contra-indications include severe sepsis, failure of a previous single stage revision, culture negative infection, where the appropriate antibiotics cannot be determined, highly virulent or multi-drug resistant organisms (especially those for which no local antibiotic options are available), fungi, and where radical debridement is not possible, for example, where the neurovascular bundles are involved, or where there is severe bone loss and soft tissue damage that would compromise primary wound closure [25].

Two Stage Revision

Two stage revision is the most common treatment for PJI in North America and involves a minimum of two operations. During the first stage, there is removal of all implants (including the patella button), sampling, debridement, irrigation, and insertion of an antibiotic-loaded spacer, followed by wound closure. The patient then receives systemic antimicrobials, as dictated by the infectious disease team, before re-implantation of the definitive prosthesis when the treating team consider the infection to be controlled, based on clinical judgement, laboratory, and radiological findings. We do not routinely aspirate the joint prior to the second stage reimplantation as culture of synovial fluid from a joint with an antibiotic-loaded cement spacer in situ has been shown to have low sensitivity for dem-

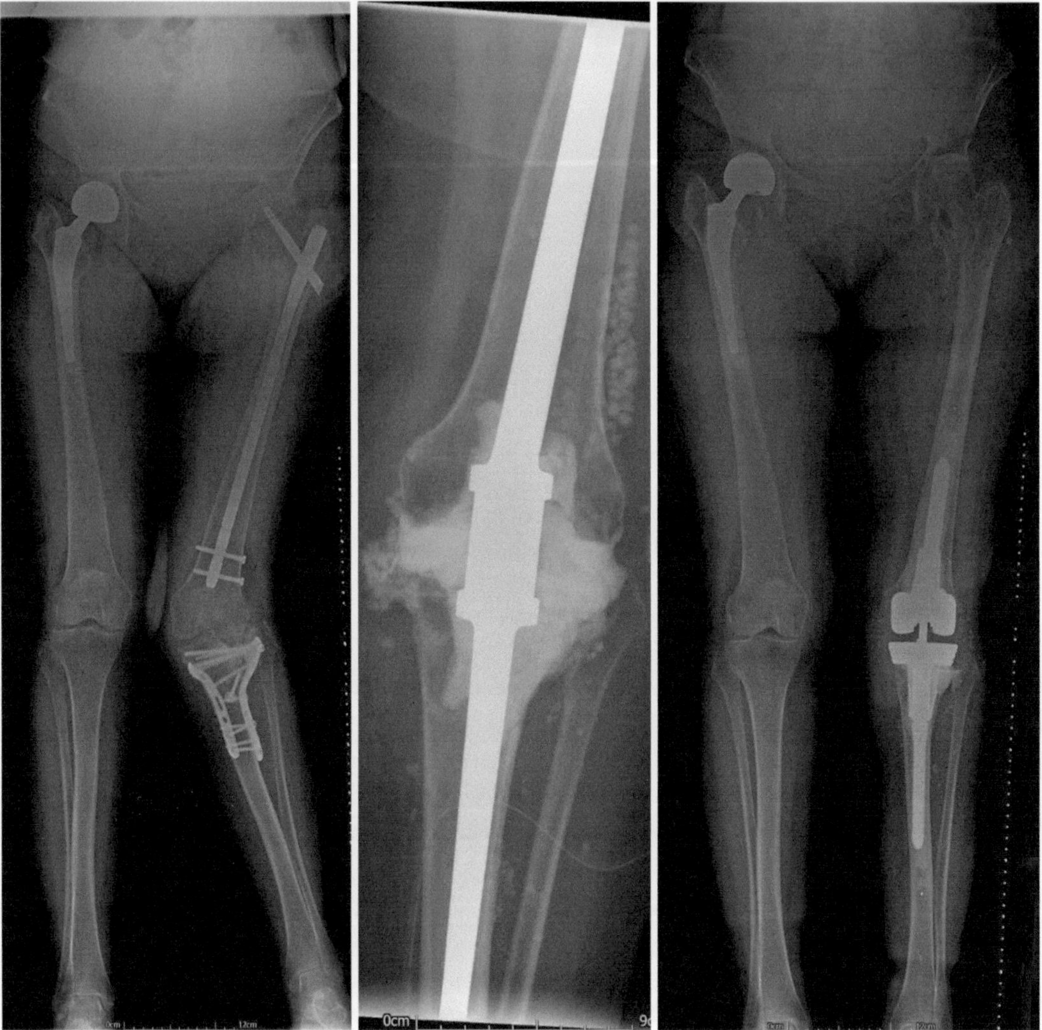

Fig. 14.3 Two Stage Revision: A 78-year-old patient presents with chronically infected metalwork and multiple sinuses of the left knee. A two stage revision was performed. During the first stage, the metal work was removed from the tibia and femur, a temporary arthrodesis nail cemented in situ with antibiotic-laden cement and medial and lateral pedicled gastrocnemius muscle flaps with split skin grafting placed. The patient received 6 weeks antibiotics after their first stage before their second stage procedure where definitive implants were placed

onstrating persistence of infection. If the infection remains uncontrolled, it may be necessary to repeat the first stage procedure.

Once the infection is considered irradicated, definitive reimplantation occurs; this is the second stage of the two stage procedure. At the time of reimplantation, it is very important that further samples are taken as previously described. Patients with positive microbiology at this point receive further antibiotics, as the presence of organisms during the second stage has been shown to correlate with higher rates of failure and early reinfection. Once sampling is complete, further formal debridement and irrigation is performed prior to implantation of the definitive prosthesis.

Two stage revision is indicated in cases of severe sepsis with haemodynamic compromise, infection with highly virulent or multi-drug resistant organisms or fungi, cases with severe bone and/or soft tissue loss that compromises primary wound closure, cases in which radical debride-

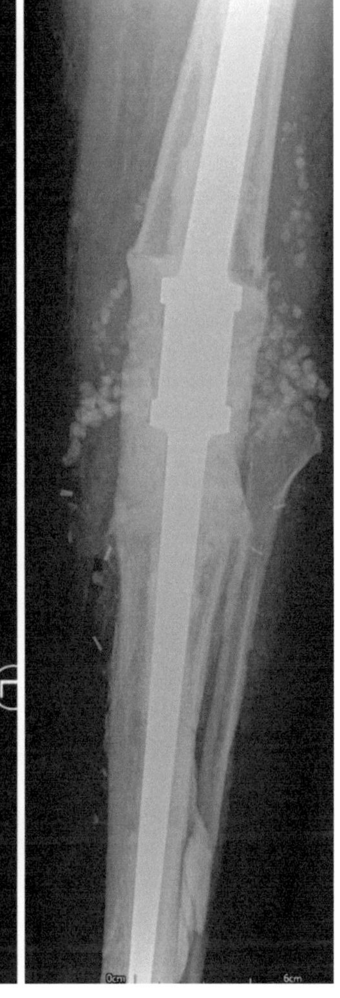

Fig. 14.4 Arthrodesis: An 87-year-old patient presented with an exposed, chronically infected, prosthesis and deficient extensor mechanism. They had declined amputation on several occasions at peripheral centres. A single stage cemented arthrodesis nail was placed with antibiotics for 6 months from the date of surgery. Primary closure was achieved by the plastic surgeons facilitated by patellectomy and medial and lateral pedicled gastrocnemius muscle flaps with split skin grafting

ment is not possible due to the involvement of neurovascular structures or when a prior single stage revision has failed [25].

Arthrodesis

Where there have been multiple attempts at infection irradiation, or where the joint is unreconstructable on account of bone or soft-tissue loss or extensor mechanism failure, arthrodesis may be considered as an option for limb salvage. The aim of the procedure is to give the patient a stable, pain-free limb on which to mobilise. There are multiple methods to achieve arthrodesis including external fixator, or internal plate fixation; however, our preference is for intra-medullary nail fixation.

Amputation

Amputation is used as a last resort for the management of PJI with both hip and knee amputation resulting in significant functional deficit. Mobilisation with a prosthetic limb (as compared to native limb) requires considerably more energy

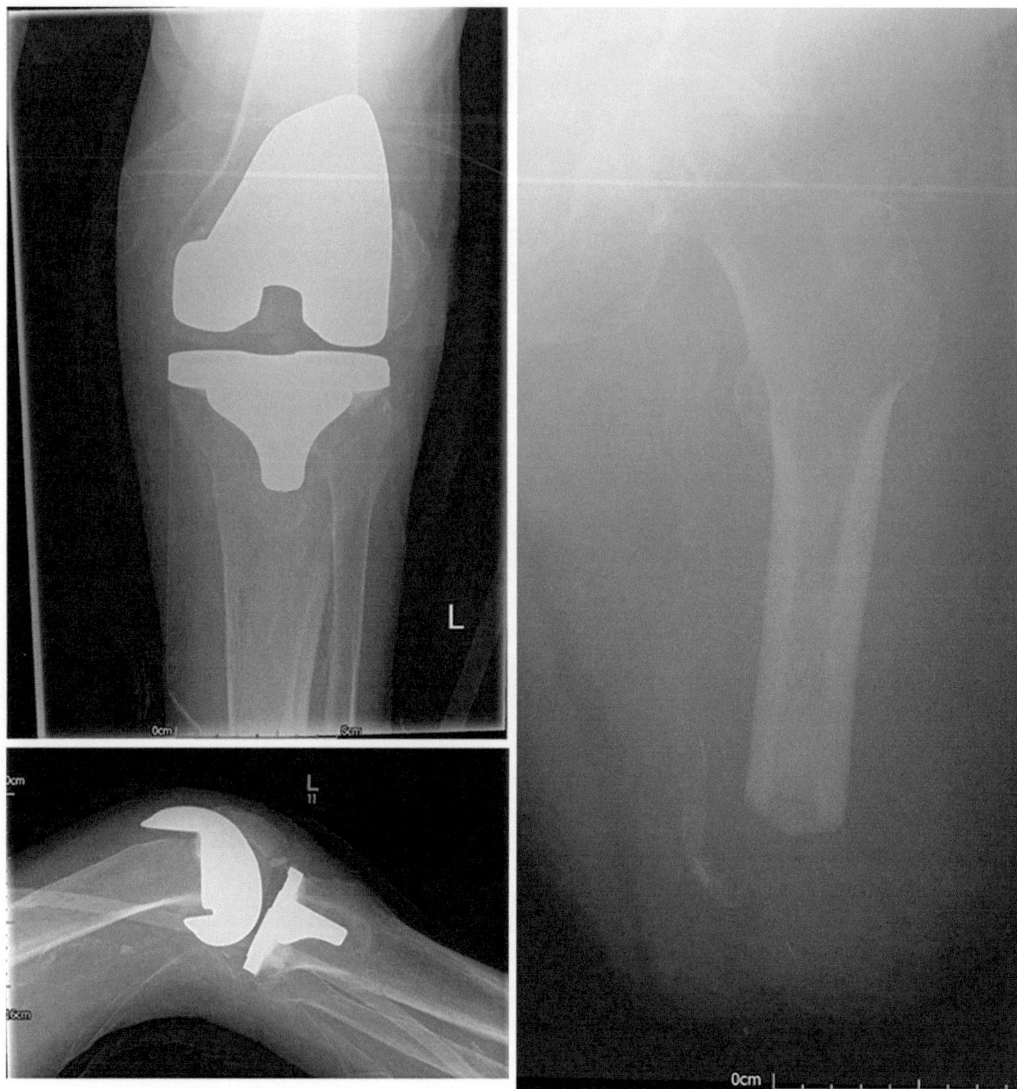

Fig. 14.5 Amputation: A 73-year-old patient with multiple comorbidities presented with bilateral chronically infected total knee arthroplasty with exposed implants and draining sinuses. Due to the multiple comorbidities, a decision was made to perform single stage revisions at separate sittings as it was not felt that they would survive multiple surgeries. During the right, contralateral, knee revision, the patient had an intra-operative myocardial infarction and cerebrovascular accident. Following MDT discussion, including discussion with the patient and their family, they were not considered fit for any further reconstructive options of the left knee and amputation was performed. The right knee distal femoral replacement remains infection-free at 1 year

and poses a significant risk of the loss of independence. Where amputation is considered, patients are pre-operatively counselled as to these risks by a doctor specialising in rehabilitation medicine. Where appropriate, review is arranged with the limb-fitting service pre-emptively to aid surgical planning and optimise rapid rehabilitation.

Key Surgical Considerations

Patients undergoing revision for infection are at high risk of morbidity and mortality. To optimise outcomes, in addition to being discussed at BIU MDT, all cases are additionally presented at a weekly joint reconstruction meeting to discuss the technical aspects of surgery. Because primary closure in the revision arthroplasty population can be challenging, and a high proportion of patients have factors that compromise wound healing, we have a low threshold for plastic surgery involvement. Overall, around 30% of our surgical cases involve plastic surgeons.

There are some key surgical considerations in patients with knee PJI, independent of the surgical strategy pursued. The following section outlines our approach.

Pre-operative

Risk Factors and Patient Optimisation

Prior to surgery, patients are assessed in a nurse-led pre-operative assessment clinic with a consultant anaesthetic review where appropriate. Additional consultations from other specialties, particularly cardiology, vascular, respiratory and endocrine are arranged where necessary. Particular attention is paid to optimising diabetic control (HBA1c <8.5%, 69 mmol/mol) and anaemia (Hb $\geq$13.0 g/dL), as well as ensuring that the patient is not malnourished. Ideally, patients are fully optimised prior to surgery, except in emergency cases [29, 30].

Staphylococcus Decolonisation

Our institution has adopted a universal decolonisation policy. Local practice is that all patients undergo nasal swab to assess for MRSA colonisation 2 weeks before surgery followed by, in all patients, decolonisation treatment. The rationale for assessing for MRSA colonisation is that it may inform the timing of surgery (MRSA colonised patients are placed last on the theatre list if possible), the choice of antimicrobial therapy and use of single rooms on the ward. Staphylococcal decolonisation usually consists of a topical nasal chlorhexidine with neomycin cream (Naseptin, Alliance Pharmaceuticals Limited) together with a chlorhexidine skin wash. For MRSA colonised patients, the topical nasal chlorhexidine with neomycin cream is applied three times daily for 5 days prior to surgery, and the chlorhexidine wash (HiBiScrub 4%, Molnlycke Health Care Ltd) is used for a similar duration twice a day. In patients with an allergy to either chlorhexidine or neomycin (or a peanut or soya allergy),

Mupirocin (Bactroban 2% cream, GlaxoSmithKline UK Ltd) is used. If patients have an allergy to the chlorhexidine, Octenisan antimicrobial wash (Schulke) is used. In patients not MRSA colonised, independent of known MSSA colonisation, topical nasal chlorhexidine with neomycin cream is applied three times daily for 1 day prior to surgery and the chlorhexidine wash (HiBiScrub 4%, Molnlycke Health Care Ltd) is used the night before and on the morning of surgery only. Patients are not routinely swabbed to confirm decolonisation.

Intra-operative

Surgical Incision

Often, this patient group has had multiple previous operations and the limb may already be significantly scarred. Careful consideration of the methods for wound closure should be considered pre-operatively and the surgical incision should not put at risk the vascular supply to the local skin or 'burn bridges' for later reconstruction. Plastic surgical advice and formal involvement in the surgical procedure should be sought for almost all cases other than the simplest wounds.

Multiple previous skin incisions should be evaluated carefully. The blood supply to the skin over the anterior aspect of the knee is fasciocutaneous. It arises from the deep perforators which are predominantly located along the medial side of the joint and provide the dominant contribution. Thus, when multiple longitudinal incisions are present, the lateral most incision should be used. In most circumstances, a medially based full thickness skin flap can then be raised to allow access to the medial aspect of the patella, medial parapatellar region and subsequent access to the joint. In some circumstances, a lateral parapatellar approach may be needed. Transverse incisions can be crossed with a new longitudinal incision at 90°, and short oblique incisions that are near the midline can be incorporated into new longitudinal incisions. Scars from prior incisions should preferentially be utilised as parallel scars can lead to skin necrosis if the skin bridge between the old and the new incisions is less than around 5 cm [31]. The length of the incision should be adequate to ensure that the apices are not under excessive tension which may impar subsequent healing.

The flaps raised to access the joint should be as thick as practical and contain skin, fat and fascia to preserve the dermal blood supply which is critical for skin healing. Skin flaps should be handled carefully, and care is taken to prevent damage from excessive retraction or pressure from bone levers.

Tissue Sampling

To maximise the chance of identifying the infecting organism, we perform a rigorous standardised sampling framework previously described [17]. Pre-operative prophylactic antibiotics are withheld until deep surgical samples have been obtained in all cases where infection is suspected. For second stage re-implantations where infection is no longer suspected, antibiotics are given at induction. The surgical samples are taken as soon as possible after the skin incision, and prior to significant manipulation of the surgical wound with the sole aim of reducing contamination of samples. We recommend five deep samples be sent for microbiology and at least two for histopathology in all cases of suspected or possible infection. Each sample is taken with a clean set of surgical instruments so that each sample is totally independent from the others and separately labelled as to its anatomical source. For the knee, we aspirate the joint after skin incision, but before arthrotomy, to minimise skin contamination. Care is taken not to violate the joint (particularly with the tip of the overly helpful assistant's suction catheter), with samples systematically taken from the following areas:

- Suprapatellar recess
- Medial and lateral gutters
- Fat pad
- Posterior capsule
- +/− Prosthetic bone membrane in the tibia and femur

Following sampling, antibiotics can be given and a formal radical synovectomy performed which improves access to the joint.

Irrigation

Following radical synovectomy, debridement and removal of prosthesis/modular components, lavage of

the joint is performed with a minimum of 6 litres of 0.05% chlorhexidine gluconate; the latter has been shown to be superior to 0.9% saline lavage in vitro [32]. In addition to chlorhexidine gluconate lavage, a 3-min dilute sterile povidine-iodine soak is routinely performed [33]. The exception is DAIR of a unicompartmental knee arthroplasty where 0.9% saline is used and delivered by syringe to protect the retained compartment from chemical or mechanical damage. Where DAIR is performed, the well-fixed components should be scrubbed with a soft nail brush to disrupt any biofilm.

Local Antibiotics

Antibiotics/anti-fungals can be delivered locally through antibiotic-loaded cement and/or absorbable antibiotic carriers. The antimicrobial therapy can be targeted at the infective organism with high local antibiotic concentrations being achieved. In cement spacers, large concentrations of antibiotics (up to 20% of total spacer mass) may be used. Hand mixing the cement (i.e., non-vacuum mix) incorporates air bubbles which increase the surface area and lead to greater antibiotic elution. The antibiotic choice is pre-operatively discussed with the infectious disease team. In addition to antibiotic-loaded cement, we also use absorbable calcium phosphate antibiotic carriers. Again, these can be tailored to the causative organism and are used to deliver antibiotics to the joint cavity at levels significantly higher than minimum bactericidal concentrations [34].

Haemostasis

Prior to closure, it is important to obtain adequate haemostasis. At induction, and prior to tourniquet inflation, patients are given 1 g tranexamic acid intravenously and a further 1 g dose of tranexamic acid intravenously is administered upon release of the tourniquet. Tourniquet release is typically performed following the initial debridement and prior to implantation of a spacer or implants as this permits access to the posterior aspect of the knee for haemostasis. At the end of the procedure, following closure of the capsule, 1 g tranexamic acid is also given intraarticularly to provide further pharmacologic and hydrostatic haemostasis. The use of drains is decided on a case-by-case basis, but overall is decreasing.

Closure

Wound closure is a critical part of the operation and should not be overlooked. If there is any doubt that simple direct closure cannot be achieved, advice is sought from the plastic surgical team *before* surgery. It may be advisable to ensure availability of plastic surgeons and accept that sometimes they will not in fact be required, rather than to struggle with the final operative step. In most patients, direct closure in standard fashion is best but commonly in knee PJI, the soft tissues can be tight and difficult to close. This is most often seen at the distal end of a midline incision over the proximal tibia, or when a sinus has been excised. We have a low threshold of using local flaps to close these wounds. This has multiple benefits: it covers metalwork, bone and tendon with well-vascularised tissue, it helps to obliterate dead space, it delivers antibiotics and helps to take tension away from local skin edges and soft tissues. In a two stage reconstruction, a flap is used in the first stage with a spacer that is larger than the proposed definitive implant. This results in easier closure and healing at the definitive second stage when wound healing needs to be optimal.

The workhorse flap is the gastrocnemius muscle flap and skin graft, delivered through a subcutaneous tunnel [35, 36]. This is robust, quick, reliable and has a low donor site morbidity. Typically, a medial gastrocnemius muscle flap is used but the lateral gastrocnemius muscle can be used for lateral wounds, or in addition to a medial flap for larger wounds. The lateral gastrocnemius flap, however, has the disadvantage of being smaller and may risk peroneal nerve damage, so is typically held in reserve. If the defect is too large, or if local flaps have been used before, then we generally move up to free tissue transfer using the latissimus dorsi muscle flap as this can cover virtually any defect around the knee. There are a wide range of other flaps available but are rarely needed in our experience. Importantly, if the distal tip of a flap fails, then we will not wait for the inevitable tip necrosis with exposure and reinfection of the implant but will aggressively proceed to further flap coverage in order to salvage the implant.

Post-operative

Negative Pressure Dressings

Negative pressure dressings do not compensate for inadequate surgical debridement or failure of meticulous wound closure. Where issues with wound healing are observed, it is paramount that the patient is clinically evaluated as to whether the underlying PJI has been cleared; we have a low threshold for repeat surgery in this patient group. The use of negative pressure dressings in the untreated PJI delays the definitive treatment, leads to extensive fibrosis of the surrounding tissues and proliferation of the underlying biofilm. The role of *closed-incision negative pressure dressings* immediately post-operatively, with the aim to reduce swelling and promote wound healing, has not been fully defined but shows promise and we are currently evaluating these in our high-risk patients.

Splinting

Stabilisation of the soft tissues around a joint in the early post-operative period is important to aid healing. In cases where the soft tissues might benefit or when flaps are used, a cricket pad splint is used for a variable period following the procedure.

Anticoagulation

Post-operatively, patients with PJI are at an increased risk of deep vein thrombosis and pulmonary embolism. In this patient group, a balance needs to be found between reducing the risk of thromboembolism yet avoiding wound complications that arise as a result of overzealous anti-coagulation [37]. The optimum regimen is determined by local and national guidelines. In this patient group, it is particularly important to assess for other bleeding risks, including medication for primary and secondary prevention of cardiac disease, particularly as the use of these medications is overrepresented in this patient population.

Conclusion

PJI is a devastating complication following joint arthroplasty. To optimise outcomes, a structured approach should be taken and delivered by a multi-disciplinary team. It is vital to appreciate that the successful management of bone and joint infections is best achieved through the combination of complete and careful surgical debridement, primary wound closure and appropriate microbiological treatment, and that failure of any of these components will compromise outcomes.

References

1. National Joint Registry for Endlgnad, Wales, Northern Ireland and the Isle of Man 16th Annual Report. 2019.
2. Ahmed SS, et al. Risk factors, diagnosis and management of prosthetic joint infection after total hip arthroplasty. Expert Rev Med Devices. 2019;16(12):1063–70.
3. Kurtz SM, et al. Economic burden of periprosthetic joint infection in the United States. J Arthroplast. 2012;27(8 Suppl):61–5 e1.
4. Investigation and Management of Prosthetic Joint Infection in Knee Replacement. British Orthopaedic Assocation (BOA)/British Assocation for Sugery of the Knee (BASK). 2020.
5. Arias Arias C, et al. Differences in the clinical outcome of osteomyelitis by treating specialty: orthopedics or infectology. PLoS One. 2015;10(12):e0144736.
6. Wasterlain AS, et al. Diagnosis of periprosthetic infection: recent developments. J Bone Joint Surg Am. 2020;102(15):1366–75.
7. McNally M, et al. The EBJIS definition of periprosthetic joint infection. Bone Joint J. 2021;103-B(1):18–25.
8. Parvizi J, et al. New definition for periprosthetic joint infection: from the workgroup of the musculoskeletal infection society. Clin Orthop Relat Res. 2011;469(11):2992–4.
9. Parvizi J, Gehrke T, I. International consensus group on periprosthetic joint, definition of periprosthetic joint infection. J Arthroplast. 2014;29(7):1331.
10. Osmon DR, et al. Executive summary: diagnosis and management of prosthetic joint infection: clinical practice guidelines by the Infectious Diseases Society of America. Clin Infect Dis. 2013;56(1):1–10.
11. Osmon DR, et al. Diagnosis and management of prosthetic joint infection: clinical practice guidelines by the Infectious Diseases Society of America. Clin Infect Dis. 2013;56(1):e1–e25.
12. Parvizi J, et al. The 2018 definition of Periprosthetic hip and knee infection: an evidence-based and validated criteria. J Arthroplast. 2018;33(5):1309–1314.e2.
13. Shohat N, et al. Hip and knee section, what is the definition of a periprosthetic joint infection (PJI) of the knee and the hip? Can the same criteria be used for both joints?: proceedings of international consensus on orthopedic infections. J Arthroplast. 2019;34(2S):S325–7.
14. Villa JM, et al. Evolution of diagnostic definitions for periprosthetic joint infection in total hip and knee arthroplasty. J Arthroplast. 2020;35(3S):S9–S13.
15. Shemesh S, et al. The value of 18-FDG PET/CT in the diagnosis and management of implant-related infections of the tibia: a case series. Injury. 2015;46(7):1377–82.
16. Bejon P, et al. Serial measurement of the C-reactive protein is a poor predictor of treatment outcome in prosthetic joint infection. J Antimicrob Chemother. 2011;66(7):1590–3.
17. Atkins BL, et al. Prospective evaluation of criteria for microbiological diagnosis of prosthetic-joint infection at revision arthroplasty. The OSIRIS collaborative study group. J Clin Microbiol. 1998;36(10):2932–9.
18. Dudareva M, et al. Sonication versus tissue sampling for diagnosis of prosthetic joint and other orthopedic device-related infections. J Clin Microbiol. 2018;56(12).
19. Dudareva M, et al. The microbiology of chronic osteomyelitis: changes over ten years. J Infect. 2019;79(3):189–98.
20. Li HK, et al. Oral versus intravenous antibiotics for bone and joint infection. N Engl J Med. 2019;380(5):425–36.
21. Byren I, et al. One hundred and twelve infected arthroplasties treated with 'DAIR' (debridement, antibiotics and implant retention): antibiotic duration and outcome. J Antimicrob Chemother. 2009;63(6):1264–71.
22. Lora-Tamayo J, et al. Short- versus long-duration levofloxacin plus rifampicin for acute staphylococcal prosthetic joint infection managed with implant retention: a randomised clinical trial. Int J Antimicrob Agents. 2016;48(3):310–6.
23. Bernard L, et al. Antibiotic treatment for 6 weeks versus 12 weeks in patients with pyogenic vertebral osteomyelitis: an open-label, non-inferiority, randomised, controlled trial. Lancet. 2015;385(9971):875–82.
24. Dzaja I, et al. Functional outcomes of acutely infected knee arthroplasty: a comparison of different surgical treatment options. Can J Surg. 2015;58(6):402–7.
25. Middleton R, Khan T, Alvand A. Update on the diagnosis and management of prosthetic joint infection in hip and knee arthroplasty. Bone Joint. 2019;360:8(5).
26. Kunutsor SK, et al. Debridement, antibiotics and implant retention for periprosthetic joint infections: a

systematic review and meta-analysis of treatment outcomes. J Infect. 2018;77(6):479–88.

27. Vaz K, et al. A guide to debridement, antibiotics, and implant retention. Ann Joint. 2020.

28. George DA, Haddad FS. One-stage exchange arthroplasty: a surgical technique update. J Arthroplast. 2017;32(9S):S59–62.

29. Moucha CS, et al. Modifiable risk factors for surgical site infection. Instr Course Lect. 2011;60:557–64.

30. Jones RE, Russell RD, Huo MH. Wound healing in total joint replacement. Bone Joint J. 2013;95-B(11 Suppl A):144–7.

31. Rao AJ, et al. Soft tissue reconstruction and flap coverage for revision total knee arthroplasty. J Arthroplast. 2016;31(7):1529–38.

32. Schwechter EM, et al. Optimal irrigation and debridement of infected joint implants: an in vitro methicillin-resistant Staphylococcus aureus biofilm model. J Arthroplast. 2011;26(6 Suppl):109–13.

33. Brown NM, et al. Dilute betadine lavage before closure for the prevention of acute postoperative deep periprosthetic joint infection. J Arthroplast. 2012;27(1):27–30.

34. Howlin RP, et al. Antibiotic-loaded synthetic calcium sulfate beads for prevention of bacterial colonization and biofilm formation in periprosthetic infections. Antimicrob Agents Chemother. 2015;59(1):111–20.

35. Osei DA, Rebehn KA, Boyer MI. Soft-tissue defects after total knee arthroplasty: management and reconstruction. J Am Acad Orthop Surg. 2016;24(11):769–79.

36. Amin NH, et al. Total knee arthroplasty wound complication treatment algorithm: current soft tissue coverage options. J Arthroplast. 2019;34(4):735–42.

37. Parvizi J, et al. Does "excessive" anticoagulation predispose to periprosthetic infection? J Arthroplast. 2007;22(6 Suppl 2):24–8.

Sports After UKA and TKA

Nirav K. Patel and Gregory J. Golladay

Introduction

Total (TKA) and unicompartmental (UKA) knee arthroplasty are highly successful operations which address pain and dysfunction, thus leading to improvements in quality of life. They are increasingly being performed on not only younger, but older and more active patients who have high expectations of post-operative physical activity especially when already playing sports [1, 2]. As such, physicians are commonly asked about return to sport (RTS) following knee arthroplasty and considering that patient satisfaction correlates with patient expectations [3], it is important to counsel them appropriately. The challenges of this process include how to classify the impact level of the sport, which sports are safe to return to and when, as well as ability to return.

Younger, more active patients involved in sports will place higher physical demands on TKA implants which were initially designed for older, low-demand patients. Despite improvements in surgical techniques and implants, these patients report more residual symptoms of pain, stiffness and swelling giving satisfaction rates of 85% or less in multiple studies [4]. Conversely, UKAs are smaller operations, with shorter surgical times, hospital stays, and recovery times compared to TKAs [5]. This, in addition to better functional scores may be relevant on the ability to RTS. Sporting impact places excessive loads on the implant causing wear and specifically the bone-implant interface, which may accelerate aseptic loosening, adversely affecting the otherwise excellent long-term outcomes [6]. In addition, there is the risk of falling and traumatic injuries such as periprosthetic fracture and dislocation.

Current recommendations for RTS, including those from a survey from the American Association of Hip and Knee Surgeons (AAHKS) and the Knee Society [7, 8], are based on physician preference and subjectively defined categories of low-, moderate- and high-impact sports. Vail et al. classified sport impact level and provided post-arthroplasty recommendations based on degree of repetition, magnitude of joint loading, and potential for violence [9]. Initial systematic reviews and meta-analyses examining sports after arthroplasty have been of varying quality mainly due to the inherent limitations of the individual studies [10]. More recently, studies have more objectively examined sport-specific outcomes following arthroplasty enabling more robust, 'umbrella type' reviews [11] providing more evidence-based guidelines.

N. K. Patel (✉)
Department of Orthopaedic Surgery, VCU Health, West Hospital, Richmond, VA, USA

Department of Orthopaedic Surgery, Johns Hopkins University, Bethesda, MD, USA
e-mail: npate134@jh.edu

G. J. Golladay
Department of Orthopaedic Surgery, Johns Hopkins University, Bethesda, MD, USA
e-mail: gregory.golladay@vcuhealth.org

Total Knee Arthroplasty

The rate of TKA is increasing dramatically, with an increasing number performed in younger and more active patients. As such, patient expectations have increased as reflected in the updated Knee Society scoring system [12], including strenuous activity and high-impact sports. The long-term success rates of TKA are over 90% in most studies [6]. Despite its excellent track record, dissatisfaction rates can be up to 20% and the failure rate is higher in younger patients, with revision twice as likely in patients less than 47 years of age [4, 13]. Arnold et al. found mixed increases in objective physical activity after TKA at 6 months to a year over healthy controls, suggesting behavioral change may bridge the gap between perceived and actual functional gain [10]. When examining sport, a large proportion of patients have been able to RTS following TKA and UKA [14–19]. However, there was significant variability between studies regarding the proportion of patients able to do so. For TKA, Barber-Westin et al. performed a systematic review of 19 studies and 5179 patients with a mostly low-impact RTS rate of 34–100%. Only two studies used an accelerometer to measure activity, and few reported whether symptoms or limitations were experienced during activity. None described exercises or rehabilitation factors that would allow patients to RTS [14]. Another systematic review and meta-analysis of 18 studies reported a 36–89% RTS rate following TKA [19].

Unicompartmental Knee Arthroplasty

UKA are predominantly performed on the medial side and 5–10% are lateral. The cruciate ligaments, patellofemoral and contralateral compartments are preserved, thus functional outcomes are superior to TKA. In addition, there are reductions in morbidity, intra-operative complications, length of stay (by 1.4 days) and readmission rates [20]. The success rates are high with survivorship of 94% in one study of patients less than 60 years of age at 12 years [21]. Like TKA, many patients were able to RTS following UKA [14–19]. In a systematic review and meta-analysis, Wiltjes et al. showed a RTS rate of 75–100%. Participation in sport is more likely after UKA than TKA with mean number of sports participation of 1.1–4.6 and 0.2–1, respectively. In addition, patients undergoing UKA performed better than TKA patients, although the type of joint and implant used is less relevant for RTS compared to pre-operative factors [15].

Timing and Predictors of Sport

Although it may take between 1 and 2 years to fully recover from a TKA, potentially sooner for a UKA, the timetable for RTS is highly dependent on the sport in question. It is reasonable to return to low-impact activities, such as walking, as tolerated at any time point. Time to RTS was found to be similar between TKA and UKA at 13 and 12 weeks, respectively, with 90% of these sports being low impact [18, 22]. Papaliodis et al. detailed a return to golf protocol and found that patients RTS without restriction at 6–10 months post-operatively. Recommendations from physician surveys aligned with this data with one-third of physicians recommending waiting at least 3 months and two-thirds recommending 6 months postoperatively before RTS [15]. However, evidence suggests that an objective return to prior physical activity levels can take up to 1-year post-operatively [1]. Therefore, for RTS that is moderate- or high impact, requiring significant coordination or muscular strength, a gradual RTS at approximately 7 months with a full return to pre-operative sporting levels no sooner than 1 year is reasonable. To ensure a safe RTS, a multidisciplinary approach involving physical therapy and trainers is recommended to lead sport-specific exercises and make the final assessment of range of motion, strength, and coordination for sport. Objective measures of strength and balance can be employed to guide appropriate timing for RTS.

Prognostic indicators for RTS have included younger age, male gender, low body mass index, the absence of other joint pain, and pre-operative sport participation [15, 19, 23], with the latter being the most important. Smaller studies have shown that patients have been able to successfully return to reasonably high-impact and high-risk sports like judo [24] and high-level tennis [25] if they have significant experience with the sport prior to arthroplasty. Prior experience can reflect a patient's motivation as well as sport-specific strength and coordination [26], thus should be considered when counseling a patient on RTS.

Those patients who did not RTS were found to be largely due to surgeon recommendation, usually based on fears of implant wear and failure [15–19, 22]. While both latter concerns are anticipated, there is a low rate of short-term complications with modern implants and bearing surfaces demonstrating low wear rates [27]. Therefore, the risks of sport in conjunction with the benefits of physical activity, such as improved mental health and quality of life should be considered. Nevertheless, low-impact sport is generally encouraged on an incremental basis according to symptoms and with realistic goal setting.

Sport

There is some general consensus that patients can return to certain sports following TKA and UKA (Table 15.1). Patients have demonstrated success returning to low- and moderate-impact sports as well as some select high-impact sports [23]. Patients were able to RTS more frequently and 1 week earlier on average following a UKA compared to TKA; however, there is no difference in the specific sport recommendations between TKA and UKA. Nevertheless, the level of sport achieved was higher in UKA compared to TKA patients, although both were low impact [19]. While there is agreement that low-impact sports are safe, there is the possibility that moderate- to high-impact sports are safer than current guidelines suggest [16, 19] (Table 15.2).

Table 15.1 Select recommendations for RTS following UKA and TKA

Recommended	• Walking • Golf • Biking
Recommended with experience	• Hiking • Doubles tennis • Downhill skiing
Not recommended	• Baseball • Basketball • Running • Soccer

Table 15.2 Complete recommendations for RTS following UKA and TKA

Impact per Vail et al	Sport	Recommendation	Vail et al	Healy et al	AAHKS
Low	Stationary Cycling	🟢	🟢	🟢	🟢
	Calisthenics	🟢	🟢	--	🟢
	Golf	🟢	🟢	🟢	🟢
	Stationary skiing	🟢	🟢	🟡	🟢
	Walking	🟢	🟢	🟢	🟢
	Ballroom Dancing	🟢	🟢	🟢	🟢
	Water aerobics	🟢	🟢	--	🟢
Potentially low	Bowling	🟢	🟢	🟢	🟢
	Fencing	🟢	🟢	No consensus	🟢
	Rowing	🟢	🟢	🟡	🟢
	Isokinetic weightlifting	🟢	🟢	--	🟢
	Sailing	🟢	🟢	--	🟢
	Speed Walking	🟢	🟢	🟢	🟢
	Cross-country skiing	🟢	🟢	🟢	🟢
	Table tennis	🟢	🟢	--	🟢
	Jazz dancing and ballet	🟢	🟢	--	🟢
	Bicycling	🟢	🟢	🟢	🟢
Intermediate	Free weightlifting	🟡	🟡	No consensus	🟡
	Hiking	🟡	🟡	🟢	🟡
	Horseback Riding	🟡	🟡	🟡	🟡
	Ice Skating	🟡	🟡	🟡	🟡
	Rock Climbing	🟡	🟡	No consensus	🟡
	Low-impact aerobics	🟡	🟡	🟡	🟡
	Doubles tennis	🟡	🟡	--	🟡
	In-line skating	🟡	🟡	No consensus	🟡
	Downhill Skiing	🟡	🟡	🟡	🟡
High	Baseball Softball	🔴	🔴	No consensus	🔴
	Basketball Volleyball	🔴	🔴	🔴	🔴
	Football	🔴	🔴	🔴	🔴
	Handball Racquetball	🔴	🔴	No consensus	🔴
	Jogging Running	🔴	🔴	🔴	🔴
	Lacrosse	🔴	🔴	--	🔴
	Soccer	🔴	🔴	🔴	🔴
	Singles Tennis	🔴	🔴	No consensus	🔴
	Water Skiing	🔴	🔴	--	🔴
	Karate	🔴	🔴	--	Undecided

Key: 🟢 = Allowed   🟡 = Allowed with experience   🔴 = Not recommended   -- = Not reported

Risks

The concerns with high-impact sports are both the potential risk for acute traumatic injury and the possibility that increased loading cycles on the implant could cause wear or aseptic loosening necessitating revision surgery. Interestingly, Jassim et al. found that while there was increased radiographic wear seen in patients participating in sport, there was no increase in revision rates. Further, due to improved bearing characteristics, polyethylene wear is a decreasing cause of revision compared to other indications such as infection or instability [27]. Further, a recent review did not find a correlation between physical activity and aseptic loosening in TKA, while male sex was an independent risk factor [28]. While aseptic loosening is multifactorial, the increased risk seen in highly active patients tends to occur before wear suggesting increased mechanical load from activity levels as the cause. Patients should be counseled about the risk of loosening and against return to high-impact sports after TKA until more evidence becomes available.

On the contrary, patients less than 50 years of age have a shorter time to failure, such as aseptic loosening, with a higher revision rate than older patients [29]. Oljaca et al. suggested that jogging and both singles and doubles tennis are safe sports from this perspective, as multiple studies have demonstrated no increase in revision rates at a mean follow-up of 4.8 years for jogging and 7 years for tennis. Despite this optimism, there is currently a lack of long-term data to recommend patients can safely return to high-impact sports. However, patients have demonstrated success returning to doubles tennis and downhill skiing with prior experience. These sports likely represent the current upper limit of impact patients can expect to return to after knee arthroplasty.

Certain sports predispose the participant to traumatic injury, and these factors are considered in the classification system in Table 15.2. This is in addition to the recommendations by Vail et al. which considers the degree of repetition and magnitude of joint loading, and the potential for violence [9]. This correlates well with recommendations from AAHKS and the Knee Society

[7, 8]. It is universally accepted that low-impact sports are safe to return to and moderate-impact sports are safe with prior experience. High-impact sports are not recommended, largely due to the risk of traumatic injury. It could be argued that patients who are participating in high-impact sports at the highest level may have the expertise to return to these sports; however, the inherent risk and unpredictability of contact sports as well as the unknown long-term outcomes may preclude safe return.

Future Directions

It is vital to understand the forces a knee implant undergoes during specific sports. Some of this has been explored by studies utilizing the "e-Knee" and implantable sensors [30, 31]. However, there is a need to expand this work to understand typical forces, maximal forces, and degree of repetitive loading in different sports. With this data, an objective classification system based on quantified impact levels can be established, followed by improved recommendations on RTS post-TKA and UKA.

Summary

As increasingly younger and more active patients undergo TKA and UKA, physicians must be able to counsel appropriately on their ability to RTS post-operatively. Based on a reasonable classification of the impact level of sport, current literature suggests that patients can return to low-impact sports irrespective of prior experience and moderate-impact sports with prior experience in that sport. These patients are more successful in returning to sport following a UKA and do so earlier; however, there is no difference in the sports in which they eventually participate. There is insufficient long-term data to provide recommendations on high-impact sports, but in general patients are unlikely to be able to tolerate this due to its inherent mechanical nature, lack of proprioception, and limited outcomes. This is in addition to the risks of aseptic loosening and traumatic injury, risking revision surgery and thus requiring close monitoring.DisclosureNone relevant.

References

1. Maradit Kremers H, Larson DR, Crowson CS, et al. Prevalence of total hip and knee replacement in the United States. J Bone Joint Surg Am. 2015;97(17):1386–97.
2. DeFroda SF, Feller R, Klinge SA. Surgical management of the aging athlete. Curr Sports Med Rep. 2016;15(6):426–32. https://doi.org/10.1249/JSR.0000000000000310.
3. Hamilton DF, Lane JV, Gaston P, et al. What determines patient satisfaction with surgery? A prospective cohort study of 4709 patients following total joint replacement. BMJ Open. 2013;3(4):e002525. https://doi.org/10.1136/bmjopen-2012-002525.
4. Bourne RB, Chesworth BM, Davis AM, Mahomed NN, Charron KD. Patient satisfaction after total knee arthroplasty: who is satisfied and who is not? Clin Orthop Relat Res. 2010;468(1):57–63.
5. Wilson HA, Middleton R, Abram SGF, et al. Patient relevant outcomes of unicompartmental versus total knee replacement: systematic review and meta-analysis. BMJ. 2019;346:l352.
6. Argenson JN, Boisgard S, Parratte S, Descamps S, Bercovy M, Bonnevialle P, Briard JL, Brilhault J, Chouteau J, Nizard R, Saragaglia D, Servien E, French Society of Orthopedic and Traumatologic Surgery (SOFCOT). Survival analysis of total knee arthroplasty at a minimum 10 years' follow-up: a multicenter French nationwide study including 846 cases. Orthop Traumatol Surg Res. 2013;99(4):385–90.
7. Healy WL, Sharma S, Schwartz B, Iorio R. Athletic activity after total joint arthroplasty. J Bone Joint Surg Am. 2008;90(10):2245–52.
8. No authors listed. Resuming Sports After Knee Replacement. https://hipknee.aahks.org/wp-content/uploads/2019/01/resuming-sports-after-knee-replacement-AAHKS.pdf. Accessed 13 Sept 2020.
9. Vail TP, Mallon WJ, Liebelt RA. Athletic activities after joint arthroplasty. Sports Med Arthrosc. 1996;4(3):298.
10. Arnold JB, Walters JL, Ferrar KE. Does physical activity increase after Total hip or knee arthroplasty for osteoarthritis? A systematic review. J Orthop Sports Phys Ther. 2016;46(6):431–42. https://doi.org/10.2519/jospt.2016.6449.
11. Sowers C, Carrero AC, Cyrus JW, Ross JA, Golladay GJ, Patel NK. Return to sport post-Total hip arthroplasty: an umbrella review for consensus guidelines. Am J Sports Med. 2021;51:271.
12. Scuderi GR, Bourne RB, Noble PC, Benjamin JB, Lonner JH, Scott WN. The new knee society knee scoring system. Clin Orthop Relat Res. 2012;470(1):3–19.
13. Wainwright C, Theis JC, Garneti N, Melloh M. Age at hip or knee joint replacement surgery predicts likelihood of revision surgery. J Bone Joint Surg Br. 2011;93(10):1411–5.
14. Barber-Westin SD, Noyes FR. Aerobic physical fitness and recreational sports participation after Total knee arthroplasty: a systematic review. Sports Health. 2016;8(6):553–60.
15. Jassim SS, Douglas SL, Haddad FS. Athletic activity after lower limb arthroplasty: a systematic review of current evidence. Bone Joint J. 2014;96-B(7):923–7.
16. Oljaca A, Vidakovic I, Leithner A, Bergovec M. Current knowledge in orthopaedic surgery on recommending sport activities after total hip and knee replacement. Acta Orthop Belg. 2018;84(4):415–22.
17. Papaliodis DN, Photopoulos CD, Mehran N, Banffy MB, Tibone JE. Return to golfing activity after joint arthroplasty. Am J Sports Med. 2017;45(1):243–9.
18. Waldstein W, Kolbitsch P, Koller U, Boettner F, Windhager R. Sport and physical activity following unicompartmental knee arthroplasty: a systematic review. Knee Surg Sports Traumatol Arthrosc. 2017;25(3):717–28.
19. Witjes S, Gouttebarge V, Kuijer PP, van Geenen RC, Poolman RW, Kerkhoffs GM. Return to sports and physical activity after total and unicondylar knee arthroplasty: a systematic review and meta-analysis. Sports Med. 2016;46(2):269–92.
20. Liddle AD, Judge A, Pandit H, Murray DW. Adverse outcomes after total and unicompartmental knee replacement in 101,330 matched patients: a study of data from the National Joint Registry for England and Wales. Lancet. 2014;384(9952):1437–45.
21. Felts E, Parratte S, Pauly V, Aubaniac JM, Argenson JN. Function and quality of life following medial unicompartmental knee arthroplasty in patients 60 years of age or younger. Orthop Traumatol Surg Res. 2010;96(8):861–7.
22. Vogel LA, Carotenuto G, Basti JJ, Levine WN. Physical activity after total joint arthroplasty. Sports Health. 2011;3(5):441–50.
23. Buza JA, Fink LA, Levine WN. Sports activity after total joint arthroplasty: recommendations for the counseling physician. Phys Sportsmed. 2013;41(1):9–21. https://doi.org/10.3810/psm.2013.02.1994.
24. Lefevre N, Rousseau D, Bohu Y, Klouche S, Herman S. Return to judo after joint replacement. Knee Surg Sports Traumatol Arthrosc. 2013;21(12):2889–94.
25. Mont MA, Rajadhyaksha AD, Marxen JL, Silberstein CE, Hungerford DS. Tennis after total knee arthroplasty. Am J Sports Med. 2002;30(2):163–6. https://doi.org/10.1177/03635465020300020301.
26. Golant A, Christoforou DC, Slover JD, Zuckerman JD. Athletic participation after hip and knee arthroplasty. Bull NYU Hosp Jt Dis. 2010;68(2):76–83.
27. Thiele K, Perka C, Matziolis G, Mayr HO, Sostheim M, Hube R. Current failure mechanisms after knee arthroplasty have changed: polyethylene wear is less common in revision surgery. J Bone Joint Surg Am. 2015;97(9):715–20.

28. Cherian JJ, Jauregui JJ, Banerjee S, Pierce T, Mont MA. What host factors affect aseptic loosening after THA and TKA? Clin Orthop Relat Res. 2015;473(8):2700–9.

29. Aggarwal VK, Goyal N, Deirmengian G, Rangavajulla A, Parvizi J, Austin MS. Revision total knee arthroplasty in the young patient: is there trouble on the horizon? J Bone Joint Surg Am. 2014;96(7):536–42.

30. D'Lima DD, Fregly BJ, Colwell CW. Implantable sensor technology: measuring bone and joint biomechanics of daily life in vivo. Arthritis Res Ther. 2013;15(1):203. https://doi.org/10.1186/ar4138.

31. Hardwick ME, Pulido PA, D'Lima DD, Colwell CW. E-knee: the electronic knee prosthesis. Orthop Nurs. 2006;25(5):326–9. https://doi.org/10.1097/00006416-200609000-00009.

Advances in Pain Management and DVT Prophylaxis

16

John Krumme, Sanjay Kubsad, and Gregory J. Golladay

Oral/Intravenous Analgesics

Opioids

Opioid analgesics have historically been the foundation of pain management following joint arthroplasty, and opioids are more heavily prescribed by orthopedic surgeons than by any other surgical subspecialty group [1]. Of note, the quantity of opioid tablets prescribed at discharge following elective total joint arthroplasty is often well in excess of that consumed [2], leading to medication waste. Immediate and sustained release oral formulations as well as intravenous opioids administered by nurse or patient-controlled bolus are frequently employed. The analgesic effect of opioids is mediated primarily through their action at the μ-opioid receptor.

Common opioid-related side effects include pruritus, nausea and vomiting, constipation, urinary retention, and sedation as well as perturbations in psychomotor and cognitive function. Respiratory depression is observed less commonly, but is responsible for the majority of adverse opioid-related outcomes [3].

Factors placing patients at greatest risk for oversedation and respiratory depression include obstructive sleep apnea, morbid obesity, advanced age, cardiopulmonary disease, and concomitant use of benzodiazepines or other sedating medications. Given the potential for severe adverse events, The Joint Commission put forth a sentinel event alert with recommendations to guide the safe use of opioids in the hospital setting. These recommendations include the creation of an individualized pain management plan with consideration for non-opioid therapies and provision of provider and patient education [4].

Opioids prescribed for surgery increase the risk of persistent opioid use and 6% of all opioid-naïve surgical patients go on to use opioids chronically [5]. Additionally, the most commonly prescribed opioids, oxycodone and hydrocodone, are responsible for the majority of opioid overdose deaths in the United States. Given the potential for adverse effects, persistent opioid use, misuse and diversion, minimization of in-hospital opioid administration, and careful prescription during discharge is prudent for post-surgical patients. Furthermore, an increasing number of

J. Krumme
Kansas City Orthopedic Alliance, Leawood, KS, USA

S. Kubsad
Department of Orthopedic Surgery, Johns Hopkins University, Baltimore, MD, USA

Department of Orthopedic Surgery, University of Washington School of Medicine, Seattle, WA, USA
e-mail: skubsad@uw.edu

G. J. Golladay (✉)
Department of Orthopedic Surgery, Virginia Commonwealth University Health, Richmond, VA, USA
e-mail: gregory.golladay@vcuhealth.org

states are enacting prescribing guidelines for acute post-surgical pain, making it imperative for surgeons be aware of such mandates [6].

Acetaminophen

Acetaminophen is an effective and widely used analgesic with strong antipyretic and limited anti-inflammatory properties. Its mechanism of action has not been fully elucidated; however, it has been suggested that modulation of serotonin and prostaglandins play a role [7]. When administered to patients undergoing total joint arthroplasty, acetaminophen reduces both opioid consumption and pain scores. Acetaminophen is generally regarded as safe; however, given the risk of hepatotoxicity, the daily dose should be limited to 3000 mg in healthy adults. Both oral and intravenous formulations exist. Evidence consistently demonstrates analgesic benefits of intravenous acetaminophen as compared to placebo; however, the results are mixed for oral acetaminophen. Given the lack of evidence to suggest definitive superiority of the IV formulation as well as its cost-effectiveness and relative safety, routine use of the oral formulation is recommended throughout the perioperative period, including post-discharge [8].

Non-Steroidal Anti-Inflammatory Drugs

Non-steroidal anti-inflammatory drugs (NSAIDs) exert their effects through inhibition of cyclooxygenase enzyme isoforms COX-1 and COX-2. NSAIDs are formulated as both non-selective (COX-1 and -2 inhibitory) and COX-2 selective. COX-2 inhibitors are further categorized as highly selective (celecoxib) or preferentially selective (meloxicam). While COX-1 is expressed throughout the body and notably in gastric mucosa, platelets, and renal tissue, COX-2 is more specifically associated with inflammatory cells and mediates the production of prostaglandin and thromboxane with a resultant inflammatory response. COX-2-specific drugs were

designed to minimize the negative side effects of non-selective NSAIDS such as gastrointestinal bleeding while retaining their anti-inflammatory advantages. Celecoxib is the only FDA-approved, highly selective COX-2 inhibitor available in the United States.

The benefits of both selective and non-selective NSAIDs in joint arthroplasty are well described and include reduction in post-operative opioid consumption and improved pain intensity scores when compared to placebo [9]. Multiple formulations of NSAIDS, including ibuprofen, meloxicam, ketorolac, and celecoxib improve analgesia. Additionally, NSAIDs do not increase the risk of commonly described analgesic side effects, including nausea, vomiting, pruritus, and sedation. The lack of expression of COX-2 in platelets and gastric mucosa may provide a safety advantage over non-specific NSAIDs; however, they should be used cautiously in patients with or at risk for renal dysfunction or when used in combination with other potentially nephrotoxic medications.

Gabapentinoids

Gabapentinoids, including pregabalin and gabapentin, modulate pain through their central nervous system effects. They inhibit central sensitization and have historically been used to treat neuropathic pain [10]. Despite more widespread adoption for the treatment of acute post-surgical pain, data supporting their routine use is limited and is considered off-label. When administered perioperatively to joint arthroplasty patients, gabapentin has not been shown to reduce opioid requirement or pain scores when compared to placebo, whereas pregabalin may reduce opioid consumption, but not pain scores. When prescribed following discharge, gabapentin has not been shown to reduce pain scores or opioid consumption, whereas pregabalin may improve both metrics [11]. Despite potential analgesic benefits of pregabalin in the total joint arthroplasty population, the US Food and Drug Administration has issued a warning for patients receiving gabapentinoids [12]. In patients with respiratory risk factors, including COPD, reduced pulmonary function, elderly patients, or those co-prescribed other central nervous system depressant drugs, there is an increased risk for sedation and respiratory depression. The risk of such side effects should be carefully balanced with the limited potential benefits of these medications.

Peripheral Regional Blocks

Peripheral nerve blockade has been a mainstay of analgesia for total knee arthroplasty patients and provides excellent analgesia [13]. Enhanced recovery pathways with a focus on early mobilization and side-effect minimization have led to a resultant shift in practice and choice of block. However, the most effective blocks for analgesia are also those most likely to cause motor weakness, leading to ineffective patient effort with physical therapy and increasing risk for falls. Complexity of knee innervation, desire for early rehabilitation, and technical challenges of peripheral regional techniques complicate the choice of block. While evidence suggests analgesic superiority of femoral and sciatic blockade [14], newer alternatives, including proximal saphenous nerve and infiltration between the popliteal artery and the capsule of the knee (IPACK) blocks, have been successfully employed in the setting of a multimodal regimen. These blocks offer analgesic advantages, while typically reducing the risk for undesired motor blockade.

The saphenous nerve is a terminal branch of the femoral nerve and supplies sensory innervation to the medial aspect of the leg as well as the knee joint. When blocking the saphenous nerve above the knee, there are several approaches involving deposition of local anesthetic proximate to the superficial femoral artery [14]. The adductor canal block is often used broadly to describe blockade of the saphenous nerve in the thigh. With more proximal placement and using larger volumes of local anesthetic, the risk of blockade of femoral nerve branches to vastus medialis increases with an associated risk of weakness. When deposited more distally and with lower volume, the likelihood of quadriceps weakness is substantially reduced when compared to femoral nerve blockade. When used alone, the adductor canal block appears to be inferior to other approaches such as periarticular infiltration. When used as a component of a multimodal approach to pain management, the adductor canal block has been shown to reduce opioid consumption and improve pain scores.

Deposition of local anesthetic between the popliteal artery and the capsule of the knee can target the articular branches of the sciatic nerve and the obturator nerve in the popliteal fossa [15]. When placed in combination with a local infiltrative injection, the IPACK block appears to confer an analgesic advantage with limited motor decrement.

Multiple other peripheral nerve blocks have been identified as potential targets in the achievement of optimal post-operative analgesia. Technical challenges, time required for placement, required expertise, and cost considerations may all limit the applicability of various approaches, including the placement of continuous nerve block catheters.

Neuraxial Block and Intrathecal Opioids

A growing body of evidence suggests there is a reduction in complications in total joint arthroplasty patients undergoing a primary neuraxial anesthetic, including spinal or epidural [16]. Current consensus recommendations include the use of neuraxial anesthesia when possible. Post-operative analgesia may be achieved through the maintenance of an epidural catheter in the post-operative period or through the use of spinal opioids such as morphine. Epidural catheters have been shown to improve analgesia in the immediate post-operative period; however, their routine use is limited by several factors, including urinary retention, limited mobility secondary to sensory and motor blockade of the lower extremities, and the potential for hypotension. Careful consideration must be given to the use of perioperative thromboprophylaxis in the setting of an indwelling neuraxial catheter.

Intrathecal opioids have been shown to provide analgesic benefits in total joint arthroplasty and may be particularly advantageous when used in low doses as part of a multimodal regimen. Morphine is the most commonly described intrathecal opioid given its duration of up to 24 h. Side effects of intrathecal morphine commonly include pruritus, urinary retention, and nausea and vomiting. Delayed respiratory depression is an uncommon but potentially catastrophic side effect, and respiratory monitoring should be used until the drug effect has waned [17]. While both indwelling epidural catheters and single-dose intrathecal morphine may improve analgesia in this population, their use is limited by the above factors.

Local Infiltrative Analgesia

Local infiltrative analgesia involves the injection of local anesthetic, often in combination with other analgesics, into the tissues surrounding the knee joint. This is typically performed under direct visualization, intraoperatively. Large volumes of injectate, often 100 cc or more, are deliberately administered at various periarticular sites. The objective is the blockade of articular nerve branches that innervate the joint space to provide post-operative analgesia while minimizing motor blockade and reducing the requirement for opioid analgesics. Ropivacaine and bupivacaine are the most common local anesthetics used for periarticular injection. Additives often include epinephrine and ketorolac with additional normal saline to increase the total volume. Despite seemingly large doses of local anesthetic, toxic-free plasma ropivacaine levels are rare, even when a continuous infusion is employed [18, 19].These blocks are relatively low risk to place and do not require special training or equipment. When compared to placebo or no injection, patients treated with periarticular injections showed improved pain scores, reduced opioid consumption, reduced post-operative nausea and vomiting and improved range of motion. These advantages were not, however, present when local infiltrative anesthesia was used as adjunct to regional anesthesia [20].

Current pain management for knee arthroplasty should be centered on a pre-emptive, multimodal, opioid-sparing approach. Use of neuraxial anesthesia, oral or intravenous acetaminophen, anti-inflammatory medication, and local infiltrative anesthetics, with or without regional block are recommended. There is limited evidence to support use of gabapentinoids in the perioperative analgesic regimen for knee arthroplasty. Limited, short-term opioids can be used cautiously.

Venous Thromboembolism in Arthroplasty

Venous thromboembolism (VTE) refers to formation of blood clots in the veins, while deep venous thrombosis refers to clots specifically in the deep veins, often in the legs. Pulmonary embolus (PE) occurs when a clot travels to the lungs and can be a fatal event. This spectrum of disease is of importance in arthroplasty surgery and is one of the most serious medical complications seen. In the absence of prophylaxis, the rates of DVT and PE are very high following arthroplasty. These numbers have decreased with routine prophylaxis, with a systematic review identifying a VTE rate of 1.09%, a symptomatic DVT rate of 0.63%, and a PE rate of 0.27% prior to hospital discharge for patients undergoing total or partial knee arthroplasty [1]. Morbidity of VTE can include chronic venous insufficiency, pain, post-thrombotic pulmonary hypertension, and even death. In arthroplasty, these complications must be seriously weighed against complications of systemic anticoagulation, particularly wound complications and infection.

Risk Factors for VTE

It is important to identify risk factors for VTE prior to surgery. Various studies have identified many different factors that may predispose patients to these complications. A large single institution review identified age, BMI, cholesterol, HDL, apolipoprotein A, history of tumor,

VAS pain score, and operative duration all as risk factors or DVT noted on routine postoperative venography [21]. Obesity has been identified as an important risk factor with patients classified as overweight having a 1.64 odds ratio of PE and also 1.03 odds increase per each increase in kg/m^2 among patients in a US national registry undergoing primary and revision hip and knee arthroplasty [22]. An understanding of these risk factors is important because many treatment algorithms rely on the risk of clotting when determining the ideal prophylactic measures.

Clinical Guidelines

Many different organizations and societies have laid out their recommendations for the prevention of VTE. The two most familiar to orthopedic surgeons are those of the American Academy of Orthopedic Surgeons (AAOS) and the American College of Chest Physicians (ACCP). It is important to highlight the differences between these two guidelines and how they have changed in newer iterations in response to changes in treatment.

ACCP Recommendations

The main goal of the ACCP recommendations is reducing the frequency of DVT which is felt to be a surrogate measure for the rate of fatal PE. The eighth edition of these recommendations, published in 2008 [23], recommended the use of low-molecular-weight heparin, warfarin with a moderate-intensity International Normalized Ratio (INR) target of 2–3, or fondaparinux for thromboprophylaxis. They recommended therapy to continue for a minimum of 10 days following knee arthroplasty. The use of aspirin and supported mechanical compression as an adjuvant therapy was specifically recommended against. The ninth edition, subsequently published in 2012 [24], awarded aspirin the same level of recommendation as other forms of chemoprophylaxis, while including newer agents such as dabigatran, apixaban, rivaroxaban as sup-

ported modalities. They, however, still maintained that a preference should be given to low-molecular-weight heparin with a low strength or recommendation (Grade 2C/2B).

AAOS Guidelines

The AAOS guidelines had a slightly different framework, where they were aimed at decreasing the incidence of clinical PE while avoiding bleeding or wound complications [5, 25]. The first version of these guidelines stratified patients based on their risks of PE and bleeding and made recommendations based on these groups (Table 16.1). Recommended therapies included aspirin, low-molecular-weight heparin, fondaparinux, and low-intensity warfarin (INR <2.0). These guidelines supported the use of mechanical compression and early mobilization for all patients. The second edition of the AAOS guidelines, published in 2011 [26], reached more common ground with the ACCP recommendations. They recommended the use of mechanical compressive devices and/or pharmacologic agents and state that they are unable to recommend for or against specific strategies at this point. They also state that they are unable to recommend a specific duration of treatment. These guidelines highlight the difficulty in coming up

Table 16.1 first edition AAOS guidelines for DVT prophylaxis after arthroplasty based on risk stratifications. PE: pulmonary embolism, LMWH: low molecular weight heparin

	Standard PE risk	Increased PE risk
Standard bleeding risk	Aspirin Fondaparinux LMWH Low intensity warfarin	LMWH Fondaparinux Low intensity warfarin
Increased bleeding risk	Aspirin Low intensity warfarin None	Aspirin Low intensity warfarin

Source: American Academy of Orthopedic Surgeons Clinical Practice Guideline on Preventing Thromboembolic Disease in Patients Undergoing Elective Hip and Knee Arthroplasty https://www.aaos.org/global-assets/quality-and-practice-resources/vte/vte_full_guideline_10.31.16.pdf (Published September 23, 2011)

with recommendations for specific treatments due to the vast heterogenicity in studies, available treatment types, and dosing along with other confounding factors.

Specific Treatment Modalities

Mechanical Compression

Mechanical compression devices, previously considered an adjuvant or an option for patients at high risk for bleeding, have been gaining an important role in VTE prophylaxis after arthroplasty. Mechanical compression is thought to work through decreasing venous stasis while also increasing endothelium-derived fibrinolysis through varied anti-thrombotic, pro-fibrinolytic, and vasodilatory effects. Mechanical compression is generally easy to administer without causing potent systemic anticoagulatory effects, and has been shown to be the most cost-effective prophylactic strategy [27]. One of the main disadvantages of mechanical compression includes the need to use these devices for prolonged periods, with the ACCP recommending at least 18 h of use per day for the duration of the hospitalization and for a minimum of 10–14 days. With such long use requirements, compliance can be an issue, with a single study showing an 18.2% compliance by post-discharge day 7 [28]. Another downside to mechanical compression devices is the variability in how they can be used such as intermittent versus sequential compression, or calf versus foot-based devices; which confounds scientific comparisons between treatment strategies.

There is some evidence supporting the use of only mechanical prophylaxis after knee arthroplasty in standard risk patients. A single institution that instituted this treatment protocol demonstrates an ultrasound identified a DVT incidence of 2.1% and a PE incidence of 1.4%, which the authors argued is similar to published rates using chemoprophylaxis [29]. Another strategy is the "stacked method," in which mechanical prophylaxis is used for the first 48 h, followed by chemoprophylaxis such as rivaroxa-

ban, which was observed to show both good prophylaxis with limited wound drainage at a single institution [30]. The more common method of using both mechanical and chemical prophylaxis has shown to be effective, with DVT rates of 2.19% in the combined group compared to 4.10% in a mechanical prophylaxis-alone group in a large systematic review [31]. With larger numbers of TKAs being performed in the outpatient setting, there has been a growing interest in the use of portable ambulatory compression devices recently. These devices have shown low rates of symptomatic VTE (0.3%) when used as part of a multimodal aspirin-based approach in the outpatient surgery setting [32].

Aspirin

Aspirin, which works as an irreversible inhibitor of cyclooxygenase-1 (COX-1) and an inhibitor of platelet aggregation, has been growing rapidly in popularity for VTE prophylaxis after knee arthroplasty. The PE Prevention (PEP) randomized trial has been credited as the first to demonstrate the efficacy of low-dose aspirin for prevention of VTE [33]. The original AAOS guidelines recommended high-dose (325 mg) aspirin twice daily. Most recent practice has leaned towards the use of low-dose (81 mg) aspirin. A large retrospective review showed that 81 mg of aspirin twice daily was not inferior to 325 mg twice daily with a lower incidence of VTE and symptomatic DVT after total knee arthroplasty [34]. This low dose aspirin has also shown a decrease in GI upset and nausea with no difference in GI bleeding when compared to the high dose aspirin [35].

Evidence in support of aspirin compared to other methods of VTE prophylaxis is growing. Two recent metanalyses showed a non-significant reduced risk of VTE compared to other prophylaxis methods with no difference in mortality or bleeding events and an improved reduction in VTE compared to placebo among patients undergoing THA and TKA [36, 37]. A retrospective review that also included risk stratification showed lower VTE, DVT, and PE rates with aspirin compared to warfarin or LMWH, even among patients with higher thromboembolic risk [38]. Aspirin has also been shown to be associated with a lower periprosthetic joint infection rate compared to more potent anticoagulants, which is thought to be related to the theoretically lower rate of bleeding and wound complications [39].

Due to these benefits, aspirin is a very attractive choice for VTE prophylaxis after arthroplasty and its preferential use has been increasing. A recent surgery on preference of VTE prophylaxis among US surgeons demonstrates 60% prefer 81 mg aspirin BID, 13.3% prefer 325 mg aspirin BID, and 22.2% prefer aspirin at either 81 mg or 325 mg QD [40].

Low-Molecular-Weight Heparin

Low-molecular-weight heparin (LMWH) is the drug of choice for VTE prophylaxis of the ACCP guidelines and is considered the standard of care in the UK and Australia. LMWH works by binding anti-thrombin III (AT-III) and then preferentially inactivating factor X. It is a more potent anticoagulant than unfractionated heparin which binds to factors X and II more equally. It is also associated with a lower risk of heparin-induced thrombocytopenia (HIT) than unfractionated heparin. LMWH is administered as an injection at fixed dosage without need for monitoring. The benefits of LMWH are primarily related to the decrease in asymptomatic DVT observed. However, a systematic review of LMWH use after total joint arthroplasty has shown increased bleeding rates compared to control (RR: 2.32), and warfarin (RR: 1.54), and trended higher than apixaban (RR: 1.27) with similar bleeding compared to rivaroxaban (RR: 0.95) [41]. Similarly, the ACCP guidelines have suggested that enoxaparin is less appealing for VTE prophylaxis in arthroplasty because of higher possible complication rates with small perceived benefits [24].

Warfarin

Warfarin is a highly utilized method of VTE prophylaxis with a long track record. Warfarin works as a vitamin K inhibitor which blocks the synthesis of clotting factors II, VII, IX, and X in the liver. It is given orally and can be reversed with Vitamin K or fresh frozen plasma (FFP). The response to warfarin can be unpredictable and requires careful monitoring of the patient's INR. Warfarin also blocks the synthesis of factors C and S, which can result in a paradoxical hypercoagulability early in its administration if not bridged appropriately with another anticoagulant, leading to warfarin skin necrosis. The ideal dosing of warfarin and target INR is an important point of differentiation between the AAOS and ACCP guidelines. The ideal time to initiate warfarin perioperatively also remains a question when considering its use in arthroplasty.

Fondaparinux

Fondaparinux is a synthetic pentasaccharide which corresponds to the heparinoid binding site on AT-III, resulting in highly selective indirect inhibition of factor X. Fondaparinux is administered by injection at fixed dosing and is approved by the FDA or VTE prophylaxis after THA or TKA. A meta-analysis found fondaparinux to have a 47% decreased risk of VTE when compared to the LWMH, enoxaparin, but with a non-significant increased relative risk of major bleeds [42].

Direct Oral Anticoagulants

The direct oral anticoagulants (DOACs) represent a new class of medications aimed at preventing VTE. Commonly used DOACs in orthopedics are rivaroxaban and apixaban which are direct inhibitors of factor Xa, and dabigatran, which is a direct inhibitor of activated factor II. Rivaroxaban and apixaban have FDA clearance for VTE prophylaxis in THA and TKA. At this time, dabigatran is only approved for VTE prophylaxis after THA by the FDA, but is approved for both THA and TKA in Europe, Australia, and Canada. Benefits of these medications are primarily that they are administered orally without required monitoring and have a rapid onset and offset. On the other hand, these drugs are relatively new, costly; and while reversal agents now exist, they are not widely available and can also be cost-prohibitive.

There is evidence supporting the use of DOACs for VTE prophylaxis after arthroplasty. A review of the joint registry data from England, Wales, Northern Ireland, and the Ilse of Man showed a significantly lower VTE risk in TKA and THA with DOACs compared to aspirin, with no differences in wound complications, surgical site infections, major hemorrhage, mortality, or short-term revision [37]. These VTE rates were, however, very small with the aspirin group at 0.73% and the DOAC group at 0.60%, supporting the efficacy of both treatments. A metanalysis also demonstrated lower VTE rates but higher bleeding risks among DOACs compared to enoxaparin after THA and TKA [42]. Also, the EPCAT randomized trial recently showed no difference in symptomatic VTE or bleeding rates when specifically comparing rivaroxaban to aspirin.

Future Directions

There are still many ongoing areas of research and optimization for the prevention of VTE after arthroplasty. Further studies are still required to compare specific modalities in hopes of identifying the ideal strategy for patients. The PEPPER trial is one such study that is currently being conducted comparing aspirin, low intensity warfarin, and rivaroxaban in patients undergoing primary and revision hip and knee arthroplasty. The increasingly outpatient nature of total joint arthroplasty is an area that may change thromboembolic prophylactic strategies. A more precise way or risk stratifying patients may develop with many different biomarkers under investigation for predicting VTE. Finally, bundled payment structures and continued cost containment in arthroplasty will likely prove to be factors driving future treatments and guidelines.

References

1. Januel JM, Chen G, Ruffieux C, Quan H, Douketis JD, Crowther MA, Colin C, Ghali WA, Burnand B, IMECCHI Group. Symptomatic in-hospital deep vein thrombosis and pulmonary embolism following hip and knee arthroplasty among patients receiving recommended prophylaxis: a systematic review. JAMA. 2012;307(3):294–303. https://doi.org/10.1001/jama.2011.2029.
2. Volkow ND, McLellan TA, Cotto JH, Karithanom M, Weiss SR. Characteristics of opioid prescriptions in 2009. JAMA. 2011;305(13):1299–301.
3. Huang PS, Copp SN. Oral opioids are overprescribed in the opiate-naive patient undergoing total joint arthroplasty. J Am Acad Orthop Surg. 2019;27(15):e702–8.
4. Wheeler M, Oderda GM, Ashburn MA, Lipman AG. Adverse events associated with postoperative opioid analgesia: a systematic review. J Pain. 2002;3(3):159–80.
5. Brummett CM, Waljee JF, Goesling J, et al. New persistent opioid use after minor and major surgical procedures in US adults. JAMA Surg. 2017;152(6):e170504.
6. The Joint Commission. Safe use of opioids in hospitals. Sentinel Event Alert 2012. https://www.jointcommission.org/assets/1/18/SEA_49_opioids_8_2_12_final.pdf
7. Smith HS. Potential analgesic mechanisms of acetaminophen. Pain Physician. 2009;12:269–80.
8. Politi JR, Davis RL II, Matrka AK. Randomized prospective trial comparing the use of intravenous versus oral acetaminophen in total joint arthroplasty. J Arthroplast. 2017;32:1125–7.
9. Fillingham YA, Hannon CP, Roberts KC, Mullen K, Casambre F, Riley C, Hamilton WG, Della Valle CJ. The efficacy and safety of nonsteroidal anti-inflammatory drugs in total joint arthroplasty: systematic review and direct meta-analysis. J Arthroplast. 2020;35(10):2739–58.
10. Verret M, Lauzier F, Zarychanski R, Perron C, Savard X, Pinard A-M, Leblanc G, Cossi M-J, Neveu X, Turgeon AF. The Canadian perioperative Anesthesia clinical trials (PACT) group; perioperative use of Gabapentinoids for the Management of Postoperative Acute Pain: a systematic review and meta-analysis. Anesthesiology. 2020;133:265–79.
11. Hannon CP, Fillingham YA, Browne JA, Schemitsch EH, Anesthesia AAHKS, Analgesia Clinical Practice Guideline Workgroup, Buvanendran A, Hamilton WG, Della Valle CJ. Gabapentinoids in Total joint arthroplasty: the clinical practice guidelines of the American Association of hip and Knee Surgeons, American Society of Regional Anesthesia and Pain Medicine, American Academy of Orthopaedic sur-

geons, hip society, and knee society. J Arthroplast. 2020;35(10):2700–3.
12. https://www.fda.gov/media/133681/download. Accessed 10 Oct 2020.
13. Hebl JR, Dilger JA, Byer DE, Kopp SL, Stevens SR, Pagnano MW, Hanssen AD, Horlocker TT. A pre-emptive multimodal pathway featuring peripheral nerve block improves perioperative outcomes after major orthopedic surgery. Reg Anesth Pain Med. 2008;33(6):510–7.
14. Kirkpatrick JD, Sites BD, Antonakakis JG. Preliminary experience with a new approach to performing an ultrasound-guided saphenous nerve block in the mid to proximal femur. Reg Anesth Pain Med. 2010;35(2):222–3.
15. Thobhani S, Scalercio L, Elliott CE, et al. Novel regional techniques for total knee arthroplasty promote reduced hospital length of stay: an analysis of 106 patients. Ochsner J. 2017;17:233–8.
16. Memtsoudis SG, et. Al. Anaesthetic care of patients undergoing primary hip and knee arthroplasty: consensus recommendations from the international consensus on Anaesthesia-related outcomes after surgery group (ICAROS) based on a systematic review and meta-analysis. Br J Anaesth. 2019;123(3):269–87.
17. Shapiro A, Zohar E, Zaslansky R, Hoppenstein D, Shabat S, Fredman B. The frequency and timing of respiratory depression in 1524 postoperative patients treated with systemic or neuraxial morphine. J Clin Anesth. 2005;17(7):537–42.
18. Brydone AS, Souvatzoglou R, Abbas M, Watson DG, McDonald DA, Gill AM. Ropivacaine plasma levels following high-dose local infiltration analgesia for total knee arthroplasty. Anaesthesia. 2015;70(7):784–90.
19. Kerr DR, Kohan L. Local infiltration analgesia: a technique for the control of acute postoperative pain following knee and hip surgery: a case study of 325 patients. Acta Orthop. 2008;79(2):174–83.
20. Seangleulur A, Vanasbodeekul P, Prapaitrakool S, Worathongchai S, Anothaisintawee T, McEvoy M, et al. The efficacy of local infiltration analgesia in the early postoperative period after total knee arthroplasty: a systematic review and meta-analysis. Eur J Anaesthesiol. 2016;33(11):816–31.
21. Zhang H, Mao P, Wang C, Chen D, Xu Z, Shi D, Dai J, Yao Y, Jiang Q. Incidence and risk factors of deep vein thrombosis (DVT) after total hip or knee arthroplasty: a retrospective study with routinely applied venography. Blood Coagul Fibrinolysis. 2017;28(2):126–33.
22. Sloan M, Sheth N, Lee GC. Is obesity associated with increased risk of deep vein thrombosis or pulmonary embolism after hip and knee arthroplasty? A large database study. Clin Orthop Relat Res. 2019;477(3):523.
23. Geerts WH, Bergqvist D, Pineo GF, Heit JA, Samama CM, Lassen MR, Colwell CW. Prevention of venous thromboembolism: American College of Chest Physicians evidence-based clinical practice guidelines. Chest. 2008;133(6):381S–453S.
24. Falck-Ytter Y, Francis CW, Johanson NA, Curley C, Dahl OE, Schulman S, Ortel TL, Pauker SG, Colwell CW Jr. Prevention of VTE in orthopedic surgery patients: antithrombotic therapy and prevention of thrombosis: American College of Chest Physicians evidence-based clinical practice guidelines. Chest. 2012;141(2):e278S–325S.
25. Johanson NA, Lachiewicz PF, Lieberman JR, Lotke PA, Parvizi J, Pellegrini V, Stringer TA, Tornetta P III, Haralson RH III, Watters WC III. Prevention of symptomatic pulmonary embolism in patients undergoing total hip or knee arthroplasty. J Am Acad OrthopSurg. 2009;17(3):183–96.
26. Mont MA, Jacobs JJ. AAOS clinical practice guideline: preventing venous thromboembolic disease in patients undergoing elective hip and knee arthroplasty. J Am Acad Orthop Surg. 2011;19(12):777–8.
27. Torrejon Torres R, Saunders R, Ho KM. A comparative cost-effectiveness analysis of mechanical and pharmacological VTE prophylaxis after lower limb arthroplasty in Australia. J Orthop Surg Res. 2019;14(1):1–7.
28. Dietz MJ, Ray JJ, Witten BG, Frye BM, Klein AE, Lindsey BA. Portable compression devices in total joint arthroplasty: poor outpatient compliance. Arthroplast today. 2020;6(1):118–22.
29. Hamilton WG, Reeves JD, Fricka KB, Goyal N, Engh GA, Parks NL. Mechanical thromboembolic prophylaxis with risk stratification in total knee arthroplasty. J Arthroplast. 2015;30(1):43–5.
30. Jiang L, Zhang S, Zhao Y. Stacked modalities' thromboprophylactic therapy for patients undergoing total knee replacement surgery. J Knee Surg. 2017;30(03):218–22.
31. Kakkos S, Kirkilesis G, Caprini JA, Geroulakos G, Nicolaides A, Stansby G, Reddy DJ. Combined intermittent pneumatic leg compression and pharmacological prophylaxis for prevention of venous thromboembolism. Cochrane Database Syst Rev. 2022;1(1):CD005258.
32. Crawford DA, Andrews RL, Morris MJ, Hurst JM, Lombardi AV Jr, Berend KR. Ambulatory portable pneumatic compression device as part of a multimodal aspirin-based approach in prevention of venous thromboembolism in outpatient total knee arthroplasty. Arthroplasty today. 2020;6(3):378–80.
33. Prevention of pulmonary embolism and deep vein thrombosis with low dose aspirin: pulmonary embolism prevention (PEP) trial. Lancet. 2000;355(9212):1295–302.

34. Faour M, Piuzzi NS, Brigati DP, Klika AK, Mont MA, Barsoum WK, Higuera CA. Low-dose aspirin is safe and effective for venous thromboembolism prophylaxis following Total knee arthroplasty. J Arthroplast. 2018;33(7S):S131–5. https://doi.org/10.1016/j.arth.2018.03.001.

35. Feldstein MJ, Low SL, Chen AF, Woodward LA, Hozack WJ. A comparison of two dosing regimens of ASA following total hip and knee arthroplasties. J Arthroplast. 2017;32(9):S157–61.

36. Haykal T, Kheiri B, Zayed Y, Barbarawi M, Miran MS, Chahine A, Katato K, Bachuwa G. Aspirin for venous thromboembolism prophylaxis after hip or knee arthroplasty: an updated meta-analysis of randomized controlled trials. J Orthop. 2019;16(4):312–9. https://doi.org/10.1016/j.jor.2019.02.032. Erratum in: J Orthop 2019;16(4):R1.

37. Matharu GS, Garriga C, Whitehouse MR, Rangan A, Judge A. Is aspirin as effective as the newer direct oral anticoagulants for venous thromboembolism prophylaxis after total hip and knee arthroplasty? An analysis from the National Joint Registry for England, Wales, Northern Ireland, and the Isle of Man. J Arthroplast. 2020;35(9):2631–9.

38. Tan TL, Foltz C, Huang R, Chen AF, Higuera C, Siqueira M, Hansen EN, Sing DC, Parvizi J. Potent anticoagulation does not reduce venous thromboembolism in high-risk patients. JBJS. 2019;101(7):589–99.

39. Huang R, Buckley PS, Scott B, Parvizi J, Purtill JJ. Administration of aspirin as a prophylaxis agent against venous thromboembolism results in lower incidence of periprosthetic joint infection. J Arthroplast. 2015;30(9):39–41.

40. Bosch LC, Beger SB, Duncan ST, Rossi SM, Sculco PK, Barnes CL, Amanatullah DF. Intraoperative practice variability in total knee arthroplasty. J Arthroplast. 2020;35(3):725–31.

41. Suen K, Westh RN, Churilov L, Hardidge AJ. Low-molecular-weight heparin and the relative risk of surgical site bleeding complications: results of a systematic review and meta-analysis of randomized controlled trials of venous thromboprophylaxis in patients after total joint arthroplasty. J Arthroplast. 2017;32(9):2911–9.

42. Venker BT, Ganti BR, Lin H, Lee ED, Nunley RM, Gage BF. Safety and efficacy of new anticoagulants for the prevention of venous thromboembolism after hip and knee arthroplasty: a meta-analysis. J Arthroplast. 2017;32(2):645–52.

Cementless Total Knee Arthroplasty

Mackenzie Neumaier, David Quinzi,
Andrew Jeong, Linda I. Suleiman,
and Rishi Balkissoon

Introduction

Cementless total knee arthroplasty (TKA) has seen a resurgence in recent years secondary to ease of implantation, decreased surgical times, preservation of durable bone stock, and decreased risk of third body wear derived from cement particles. Furthermore, the volume of TKA performed in the world continues to rise, including an increase in younger patients pursuing TKA who will likely require more complex future revision procedures as a result of failed implant fixation. Thus consideration of alternative fixation to cement for patients undergoing TKA that may provide lasting osseointegration and durable direct fixation of implant to bone remains of interest, particularly as this is already seen with overwhelming success in cementless total hip arthroplasties. Regardless, cemented TKA is the standard that is most commonly utilized and to which cementless TKA will be perpetually compared. The 2013 European registry data suggests that 6.1% of TKAs performed utilize fully cementless or hybrid fixation [1]. This number has likely grown since. U.S. market data indicates that there has been a growth in the use of coated cementless TKA constructs between 2016 and 2019 from 3.1% to 8.2% of all cases. When also considering hybrid TKA cases using cementless femoral and cemented tibial components that comprise 2.7% the market share in 2019, 10.9% of all TKA cases in the U.S. utilized some form of cementless fixation in 2019 [2]. These estimates are consistent with those reported by the American Joint Replacement Registry (AJRR) 2020 Annual Report, indicating that in 2019, 9.9% of TKAs were fully cementless and 2.5% of TKAs were implanted using hybrid fixation [3]. And, the Australian National Joint Replacement Registry 2020 Annual Report indicates that, in 2019, 12.3% of TKAs were fully cementless, while approximately 20% of TKAs were implanted using hybrid fixation, such that nearly one-third of the TKAs being performed in Australia today utilize some form of cementless fixation [4]. However, with regard to outcomes

M. Neumaier · D. Quinzi · A. Jeong
Department of Orthopedics and Rehabilitation,
University of Rochester Medical Center,
Rochester, NY, USA
e-mail: Mackenzie_Neumaier@URMC.Rochester.
edu; David_Quinzi@URMC.Rochester.edu;
Andrew_Jeong@URMC.Rochester.edu

L. I. Suleiman
Department of Orthopedic Surgery and Medical
Education, McGaw Medical Center of Northwestern
University, Northwestern University,
Chicago, IL, USA
e-mail: lsuleima@nm.org

R. Balkissoon (✉)
Department of Orthopedics and Rehabilitation, Adult
Reconstructive Orthopaedic Surgery, University of
Rochester Medical Center, Rochester, NY, USA
e-mail: Rishi_Balkissoon@URMC.Rochester.edu

and patient satisfaction after TKA, there still remains room for improvement with cementless fixation as playing a potential role in increasing long-term success. Historically, cemented fixation has provided more reliable results when compared to cementless fixation and early failures of cementless constructs provided for skepticism preventing their widespread use [5, 6]. Overall, cementless fixation remains a promising technique when appropriately indicated and technically executed. Advances in implant technology such as hydroxyapatite-coated integration surfaces, a wide array of commercially available porous metal constructs, and newer manufacturing techniques including "3D" printed biomaterials have shown promise and potential for excellent survivorship in the appropriate patient, and thus cementless fixation for TKAs will continue to be utilized moving forward [7, 8].

History and Implant Design

With reports dating back to the late 1970s with the Kodama-Yamamoto prosthesis, evolution of the cementless total knee arthroplasty has been an ongoing process. Over the ensuing four decades from initial development, uncemented implants have undergone modifications with regards to implant design, material technology, and technical knowledge to rival outcomes associated with more traditional cemented components. Reflection on early failures has paved the way for more reliable instrumentation to maximize highly sought theoretical advantages of cementless fixation, including preservation of bone stock and improved longevity of the implant–bone interface. These advances are perhaps best illustrated by focusing on each TKA component individually.

Historically, the femoral component has demonstrated the most success in terms of osseointegration [1, 5, 9]. This allows for reliable usage in both fully uncemented and hybrid knees. At the core of a successful outcome lies technical precision when performing the axial, coronal, and chamfer cuts, as elimination of cement also eliminates some margin for error. Taking care to do so allows for a natural press-fit of the component.

Most components have also been developed to contain pegs to control for rotational stability. It has been determined that these pegs are best left smooth as coated pegs can alter bone ingrowth patterns contributing to stress shielding of the anterior femoral cortex. This can be problematic as it may increase the risk for fracture as well as compromises remaining bone stock should revision be required.

Previous studies have demonstrated that the patellar component is typically one of the more problematic components, especially earlier in development [1, 5, 9]. Initially designed as a thin, metal-backed polyethylene surface, (Fig. 17.1), these early designs were fraught with complication. Failure of this design was multifactorial, including polyethylene wear, polyethylene-metal dissociation, shearing at the peg-baseplate interface, and loosening (Figs. 17.2 and 17.3). Near-complete polyethylene wear is especially problematic in this case as it creates a metal-on-metal articulation between the baseplate and femoral component. This can result in a metallosis-type adverse local tissue reaction as well as direct damage of the femoral trochlear groove, requiring revision of an otherwise well-fixed femoral component (Fig. 17.4). A 2001 study by Berger et al. cited the 10-year all-cause survivorship of this type of implant at 67.9%. Outcomes have improved quite dramatically with use of an inlay-type patella component. This allows for the ability to maintain the metal-backed ingrowth surface while allowing for accommodation of a thicker polyethylene component. Alternatively, an all-

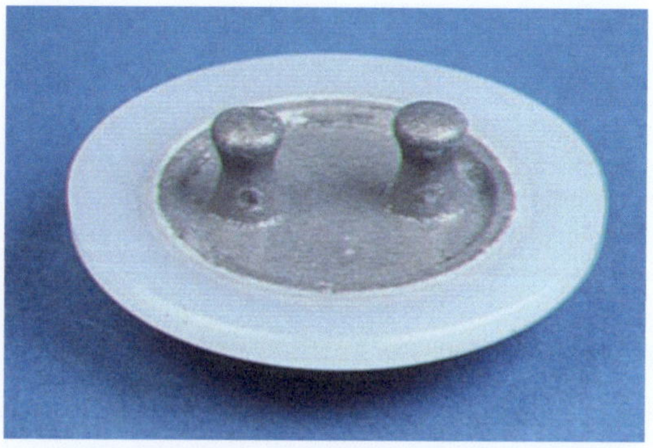

Fig. 17.1 Clinical Photo of Patella Component. Clinical photograph of undersurface of polyethylene on metal implant. (Image courtesy of Richard Berger, MD)

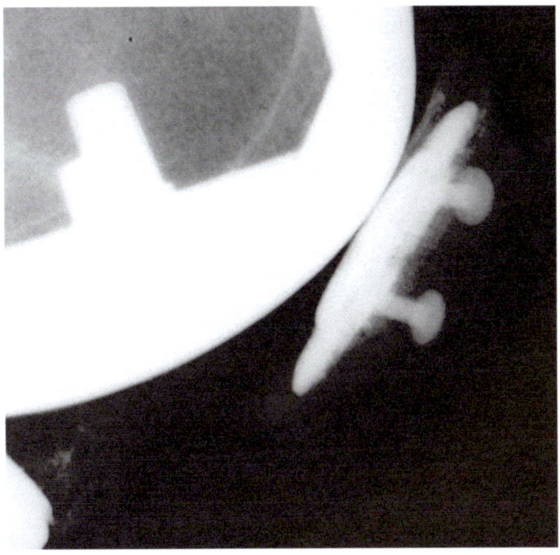

Fig. 17.2 Patella Failure Through Wear. Lateral view of the knee demonstrating complete wear of the polyethylene component resulting in metal-on-metal articulation through the patella ingrowth surface. (Image courtesy of Richard Berger, MD)

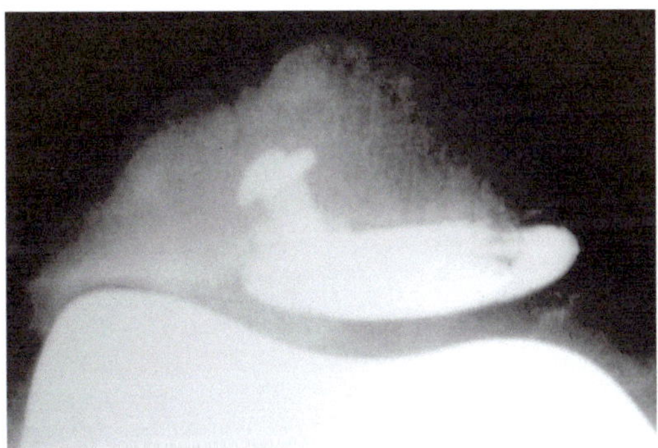

Fig. 17.3 Patella Failure Through Shearing. Merchant view of the knee demonstrating shearing of the metal peg from the patella component resulting in displacement and failure of the component. (Image courtesy of Richard Berger, MD)

polyethylene component can be cemented; however, this may increase operative time and introduce potential third-body cement particles, negating some benefits of the cementless model.

Since the initial development of the cementless concept, the most attention has been dedicated to optimizing the tibial component. It has been demonstrated that once osseointegration occurs, the uncemented total knee arthroplasty has the potential to match or outperform the outcomes and longevity of the cemented TKA. However, the challenge for some models has been reaching this

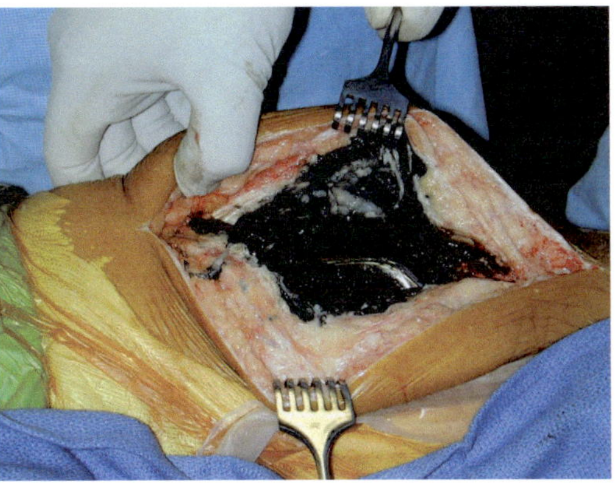

Fig. 17.4 Metallosis After Patella Failure. Clinical photograph of metallosis-type reaction resulting from polyethylene wear and subsequent metal-on-metal articular as also depicted in Fig. 17.1. (Image courtesy of Richard Berger, MD)

point, with most failures occurring in the first 2 years [10]. From a theoretical standpoint, this entails limiting early micromotion with component features that best minimize potential failed osseointegration. The earliest tibial tray designs were exclusively polyethylene and relied on pegs or fins to stabilize the component. It is perhaps obvious that these failed due to a lack of integration surface. Metal trays and modularity were soon incorporated, initially with a smooth or matte undersurface and eventually with partial porous coating. While the addition of porous coating was beneficial, failures continued to be seen for lack of integration. It has been postulated that the non-coated portions of the implant allowed for violation of the implant-bone interface with synovial fluid and joint debris, hindering successful integration of porous segments. This prompted transition to a fully coated implant, with some favoring asymmetric designs with larger medial footprints to mirror the native tibia and allow for greater surface area for ingrowth. Despite this, the concern of initial stabilization remains.

As the tibial component evolved, as noted above, ongoing experimentation with stems, keels, and pegs was also occurring. Initial peg designs were deemed too short and ineffective (Fig. 17.5). Therefore, more modern designs favor deeper pegs, stems, or keels. These are typically not coated for ingrowth. Additionally, another means of initial fixation (and source of

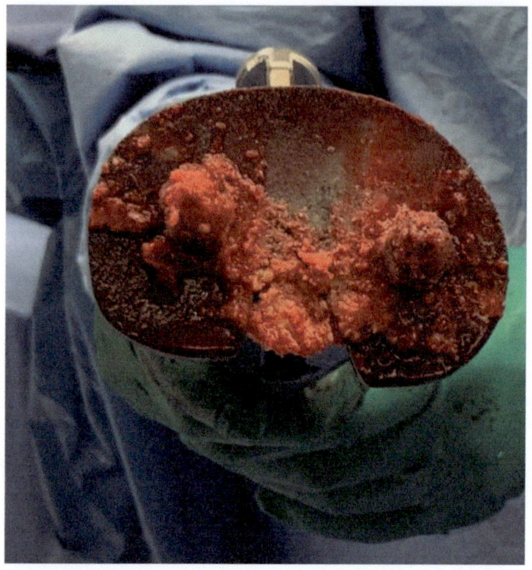

Fig. 17.5 Tibial Tray Failure. Clinical photograph depicting the osseointegration surface of an explanted tibial tray. Note the bony ingrowth centered around the short pegs

ongoing debate) is the use of screws. Both opinions and outcomes have been split as the trade-off of increased early fixation is met with the risk of developing screw track osteolysis. A 2008 study by Ferguson et al. did not find any evidence of screw track osteolysis or loosening compared to a control group using an identical fully porous coated tibial tray without screws. This idea was further analyzed on a molecular and biomechanical level in 2019 by Klutzny et al. [11].They analyzed 88 patients, roughly 8% of their cohort, and found that tibial screw track osteolysis was more likely to occur medially. There was a correlation between severity of osteolysis on imaging and varus positioning of the tibial tray as well as suboptimal positioning of the medial screw. While these trends were not thought to contribute to poorer outcomes, they do contribute to bone loss, which could complicate revision surgery (Figs. 17.6 and 17.7). The osteolytic cavities

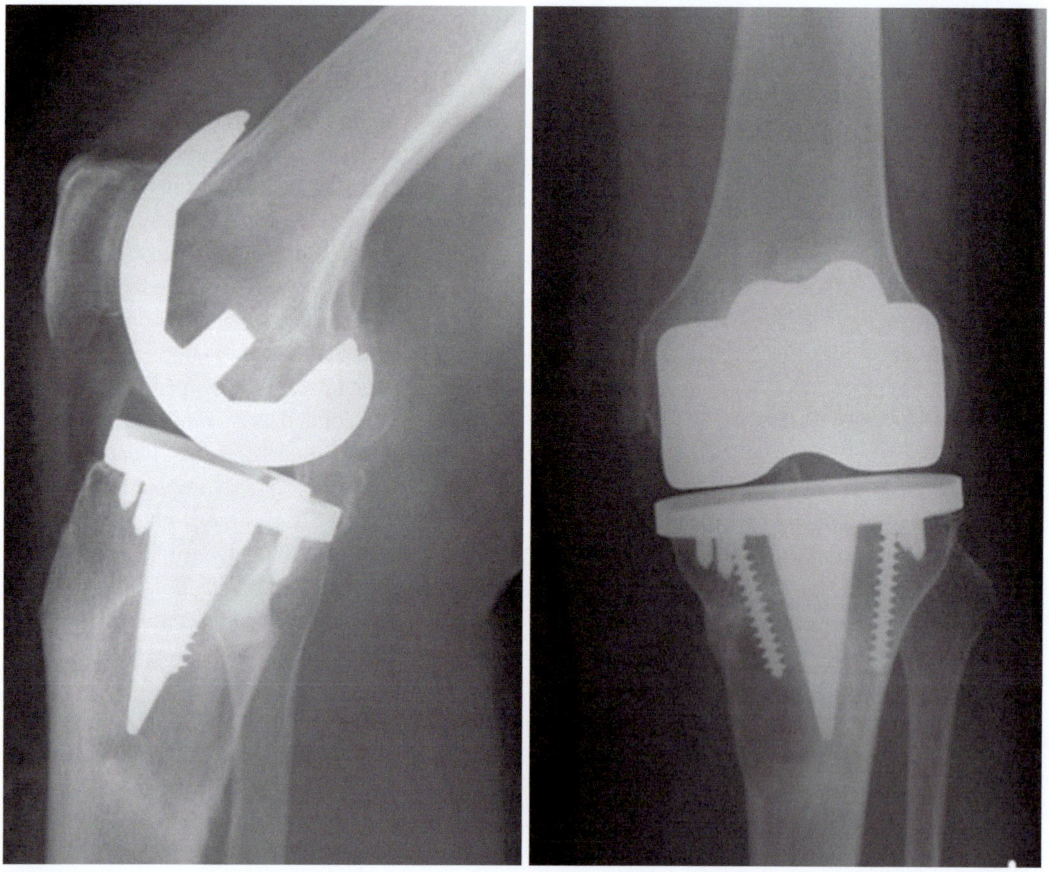

Fig. 17.6 Radiographic Depiction of Screw Track Osteolysis. AP and lateral X-rays depicting screw track osteolysis, localized around the medial screw. (Image originally published by Klutzny et al. [11])

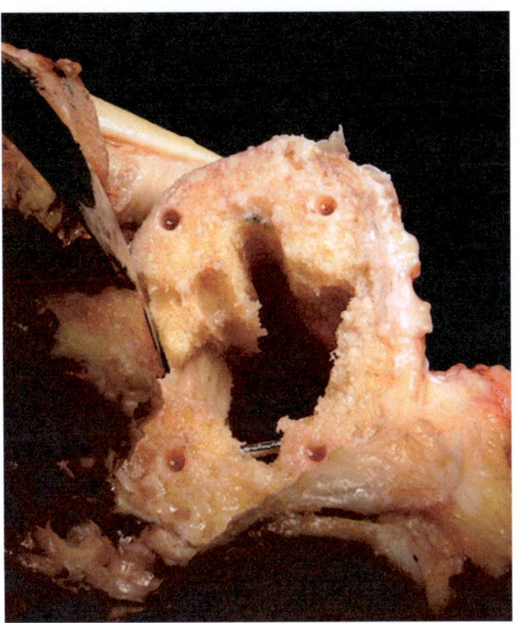

Fig. 17.7 Clinical Photo—Screw Track Osteolysis. Intra-operative demonstration of bone loss caused by screw track osteolysis. (Image originally published by Klutzny et al. [11])

were also studied on a molecular level, revealing metal ions, specifically titanium, as the likely culprit. This contradicted early thinking that this was primarily caused by polyethylene and joint debris escaping into the screw tracks. While there was some deformation on the undersurface of the recovered polyethylene components in the regions overlying the screw holes, there was no evidence of polyethylene on a molecular level. It was concluded that screw track osteolysis is primarily caused by the interaction at the screw-tray interface, specifically an outer layer used in the packaging and preservation process. With this information in mind, the utility of screw usage is likely supplemental fixation when concerned for poor bone quality or in situations where there may be some irregularity of the tibial surface due to either technique or pre-existing cysts. With lack of agreement about optimal design features necessary to achieve excellent early fixation that will enable stable long-term osseointegration, there certainly remains room for design improvement and consistency for the cementless tibial component.

Aside from the attributes of the components themselves, component philosophy has also been studied. Historically, many of the cementless implants had been cruciate-retaining (CR) by design. While this remains true today, posterior stabilized (PS) designs have also been assessed. Initially, there was a theoretical barrier to these implants as it was feared the interaction between the cam and post would cause excess micromotion at the implant–bone interface and interfere with osseointegration. This concern has since been debunked [12]. Likewise, there was also thought of theoretical benefit to use of mobile-bearing implants to offload micromotion at the implant–bone interface. Results of these studies have not been as convincing.

Lastly, it is the evolution of porous coating technology that has most significantly contributed to the advancement of cementless implants. Initial implants were typically cobalt–chrome or titanium and ranged from smooth to grit-blasted to porous. More recent advances have gravitated more towards increased porosity to increase surface area for ingrowth. Popular options today include highly porous titanium as well as tantalum. The advancement of 3D printing has allowed for micron-level modification of these designs to more adequately resemble trabecular bone and provide a more smooth transition biomechanically at the implant-bone interface compared to more traditional cemented options [8]. Additionally, coatings, such as hydroxyapatite, have been well studied as useful adjuncts. Manipulation of the bone-cement interface remains at the forefront of future research and is a vital variable in current and future successes of cementless technologies.

Outcomes

As the number of cementless TKAs performed continues to rise, an increasing number of studies demonstrate early positive results of cementless TKAs that utilize newer model implants both across various subgroups of patients, and also in comparison to cemented TKA implants [9, 13–18]. The emergence of these newer studies contrasts past reports illustrating poorer performance of cementless fixation outcomes over time. Notably, Berger et al. reported in 2001 that cemented fixation was the "gold standard" and that his group was abandoning PCL retaining cementless TKA fixation due to a lack of consistent bony ingrowth of the tibial component (8%), osteolytic lesions around screws or screw holes in the tibial components (12%), and an excessively high revision rate of the metal-backed patellar components (48%). The advent of more advanced techniques, biomaterials, and instrumentation has shown that cementless TKAs can afford greater durability and bony ingrowth, allowing them to potentially serve as a more viable alternative to cemented TKA. This is especially relevant in light of the known limitations of cemented TKA in certain patient subgroups, including the obese, young, and active patients.

Boyle et al. reported the incidence of revision due to aseptic loosening of the tibial baseplate in patients undergoing either uncemented or cemented cruciate-retaining TKA specifically in patients with a body mass index (BMI) greater than 30. They found no statistically significant difference between the groups in survivorship for aseptic loosening (99.4% uncemented, 99.3% uncemented, $P = 0.94$), as well as overall survivorship (98.1% uncemented, 98.3% cemented, $P = 0.90$) at an average of 5.7 years follow-up. Furthermore, they comment on the clinical and radiographic short- to mid-term outcomes, indicating comparable Lower Extremity Activity Scale (10.2 ± 3.7 uncemented vs. 9.7 ± 3.4 cemented, $P = 0.33$), Forgotten Joint Score (66.1 ± 28.2 vs. 64.9 ± 24.3, $P = 0.78$), and postoperative knee flexion (114.6 ± 9.3 vs. 114.1 ± 9.3, $P = 0.67$) [13]. More recently, Sinicrope et al. similarly reported on the survivorship of 108 cementless vs. 85 cemented posterior stabilized TKAs in morbidly obese patients (BMI > 40) with a minimum of 5-years follow-up, with aseptic loosening as the primary endpoint. They found that in this patient subgroup, there was greater survivorship amongst patients with cementless vs. cemented implants (99% vs. 92.9% at 5-year follow-up, 99.1% vs. 88.2% at 8-year follow-up) [14]. They theorize that this relatively steady state survivorship of the cementless implants over time is secondary to a more durable implant-bone interface that can better withstand the added mechanical stress in the morbidly obese population.

Kim et al. evaluated outcomes, including clinical results, radiographic findings, complications, and revision and survivorship rates in patients younger than 55 years old at a minimum of 16 years follow-up after undergoing bilateral, sequential, simultaneous, cemented, and cementless TKAs in the same patients [15]. In their prospective and randomized study, they evaluated 80 patients (160 knees) who received a cementless implant in one knee, and a cemented implant in the contralateral knee. They found that at mean follow-up of 16.6 years, the mean Knee Society knee score (95.8 cementless, 96.9 cemented), Western Ontario and McMaster Universities (WOMAC) osteoarthritis (OA) index (25.4 cementless, 25.9 cemented), range of motion (ROM) (125° cementless, 128° cemented), patient satisfaction (8.1, cementless, 8.3 cemented) and radiological results were similar in both groups. At 17 years follow-up, the femoral component survival rate was 100% in both groups, and tibial component survivorship was 98.7% in the cementless group, and 100% in the cemented group. The authors note that the average low patient weight, good pre-operative ROM, and young age of the group may limit general applicability to other patient groups. However, the comparable outcomes between cementless and cemented TKAs in their study highlight the potential feasibility of utilizing newer cementless implants with success in younger patients requiring TKA.

Dixon et al. demonstrated that the success of uncemented instrumentation is not exclusive to the young population. In a 2004 study comparing a young (<75y) and older (>75y) cohort of patients undergoing cementless TKA, there was no difference in functional outcomes and range of motion at 5 years. Complication profiles were also comparable, aside from deaths during follow up being higher in the older group. This was not attributed to be a result of the surgery.

Bingham et al. reported a systematic review of the literature to evaluate clinical outcomes, revision rates, and survivorship of patients undergoing cementless TKA using contemporary implants [9]. They evaluated 43 studies with 10,447 TKAs, of which 8187 were primary cementless TKAs, with a mean follow-up of

7 years. The authors note that contemporary cementless designs have yielded excellent survivorship and clinical outcomes, with results comparable with modern cemented designs. They highlight several studies to this effect, including additional systematic reviews such as that from Mont et al. [16], which demonstrates similar survivorship between cementless and cemented TKAs in a study comparing cementless vs. cemented TKAs in 2940 patients (mean survivorship at 10 years follow-up of 96% in the cementless group, and 95% in the cemented group). Of note, Bingham et al. observe that in their review, there was variability in survivorship within the review of the cementless implants based on design (i.e., cementless implants from myriad manufacturers may produce varying results), and that only mid-term follow-up is available for the more contemporary designs. They also emphasize the need for additional clinical randomized clinical trials that specifically examine more contemporary implant designs to delineate the potential benefits of cementless TKA fixation.

The aforementioned studies demonstrate similar outcomes between cementless and cemented TKA implants, especially at short- to mid-term follow-up. On the basis of clinical outcomes such as patient satisfaction, functional outcomes, and radiographic studies, cementless TKA appears to be a viable option in comparison to cemented TKA across a variety of patient subgroups. However, multiple studies have pointed to the need for further long-term trials to truly delineate the potential of these newer generation cementless implants.

Benefits and Complications

When considering the most appropriate mode of fixation and implant choices for knee arthroplasty, the risk–benefit profile must be critically analyzed, as is true for any surgical procedure. For many, this will include an analysis of patient factors such as age, bone quality, comorbid conditions, and pre-operative deformity, paired with surgeon factors, including implant comfort level, previous training, philosophical beliefs and access to resources, including implants and instrumentation for their implantation. Theoretical advantages of cementless TKA components include a biologic bond at the implant-bone interface with the potential promise of longevity greater than may be afforded by cemented implants, preservation of bone stock for revision surgery, and decreased surgical time. Indirect benefits, including elimination of potential for third-body wear derived from cement usage. While it may seem difficult to dispute these potential advantages, they must be tempered against the risk of failed implant integration, the costs of cementless implants, and further less understood factors—such as whether patient symptoms may occur before implant osseointegration is complete, true ease of revision procedures, and the effects imparted to surrounding bone with long-term fixation, including areas of stress shielding and bone remodeling, among others.

Despite the end goal of cementless fixation being a more natural, robust osseous bond at the implant-bone interface, there remains concern regarding aseptic loosening, especially prior to maturation of this bond. As noted in the "History and Design" section, this concern in modern implants remains focused on the patellar and tibial components. Radiostereometric analysis (RSA), which involves implantation of radio-opaque markers that can be used to monitor radiographic component migration over time, has aided significantly in our understanding of the degree of migration that may be expected or whether a component may be at risk for failure [7]. It is now understood that uncemented TKA components have an earlier window for both migration and failure compared to cemented counterparts. Migration of cementless TKA components has been demonstrated with greater displacement than cemented components for up to 2 years post-operatively [10], although typically reaching stability by 3 months compared to 5 years of micromotion that may occur for cemented components [6]. For uncemented components, if this migration exceeded 0.2 mm between the first and second year, the patient was more likely to experience failure secondary to aseptic loosening. Furthermore, a potential relationship has been established whereby greater migration may occur in patients with lower bone mineral density, suggesting use of cementless fixation may be at greater risk for failure in the elderly population [1].

Randomized studies have suggested that once outside the initial window for failure, cementless components have (up to) a 4.7 times lower risk for future loosening compared to cemented [10]. These results are supported by several long-term studies demonstrating near-unanimous 100% survival of femoral components and tibial tray survival ranging from 94 to 98% in studies looking at 10 years of follow up or more [9, 19, 20]. While many lacked a direct comparison to cemented knees, most concluded there was at least non-inferiority compared to cemented previously published standards. A more detailed analysis of some of these studies can be found in the "Outcomes" section. This data is met with resistance from international registry studies, specifically from Australia, New Zealand, and Sweden, where outcomes are not as favorable with regards to revision for loosening. Specifically, the Swedish registry notes a 1.6 times higher risk of revision with regards to the tibial component [1]. While some of this variability may be explained by the innate disadvantages of registry data compared to single surgeon or group data, there remains a need for more convincing studies in support of cementless fixation for TKAs.

Integral to the assessment for loosening of uncemented TKA components is radiographic evaluation for component stability. Radiolucencies surrounding implants have long been noted at various time points after uncemented TKA with some reporting an incidence in upwards of 50% of cases [21]. The development of these radiolucencies can be attributed to a lack of cement that may account for subtle non-conformity between implant and bone versus stress-based bony remodeling over time. The natural history of these radiolucent lines was investigated by Costales et al. in a 2020 study following patients over 9 years post-operatively. They concluded that these lines were noted as early as 6 weeks post-operatively and continued to appear for up to 1 year. No new radiolucencies were noted between 1 year and final follow up. These were found on both the femur and tibia, with the femoral lines noted at the chamfer cuts and the tibial lines at the medial and lateral peripheral margins. Characteristics of these lines were < 2 mm, incomplete, and non-progressive over time [21]. These patients experienced improved outcomes compared to pre-operative scores without an increased risk of failure, therefore it was concluded that similar radiolucent lines should not be grounds for concern.

An additional risk unique to performing uncemented TKA is that of increased blood loss. Due to a lack of the tamponade effect of cement on the bony cuts, there is some evidence that those undergoing uncemented TKA may be at increased risk for requiring a blood transfusion within 48 hours of surgery. While some have refuted this, it remains a serious consideration, especially with the increased push for outpatient arthroplasty models [1].

Cementless TKA has also been evaluated for prosthetic joint infection rate as well as other medical complications. A 2020 meta-analysis by Bingham et al. noted that infection occurred in 1% of the total cohort and accounted for <1% of all revisions performed. As noted above, the true benefit of cementless TKA is not in preventing infection; however, it could prove advantageous with regards to revision options and bone stock after implant removal. Other noted complications included deep vein thrombosis (3%) and stiffness (1%), which are commonly reported events and may be expected following total knee arthroplasty in general [9].

Future Directions

The future of cementless fixation will likely hinge on the expectations and patient-reported outcomes regarding the TKA patient of the future as younger and more active patients continue to enter the clinical marketplace for TKA. Contemporary implants, instrumentation, and emerging technologies such as computer navigation and robotics potentially reduce technical issues that may have previously limited more widespread adoption of cementless TKA constructs. Currently, the global cementless TKA marketplace is rapidly growing and with the increase in total TKAs performed yearly, orthopedic implant companies have been aggressive in their development of cementless technologies for primary and revision TKAs. Ultimately, it will be of great future significance for the treating orthopedic surgeon to determine the true role for cementless TKA with high quality evidence derived from long-term randomized controlled trials, cost analyses (including factors such as implant costs, time saved during surgery, costs of reoperation, etc), and costs of adjunctive measures that may be necessary to achieve success in their implementation (such as the use of robotic-assisted surgery).

Conclusion

The development of the cementless TKA has improved quite impressively since its entry into market over four decades ago. While we are still within a renaissance period of implant development, current implants have demonstrated the longevity and performance to compete with more traditional cemented models. While outperformance of cemented implants has yet to be proven, reliable studies have at least demonstrated non-inferiority. It is evident that the advantages of cementless TKA are no longer purely theoretical and may be considered in the armamentarium of solutions of the treating orthopedic surgeon tailored to the appropriate patient to improve the quality of life in both traditional and less traditional (perhaps young or obese) TKA candidates.

References

1. Dalury DF. Cementless Total knee arthroplasty. Bone Joint J. 2016;98-B:867–73.
2. Mendenhall S. OrthoTrends 2011-Q1/2020. Orthop Netw News. 2020;31(3):1–24.
3. American Joint Replacement Registry (AJRR). 2020 Annual Report. Rosemont, IL: American Academy of Orthopaedic Surgeons (AAOS); 2020.
4. Australian Orthopaedic Association National Joint Replacement Registry (AOANJRR). Hip, Knee & Shoulder Arthroplasty: 2020 Annual Report. Adelaide: AOA; 2020. p. 1–474.
5. Newman JM, Sohdi N, Khlopas A, Sultan A. Cementless Total knee arthroplasty: a comprehensive review of the literature. Orthopedics. 2018;41(5):263–73.
6. Aprato A, Risitano S, Sabatini L, Giachino M. Cementless total knee arthroplasty. Ann Transl Med. 2016;4(7):1–7.
7. Haddad FS, Plastow R. Is it time to revisit cementless total knee arthroplasty? Bone Joint J. 2020;102-B:965–6.
8. Sultan A, Mahmood B, Samuel L, Stearns K. Cementless 3D printed highly porous titanium-coated baseplate Total knee arthroplasty: Suvivorship and outcomes at 2-year minimum follow-up. J Knee Surg. 2020;33(3):279–83.
9. Bingham JS, Salib CG, Hanssen AD, Taunton MJ. Clinical outcomes and survivorship of contemporary cementless primary total knee arthroplasties. JBJS Rev. 2020;8(8):1–8.
10. Nakama GY, Peccin MS, Almeida GJM, Lira Neto ODA. Cemented, cementless or hybrid fixation options in total knee arthroplasty for osteoarthritis and other non-traumatic diseases. Cochrane Database Syst Rev. 2012;10:1–44.
11. Klutzny M, Singh G, Hameister R, Goldau G. Screw track Osteolysis in the Cementless Total knee replacement design. J Arthroplast. 2019;34:965–73.
12. Harwin SF, Levin JM, Khlopas A, Ramkumar PN. Cementless posterior stabilized Total knee arthroplasty: seven-year minimum follow-up report. J Arthroplast. 2018;33:1399–403.
13. Boyle KK, Nodzo SR, Ferraro JT, Augenblick DJ, Pavlesen S, Phillips MJ. Uncemented vs cemented cruciate retaining total knee arthroplasty in patients with body mass index greater than 30. J Arthroplast. 2018;33(4):1082–8.
14. Sinicrope BJ, Feher AW, Bhimani SJ. Increased survivorship of cementless versus cemented tka in the morbidly obese. A minimum 5-year follow-up. J Arthroplast. 2019;34(2):309–14.
15. Kim YH, Park JW, Lim HM, Park ES. Cementless and cemented total knee arthroplasty in patients younger than fifty five years: which is better? Int Orthop. 2014;38(2):297–303.
16. Mont MA, Pivec R, Issa K, Kapadia BH, Maheshwari A, Harwin SF. Long-term implant survivorship of cementless total knee arthroplasty: a systematic review of the literature and meta-analysis. J Knee Surg. 2014;27(5):369–76.
17. Hampton M, Mansoor J, Getty J, Sutton PM. Uncemented tantalum metal components

versus cemented tibial components in total knee arthroplasty: 11- to 15- year outcomes of a single-blinded randomized controlled trial. Bone Joint J. 2020;102-B(8):1025–32.

18. Miller AJ, Stimac JD, Smith LS, Feher AW, Yakkanti MR. Results of cemented vs Cementless primary Total knee arthroplasty using the same implant design. J Arthroplast. 2018;33:1089–93.

19. Kim YH, Park JW, Lim HM, Jang YS. The 22 to 25-year survival of cemented and Cementless Total knee arthroplasty in young patients. J Arthroplast. 2021;36:566–72.

20. Chen C, Li R. Cementless versus cemented total knee arthroplasty in young patients: a meta-analysis of randomized controlled trials. J Orthop Surg Res. 2019;14:1–11.

21. Costales TG, Chapman DM, Dalury DF. The natural history of Radiolucencies following Uncemented Total knee arthroplasty at 9 years. J Arthroplast. 2020;35:127–31.

The Future of the Modern Total Knee Arthroplasty

Bo Zhang, Julius K. Oni, and Savyasachi C. Thakkar

Introduction

Total Knee Arthroplasty (TKA) has advanced significantly both in technique and in perioperative management. By 2030, the number of TKAs performed in the United States annually is expected to reach between 1.26 and 3.48 million. At the same time, both hospital cost and cost of implants have increased, attributable to technology such as robotics, navigation, and custom implants. Rising demand coupled with increasing cost of TKA has led to the bundled payment program and driven efforts to decrease cost and increase capacity. As a result, perioperative protocols have become more streamlined, length of stay has significantly decreased, and new techniques and technology have been incorporated to maximize efficiency. At the same time, every aspect of TKA has been advanced to improve outcomes. Together, cost reduction and quality improvement aim to increase the value of TKA for insurance, hospitals, and surgeons alike. This chapter outlines the recent trends and future outlook of TKA.

B. Zhang (✉) · J. K. Oni · S. C. Thakkar
Department of Orthopedic Surgery, Johns Hopkins, Baltimore, MD, USA
e-mail: bo@jhmi.edu; joni1@jhmi.edu; savya@jhmi.edu

Economics of Total Knee Arthroplasty

Increasing Demand

Total Knee Arthroplasty (TKA) is one of the most commonly performed surgeries in the United States, and its volume is expected to rise rapidly. If growth continues at the current trend, the annual number of primary TKAs performed is projected to reach 1.37 million by 2020 and 3.48 million by 2030 [1]. This is further supplemented by a similar increase in revision TKA. While advancements in TKA has decreased certain modes of failure, the primary culprits of aseptic loosening and prosthetic joint infection have maintained a stable overall revision rate. More recent models have suggested that this exponential growth may not be likely [2]. While the growth of total hip arthroplasty has remained stable, growth in TKA has plateaued in recent years. Other modulators of growth, such as health care changes, prevalence of arthritis, and shifting surgical indications are difficult to predict. Although the economic turbulence of the 2000s did not significantly impact the trends in TKA [3], the long-term effect of the Coronavirus pandemic on elective surgical volume is unknown, given its profound impact to the TKA patient population.

Decreasing Cost

The rapidly rising demand for TKA places a significant financial burden on the U S health care system and is driving the implementation of cost containment strategies. Internationally, 37 countries in the Organization for Economic Co-operation and Development have also reported increases in TKA utilization. Obesity, increasing age, economic growth, and lower baseline TKA utilization were drivers of this growth [4]. In 2014, Medicare paid for 55% of TKAs in the United States, with hospitalization of lower extremity joint replacements costing Medicare over $7 billion [5]. Key strategies for limiting costs have involved decreasing length of stay and maximizing outpatient surgery, which may yield 30% cost savings compared to inpatient TKA [6]. Despite down-trending length of stay, mean hospital cost for TKA increased from roughly $15,000 to $23,000 between 2002 and 2013, signaling a need for additional reform. In April 2016, the Comprehensive Care for Joint Replacement Model enacted a bundled payment model for TKA and THA [7]. In this model, the reimbursement is fixed for the surgery and the 90-day global period afterwards, which incentivizes the hospital to reduce cost and complications which may significantly increase costs. In the first two years of its enactment, cost per surgery declined 3% without significant changes in complications or selection of high-risk patients [8]. In the full bundle of care, TKA cost is primarily driven by consumables (44%) and personnel (50%), with space and equipment making up the rest [9]. In addition to shortening hospitalization and minimizing complications, reducing implant cost and efficient use of staff per case may be the most effective next steps toward a substantial cost reduction. Strategies may include utilizing personnel to capacity at the "top of their license" and minimizing redundancy in staffing of cases.

Traditionally, reimbursements are either through private insurance, government insurance, or self-pay. However, a new pathway has become popular where large companies take insurers out of the equation and directly contract with large health systems to provide joint replacement for its employees [10]. This requires patients to travel to designated surgery sites, Centers of Excellence, with the goal of decreasing costs. So far, results are promising, with no increased complications despite long distance travel [11]. With the financial incentives for the companies, this model may become a significant part of future joint replacement practice.

Patient Selection and Perioperative Optimization

Patient Selection

Selecting appropriate patients for TKA has gained wide acceptance as increasing evidence demonstrates worse outcomes and higher complication rates in patients who do not meet criteria. More recently, certain risk factors have been found to drive increased costs beyond reimbursement from the bundle payment plan [12]. For example, infection rates are higher in morbidly obese patients, and an infection triples the cost of a primary joint replacement [13, 14]. The trend is expected to continue; with the identification of additional risk factors, new guidelines will be enacted. If demand for TKA exceeds capacity, there may be an incentive to screen more qualified patients, as patient outcome has become a part of physician reimbursement models. The focus will be maximum on surgical improvement with minimum risk of readmission, reoperation, and revision. These selected patients are expected to gain the most quality-adjusted life years and have the least complications, therefore the most cost-effective for surgery. Patient selection will also be critical as the number of outpatient surgeries increase. Ambulatory centers often have limited capacity to manage perioperative complications or monitor patients overnight. Thus, choosing patients that are most likely to undergo a complication-free TKA and recover quickly for a same-day discharge maybe the most important aspect of a successful outpatient surgery center. On the other hand, those with significant comorbidities still benefit substantially from TKA and should be treated on an inpatient basis.

Patient Education and Perioperative Care

Preoperative education and setting expectations have been an increasing point of emphasis in current TKA pathways. This starts at the first clinical visit and may include instruction from the surgeon, nursing staff, or physical therapists. Due to time restrictions in clinic, patients may benefit from an educational class to guide them through the entire surgical process. Improving patients' knowledge and confidence increases patient activation, the ability to manage one's own care. Higher patient activation can reduce cost, improve outcomes, and better prepare the patient for outpatient surgery [5]. The same applies to the patients' family members. Reducing their anxiety through education can have a direct and positive impact on the patients' emotional state. For both the patient and family, having a preoperative checklist ensures that necessary preoperative steps are completed so that the surgical pathway can run smoothly. Optimizing home environment and devising a plan for support ahead of time allows for a smooth and timely discharge. In the perioperative and postoperative periods, patient education should continue in order to relieve anxiety associated with expected symptoms, and to provide expectations regarding recovery.

Traditionally, TKA patients are seen in clinic, booked for surgery in person, and are followed up again in clinic. But with technological advancements and the TKA population becoming more adept with technology, every phase of care, short of surgery itself, can be achieved without seeing the patient in person. In the Center of Excellence model, preoperative visits may be performed by advanced practitioners anywhere across the country, and have records electronically reviewed by the surgeon for booking. Postoperative visits have been able to be almost entirely replaced by a virtual clinic. Patients can obtain X-ray at any location, avoid long wait times, and improve satisfaction. If any complication is suspected, they can be referred to an in-person visit as needed. This model has resulted in cost reduction without the increased risk of missing complications [15, 16]. Virtual visits may be more difficult for preoperative visits due to its complexity and the relationship building aspect for a new patient. However, it may be a good option for non-local patients and those with difficulty in traveling. Due to the Covid-19 epidemic and social distancing, especially important for the TKA population, the transition to virtual visits may be accelerated to become the norm in the near future.

Telemedicine has been an expanding option even before its popularization after the Coronavirus epidemic. Virtual clinics were well received by both physicians and patients. In fact, nearly half of patients preferred this method over an in-person visit. A caveat is that while patients who were doing well liked telemedicine, those with concerns were less satisfied [17]. Thus, it may be beneficial to screen those patients beforehand as an indication for an in-person visit. Successful implementation of telemedicine may reduce cost and increase capacity while improving patient satisfaction. This is especially relevant in the 90-day global period, where postoperative visits are not reimbursed.

Medical Optimization

Preoperative medical optimization is crucial for improving outcomes. Current practice typically involves a streamlined preoperative clearance, including primary care for medications and comorbidities, as well as specialist evaluation such as cardiology, oncology, and rheumatology when indicated. Laboratory thresholds associated with increased complications include lymphocyte below 1500 cells/mm, albumin under 3.5 g/dL, transferrin less than 200 mg/dL, and prealbumin less than 22.5 mg/dL [18, 19]. Falling below these levels is associated with poor wound healing and should be nutritionally optimized. Same applies to anemia below 13 g/dL, which increases risk of transfusion and resultant infection. Various thresholds for BMI and hemoglobin A1C have also been proposed, typically less than 40 kg/m^2 and 7.5%, respectively.

Additional considerations include stopping medications such as NSAIDs, Aspirin, anticoagulation, hypoglycemic agents, certain rheumatoid medications, and certain cancer treatments. Detrimental social habits must be stopped and confirmed. Alcohol abuse increases the risk of dislocation, and should be abstained from for at least 1 month preoperatively. Smoking is associated with infection and wound complications, and should be stopped 6–8 weeks preoperatively. Illegal drug use, especially intravenous, increases the risk of infection and should be cleared 2 years prior to TKA [18].

Achieving all of the above may be a significant challenge for some patients and surgeons alike, as a single missed threshold can cause unexpected delay or cancellation. Methods to streamline the process include providing checklists to prevent missing requirements, utilizing electronic monitoring to track progress and send reminders, and integrating primary care practitioners for efficient medical optimization and timely clearance.

Prehabilitation and Rehabilitation

Prehabilitation (prehab) is typically done for 1 visit to familiarize the patient with postoperative mobilization, or for multiple visits to improve function. Prehab has been shown to improve function before surgery, as well as decreasing length of stay and improving outcomes postoperatively [20, 21]. Improving preoperative function may also decrease inpatient rehab utilization. With the advent of virtual rehabilitation, prehab can be performed at home with low cost, high efficacy, and convenience.

Postoperative rehabilitation has undergone similar advancements. Immediately after surgery, accelerated physiotherapy typically done the same day reduces length of stay [22]. This is crucial for outpatient surgery and next-day discharges. There is also a push for decreasing discharge to inpatient rehab facilities, which has shown no benefit compared to a home discharge [23]. Inpatient rehab may be reserved for only patients with no support at home and unable to take care of themselves. After discharge, therapy visits can be done at home or outpatient. One-on-one sessions have not been found to be superior

to group sessions and monitored home programs, which are more cost- and resource-friendly [24]. Virtual therapy, or telerehabilitation, has also become an option with similar efficacy as in-person rehabilitation while reducing cost and improving adherence [25]. Results have been mostly positive, with high levels of patient satisfaction. Range of motion, functional improvement, and physical activity level were all found to be comparable between virtual and in-person therapy. Virtual rehabilitation, both preoperatively and postoperatively, may prove to be easily implemented into TKA pathways for widespread use, with potential cost savings without loss of efficacy.

Anesthesia and Analgesia

In line with the trend to quicker recovery and fast discharge, anesthesia for TKA has shifted to neuraxial anesthesia. In an outpatient joint replacement program, anesthesia that allows rapid recovery is even more important. Application of regional anesthesia with ultrasound guidance is clinically effective and cost-friendly [26]. Compared to general anesthesia, it is also less morbid, with less significant medical complications, reduced 30-day mortality, less blood transfusions, and fewer superficial wound infections [27]. Furthermore, regional anesthesia significantly reduces side effects such as nausea, respiratory compromise, delirium. As a result, patients are able to recover faster with a shorter length of stay compared to using general anesthesia. Traditionally, regional anesthesia techniques include femoral and sciatic nerve blocks, as well as epidural blocks. However, these methods also result in muscle weakness postoperatively, which delays ambulation and increases the risk of falls. Epidurals have their own set of risks, such as epidural hematoma, epidural abscess, and urinary retention. To further improve postoperative recovery, the IPACK (interspace between the popliteal artery and posterior capsule of the knee) block and adductor canal blocks have been described with efficacious results for pain without compromising muscle function. As pain is likely to persist beyond the duration of a single anesthetic injection, an adductor canal catheter may be placed for intermittent boluses for 1–2 days postoperatively before removal. A single IPACK injection with adductor canal continuous catheter block has comparable efficacy as a femoral and sciatic combined block, with less weakness, better performance in physical therapy, and quicker discharge [27]. This technique will likely become the standard for both inpatient and outpatient knee arthroplasty.

Postoperatively, pain control is also critical for a quick recovery, clearing physical therapy, progress in rehabilitation, and patient satisfaction [28]. Evidence supports the use of a multimodal approach to minimize opioid intake, which may include acetaminophen, NSAIDS, including COX2 inhibitors like celebrex and pregabalin. In addition, they have shown effectiveness given prior to incision. These medications can be further augmented by periarticular injections and peripheral nerve blocks as previously described, which has been shown to decrease postoperative opioid use in an opioid-sparing approach to pain control. However, local anesthetic infiltration (LAI) has not been shown to be more efficacious than an IPACK block. As the IPACK becomes more popular, further research is necessary to determine if additional LAI is beneficial [27]. A combination of regional anesthesia with a comprehensive multimodal pain regimen may lead to a more efficient discharge while minimizing opioid consumption and the side effects of anesthesia and analgesia.

Surgical Setting

Inpatient Surgery

Inpatient TKA remains a critical component of any joint arthroplasty practice despite more TKAs being transitioned to an outpatient basis. The goal of outpatient surgery is to improve efficiency without sacrificing outcome. However, a significant proportion of TKA candidates are not healthy enough to qualify for outpatient surgery. Patients older than age 75 have increased risk for falls, stiffness, pain, urinary retention, and readmission [5]. Those with significant comorbidities require additional monitoring, ICU availability, and anticipated admission only afforded on an inpatient basis. Those with poor baseline function or limited support system may need multiple therapy sessions or potential placement to rehab. Furthermore, any indication other than primary TKA is best performed inpatient to prepare for unexpected complications. Streamlined postoperative protocols after TKA has led to decrease in length of stay, from just over 4 days on average in 2002 to just under 3 days in 2013 [29]. In the modern inpatient setting, most TKA patients can still be discharged the following day, with the possibility of even a same day discharge. Despite decreased length of stay, there have been no increased risk of adverse events or complications [5].

Outpatient Surgery

Outpatient TKA has been increasingly popularized, enabled by improved pain protocols, more efficient clinical pathways, and advancement in techniques. There are many benefits to a successful outpatient joints program. Patients are most satisfied with same-day discharge, as most prefer to recover at home, which can be a competitive advantage during a patient's selection process vs. a traditional inpatient joints practice. In addition, ambulatory surgery centers are typically more efficient and cost-effective, with an estimated savings of $9000 per TKA over a 3–4 day hospitalization. This has become especially important for the revenue of a practice under the bundled payment plan.

Although there are limited high quality data on determining who is safe for outpatient TKA, patients qualifying for outpatient surgery are usually under 65–75 years old and indicated for primary arthroplasty [5]. Atypical cases such as fracture, retained hardware, bilateral TKA, or other complexity should be performed inpatient. Bilateral TKA and revision surgery have been associated with increased risk of ICU admissions [30]. Other described criteria include uncontrolled diabetes, BMI greater than 30–35 kg/m^2, bleeding disorders, ASA scores higher than II, significant cardiac or pulmonary comorbidities, chronic renal failure, chronic opioid use, mobility deficit, voiding difficulty, and cognitive or neurological impairments [31, 32]. These patients either have an unacceptable risk of complications requiring higher level of care, or less likelihood of achieving same-day discharge.

A successful outpatient program requires streamlined and regimented protocols. Preoperatively, a cocktail may include ranitidine, midazolam, and scopolamine in preparation for surgery and to minimize postoperative acid reflux and nausea. Regional anesthesia is used combined with IV pain medication and local infiltration. Surgery should minimize skin incision and disruption of the extensor mechanism as much as possible. Postoperatively, a multimodal pain regimen consisting of both IV and orals may be combined with cold therapy. When the patient is awake, alert, medically and vitally stable, and pain controlled, they may be cleared by anesthesia for discharge. They are generally fully weight bearing after a therapy session [5]. In rare cases, when those goals are not met, the patient may need overnight nursing care or transfer to an inpatient facility.

Combined and Bilateral Arthroplasty

Performing more than a single total joint arthroplasty, whether under a single anesthesia or during the same admission, has long been proposed as a method increasing efficiency and decreasing cost. Typically, any type of knee arthroplasty is followed by a period, usually 6 weeks, of recovery to ensure that a patient has recovered and is physically ready for another joint replacement. However, recent advancements in patient selection, perioperative management, and surgical technique has made this a viable option.

The most common variation is to perform bilateral TKAs under a single anesthesia (saTKA), as primary TKAs are relatively short surgeries that can be easily draped together into the surgical field. This could be done simultaneously by two surgeons or one after the other by the same surgeon. The benefits of saTKA include only one anesthesia event, a single recovery period, and decreased costs from one hospitalization and surgery as opposed to two. However,

risks have been reported compared to a staged approach, including increased mortality and venous thromboembolic events [33], but lower rates of deep infection and respiratory complications. Other studies have contradicted this finding, and appropriate selection of younger, healthier, less obese patients may further mitigate these risks [34–36]. Cost is another area of controversy in saTKA, with conflicting projections regarding its effectiveness in reducing costs [37, 38]. In contrast, early findings on single anesthesia bilateral UKA (saUKA) have been mostly positive, with cost savings but no increased complications [39, 40]. We believe that with a strict patient selection criteria and an improved perioperative pathway, saTKA and saUKA have the potential to significantly reduce costs, while maintaining comparable outcomes to staged surgery. In addition to cost, limitations to operating room space, nursing and anesthesia staff, and surgeon time in the future may be mitigated by saTKA in lieu of simultaneously operating two rooms.

Another proposed approach is the combined arthroplasty, which involves performing a total hip arthroplasty (THA) in addition to a TKA on the same day or staged within the same admission. This is a less common scenario as THA is less commonly performed than TKA, which may lead to unfamiliarity in executing the surgical and perioperative pathway. Both methods of combining THA with TKA has resulted in increased in-hospital complications, length of stay, and cost [41]. This approach may have room for improvement and more data is needed to justify its use.

Alternatives to Traditional Total Knee Arthroplasty

Unicompartmental Knee Arthroplasty

With advancements in implant design and technique, unicompartmental knee arthroplasty (UKA) has become an increasingly popular alternative to TKA for those with isolated compartment arthrosis. UKA may be performed for isolated medial, lateral, or patellofemoral (PF) compartment arthrosis. In addition, bicompartmental arthroplasty (BCA, medial and lateral UKA with PF arthroplasty [PFA]) and bi-unicompartmental arthroplasty (Bi-UKA, medial and lateral UKA) are also options (Figs. 18.1 and 18.2). In the short to mid-term, UKA offers similar outcomes and complications to TKA with the distinct advantage of lower cost, faster surgery, and quicker recovery [42]. As UKA is more commonly indicated in younger healthier patients, it is the perfect operation for the ambulatory surgery center. Combined with regional anesthesia, one group found 100% success in same day discharge for UKA [43]. BCA and Bi-UKA retain many of the benefits of UKA, including smaller incisions, preservation of ligaments and native kinematics, less bone resection, and easier revision. As with UKA, BCA and Bi-UKA are best for younger patients with higher functional demands. In addition, they have also been shown to have similar functional outcomes, shorter hospitalizations, and quicker rehabilitation compared to TKA [44]. However, they have also been associated with increased complications and significantly higher revision rates compared to TKA [45, 46].

Minimally Invasive Surgery and Alternate Alignment

The medial parapatellar approach is the most commonly used, with excellent exposure, but destabilizes the patella and extensor mechanism at the distal insertion of the vastus medialis. The subvastus or modified subvastus approach preserves the quad tendon and reduces blood loss. Although exposure may be more challenging, it can be used in select patients with quicker recovery of quad strength and less pain [47]. Quicker rehabilitation was also found in the midvastus technique compared to the medial parapatellar approach [48].

The minimally invasive approach involves using a skin incision shorter than 12–14 cm, avoiding patella eversion, and limiting dissection

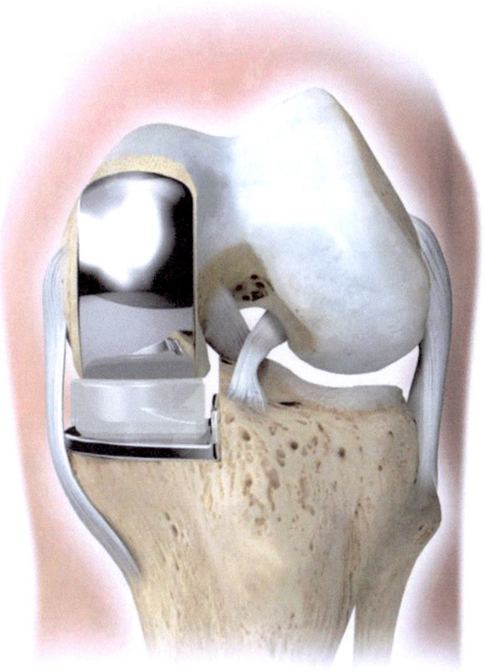

Fig. 18.1 Zimmer Biomet Oxford® Medial Compartment Arthroplasty

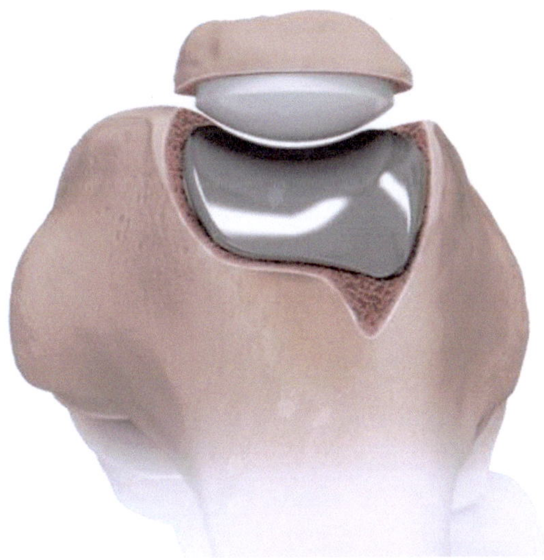

Fig. 18.2 Arthrex iBalance® Patellofemoral Joint Arthroplasty

into the suprapatellar pouch. It aims to reduce complications, improve pain, and achieve quicker return of muscle strength. The result is almost universally achieved same-day discharge with comparable outcomes to an inpatient cohort [49]. Minimally invasive and quad tendon sparing approaches should be avoided in patients at risk for difficult exposure, such as those with obesity, contracture, or patella baja. However, when indicated, they may be valuable tools for an outpatient joints program.

The traditional mechanical alignment (MA) technique has resulted in good long-term survivorship, but its functional outcomes could be improved. Thus, alternate coronal alignment techniques have been proposed. In anatomic alignment (AA), an oblique joint line in 2–3 degrees of valgus is obtained, with good mid- to long-term results. Adjusted mechanical alignment (aMA) involves undercorrecting coronal deformity by up to 3 degrees. In varus and valgus knees, this technique has resulted in good functional outcomes and long-term survivorship. In contrast, kinematic alignment (KA) essentially resurfaces the knee while maintaining native joint alignment and ligament balance. Restricted kinematic alignment (rKA) is similar; however, patients with significant coronal deformity undergo corrections to the bone cuts. In the early term, KA has demonstrated improved recovery and function compared to MA [50]. However, evidence for long-term outcomes comparing each technique is limited.

Technology in Total Knee Arthroplasty

Computer-Assisted Navigation

Computer assisted TKA (CATKA) provides greater surgical precision and prevents outliers (Fig. 18.3). Depending on the system, it can provide tight control over lower leg alignment, component positioning, and soft tissue balancing [51]. Its popularization is based on the belief that

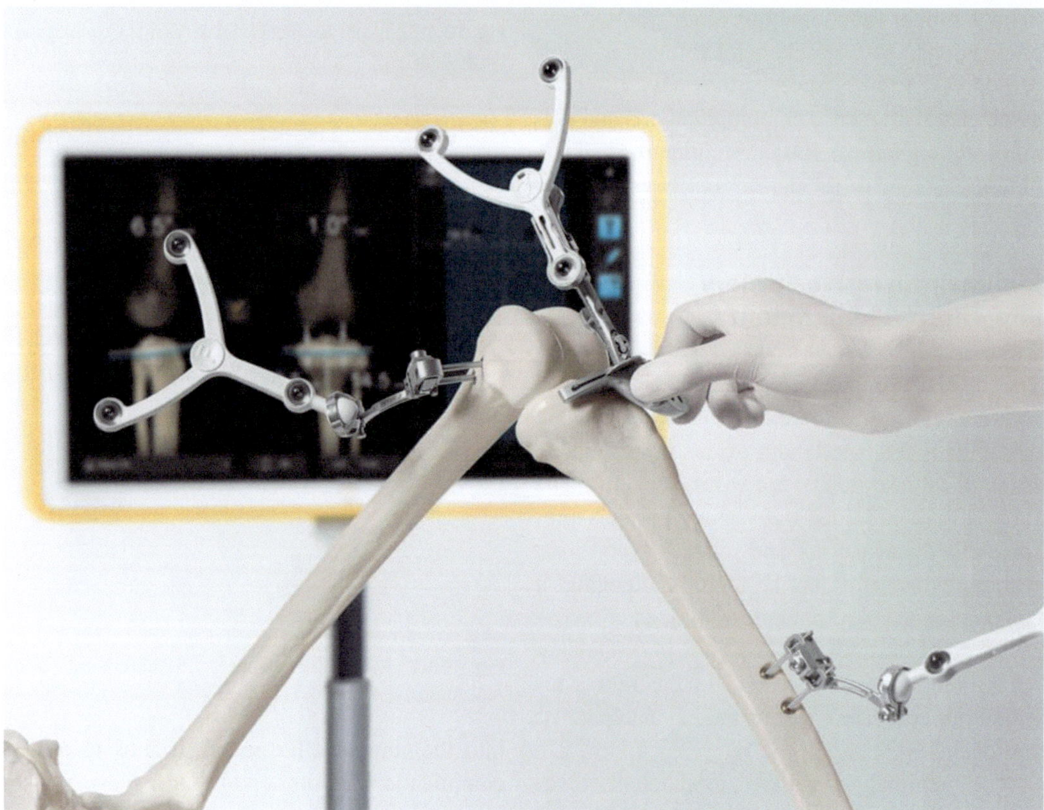

Fig. 18.3 Smith and Nephew Brainlab® Computer-Assisted Navigation

accuracy in these surgical steps leads to improved outcomes. As well, patients may also share the bias that computer-assisted surgery is better, driving the shift from traditional TKA. However, most of the evidence has been consistent that there is no difference in outcomes, complications, satisfaction, and length of stay between traditional TKA and CATKA [52]. As a result, the 2016 AAOS clinical practice guidelines recommended against CATKA. There are reports suggesting navigation systems that includ e soft tissue balancing are superior to non-navigated TKA [53]. In addition, minimally invasive CATKA was found to be superior to traditional CATKA with shorter length of stay and improved outcomes, similar to the minimally invasive effect in non-navigated TKA [54]. Navigation has also been studied in UKA, with no significant difference in outcomes compared to traditional UKA, especially regarding conversion rates to TKA [55]. Although joint replacement is trending toward navigation, cost and time limitations may affect its widespread adoption unless tangible benefits can be demonstrated by high quality data. Exceptions would include complex cases with extra articular deformity that would be difficult to manage using conventional techniques. Navigation can reliably achieve neutral mechanical alignment and optimal implant position in these patients [56]. Additionally, it can assist in achieving kinematic alignment as well as guiding adjustments in restricted kinematic alignment.

Robotic-Assisted Surgery

Robotic arm-assisted TKA (RATKA) further builds on navigation with greater accuracy and precision of component placement (Fig. 18.4). RATKA is classified as passive, where the surgeon maintains direct control; active, where the system performs independently from the surgeon; and the most popular semi-active or haptic, where the system provides feedback to augment surgeon control [57]. Implants may be specific to the particular system, packaged together for healthcare systems to invest in. The robotic cutting process is safer for soft tissues, decreases

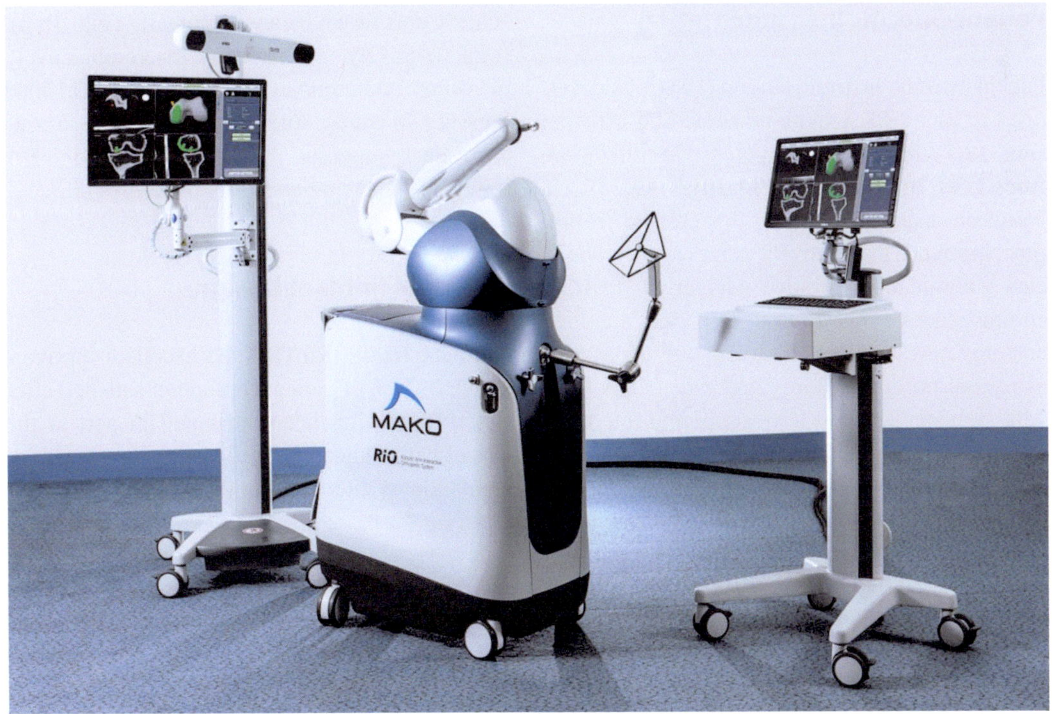

Fig. 18.4 Stryker Mako® Robotic-Assisted TKA

surgeon fatigue, and is reported to have high patient satisfaction [58]. Quicker recovery and reduced length of stay were also observed with RATKA [59]. The higher cost of the system and additional time involved in preoperative planning may be offset by reducing intraoperative instrument utilization and number of surgical trays. Specifically for haptic RATKA, studies have demonstrated lower 90-day cost compared to manual TKA [60]. Similar to navigation, RATKA may be beneficial in cases with extra articular deformity [61]. Although early outcomes appear promising and superior to that of manual TKA, because of the novelty of this technology, there is a lack of long-term outcome data [62]. If long-term data is comparable or better than manual TKA, RATKA may be a valuable tool, especially for high volume outpatient surgery. However, it has not been shown to be cost-effective for low to medium-volume arthroplasty centers at this time [63]. As with most technological advancements, robotics will likely become more affordable over time.

Patient-Specific Instrumentation

Patient-specific instrumentation (PSI) was developed to make TKA more accurate and efficient (Fig. 18.5). It has seen an increase in utilization, from 1.3% in 2009 to 6% in 2012 [52]. PSI is based on disposable cutting jigs created from a preoperative CT, effectively achieving navigated cuts without intraoperative navigation. Custom cutting guides aimed to fit each patient's unique anatomy may decrease alignment outliers as well as restore normal anatomy and kinematics [64]. Although some studies have supported improved overall alignment with PSI, others have found no difference compared to conventional instrumentation, and there is concern that tibial malalignment may be higher in PSI [65]. Data on outcomes are also varied, with generally similar outcomes, operating time, and complications as standard TKA [66]. In UKA, PSI produces similar short-term outcomes, with mixed data regarding the accuracy of its cutting guides [67]. At this time, the lack of clear benefit and higher cost of PSI does not justify its use for most patients.

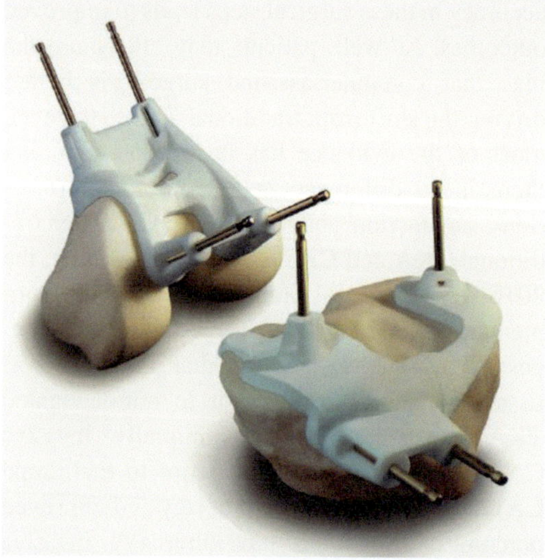

Fig. 18.5 Zimmer Biomet Persona® patient-specific instrumentation

Pressure Sensor Technology

Sensor-assisted TKA was developed on the basis that soft tissue balancing is critical to outcomes and that surgeons are unable to consistently achieve soft tissue balance manually (Fig. 18.6). Intraoperatively, a tibial trial insert objectively measures intercompartmental tibiofemoral load pressure to guide soft tissue balancing. Short-term data suggests that sensor-assisted TKA improves balancing and early outcomes [68].

Alternate Implant Designs

Although traditional TKA has excellent survivorship, 20–30% of patients remain unsatisfied after surgery. This has been attributed in part to the loss of native knee kinematics, driving the implementation of alternate implant designs. Rotating Platform, or mobile-bearing (MB), TKA aims to improve congruity and mobility at the tibiofemoral bearing surface. This decreases contact stress as well as constraint, which theoretically decreases loosening and poly wear. Lower wear in MBTKA has been shown in biomechanical studies as well as clinically. However, these benefits also come with complications, including smaller particle induced osteolysis, patellar

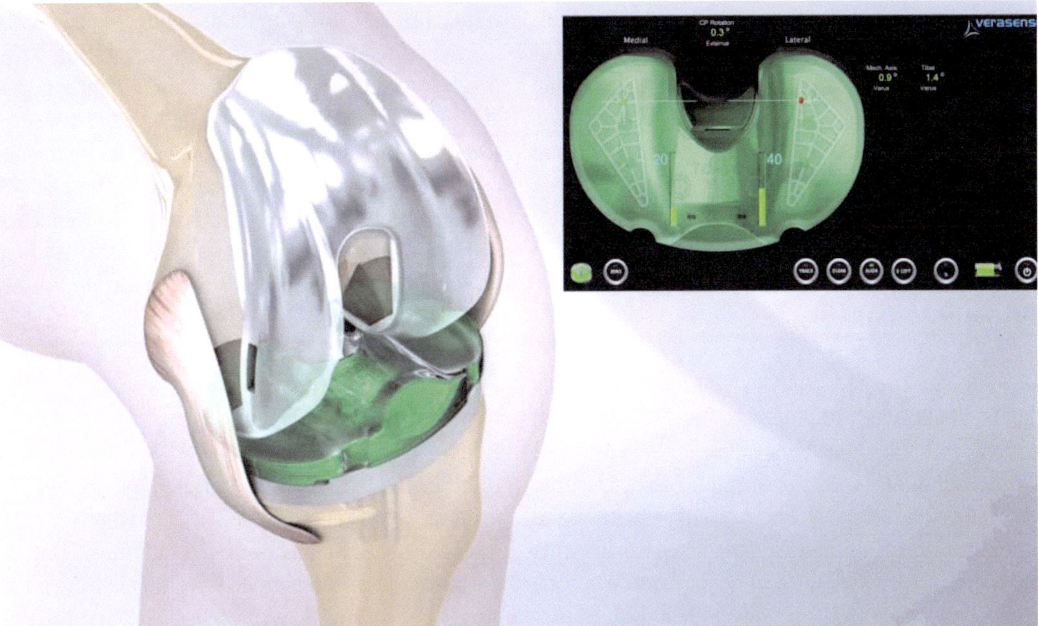

Fig. 18.6 Stryker Verasense® pressure sensor-assisted TKA

clunk, and implant dislocation. Additionally, MBTKA has not been shown to extend implant longevity compared to fixed bearing TKA. Thus, the overall benefit and indications for MBTKA is unclear. In young patients, MBTKA may be beneficial for potentially decreasing wear and improving kinematics [69].

Medial Pivot designs utilizes a medial congruent poly insert to recreate a normal, medial pivot biomechanics in TKA. In contrast, traditional TKA involves anterior sliding of the femoral component, or "paradoxical motion." This has been associated with abnormal sensation, subjective instability, decreased motion, and inferior outcomes [70]. In short-term studies, medial pivot TKA results in superior outcomes than traditional TKA [71].

Asymmetric designs have been studied in tibial baseplates and polyethylene inserts. The asymmetric baseplate was designed to improve coverage, but was shown to be inferior in cadaveric testing [72]. Asymmetric polyethylene is coupled with MBTKA and aims to improve implant conformity and thereby decrease stress and wear. These advantages were confirmed with biomechanical analysis, with good short-term clinical outcomes [73].

Bicruciate-retaining (BCR) implants have been around since the 1960s with mixed results

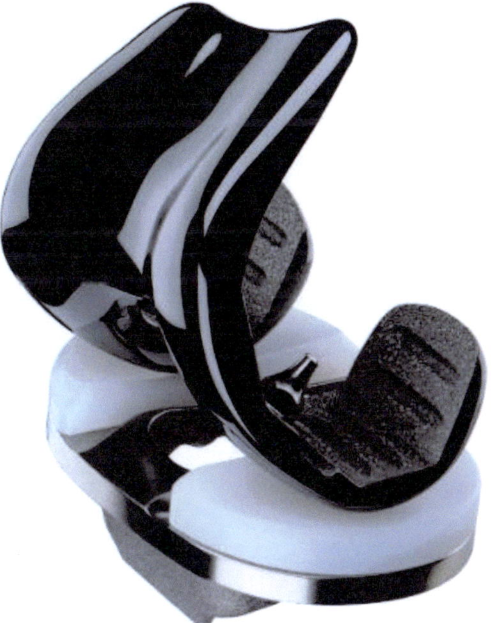

Fig. 18.7 Smith and Nephew Journey II XR® Bi-Cruciate Retaining TKA

(Fig. 18.7). However, it has seen a resurgence due to technical advancements and interest in restoring native knee kinematics. Retention of the ACL preserves native anteroposterior laxity and should feel closer to a normal knee. Still, there are challenges to BCR TKA, including technical difficulty, challenging exposure, less implant to bone contact surface, and potentially higher revision rates. Nonetheless, many studies have found improved satisfaction after BCR TKA compared to traditional TKA.

Augmented Reality

To date, augmented reality (AR) technology has not been clinically implemented into knee arthroplasty. AR involves generating and projecting virtual elements into the surgical field to guide the user. The process begins with tracking the operative limb, computing the necessary information from raw data, and visualization which may come from a headset or another form of display [74]. In one study of AR, a smartphone application superimposes target cutting angles onto the operative extremity via the display (Fig. 18.8). This allows the surgeon to maintain

focus on the surgical field, while significantly decreasing costs compared to navigation. The bone resections were less than 2 degrees and 1 mm off from displayed targets, suggesting AR to be reliable and accurate [75]. No clinical outcomes exist for AR at this stage. Nonetheless, AR is expected to be integrated in many fields of orthopedics, including knee arthroplasty, given its potential benefits of lower cost and user-friendly interface.

Summary

Increasing demand and bundled payments are driving TKA to be more efficient and more cost-effective without sacrificing outcomes. One of the primary methods to achieve this is by significantly decreasing length of stay and maximizing the potential for outpatient surgery. The future of TKA involves refining the clinical pathway in addition to incorporating new technology so that the best outcomes can be achieved with the least

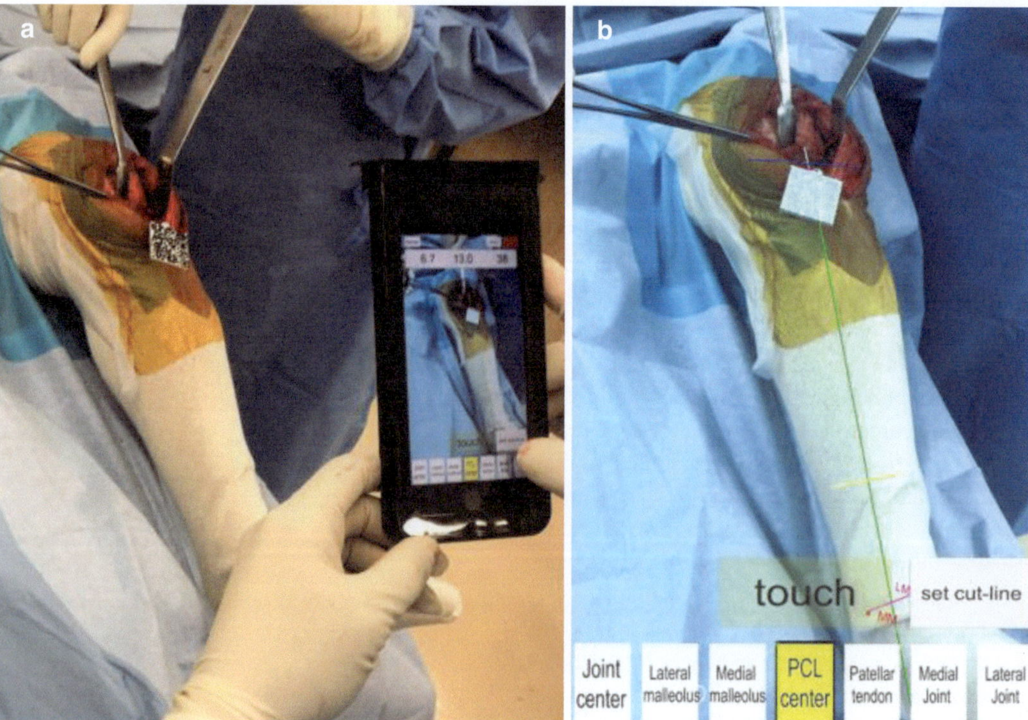

Fig. 18.8 (a, b) AR-KNEE Augmented Reality TKA [75]

resources. Appropriate patient selection, preoperative optimization, and patient education are already critical to modern practice, with proven benefits. Perioperative protocols, including regional anesthesia techniques, opioid minimizing multimodal regimens, and accelerated recovery are being incorporated to both inpatient and outpatient settings with drastic reduction in length of stay. Newer techniques and technology, such as minimally invasive surgery, bilateral surgery, navigation, robotics, custom implants, and augmented reality, are rapidly expanding. In addition, a push to restoring native knee kinematics has led to novel implant designs. While some show promising results, others have not demonstrated significant benefit. Nonetheless, these technologies will continue to evolve and establish themselves with emerging data. These surgical advancements, along with virtual education, therapy, and clinic, will likely be a significant part of TKA in the future.

Key Points

- TKA is one of the most commonly performed surgeries with significant projected growth.
- Cost of TKA has increased despite decreasing length of stay and efforts to reduce cost.
- Bundled payments incentivize cost reduction by placing the burden on the hospital and surgeon.
- Appropriate patient selection and medical optimization is key to improving outcomes and decreasing complications.
- Patient education can improve perioperative efficiency and surgical outcome.
- Perioperative visits and physical therapy are increasingly performed virtually.
- Regional anesthesia and an opioid minimizing multimodal pain regimen can decrease side effects and length of stay.
- Inpatient surgery is necessary for patients with comorbidities and complex cases.
- Outpatient surgery is becoming more popular for younger, healthier patients, and can decrease costs significantly.
- Bilateral TKA can be an option in select healthy patients to increase efficiency and decrease cost. But combined TKA and THA has increased complications.
- UKA and minimally invasive TKA allows faster recovery and excellent short-term outcomes, ideal for outpatient surgery.
- Computer assisted navigation, robotic assisted surgery, and patient-specific instrumentation increase accuracy, but have not consistently demonstrated benefit over traditional TKA.
- Alternate implant designs mimic native knee kinematics, and may improve patient satisfaction.

Disclosure

Bo Zhang: No disclosures
Julius K. Oni: Disclosures: AAOS disclosures
AAOS: Board or committee member
American Association of Hip and Knee Surgeons: Board or committee member
Zimmer: Paid consultant
Savyasachi C. Thakkar: Disclosures: AAOS disclosures
American Association of Hip and Knee Surgeons: Board or committee member
Arthroplasty Today: Editorial or governing board
Journal of Arthroplasty: Editorial or governing board
KCI: Unpaid consultant
OrthAlign: Unpaid consultant

References

1. Kurtz S, Ong K, Lau E, Mowat F, Halpern M. Projections of primary and revision hip and knee arthroplasty in the United States from 2005 to 2030. J Bone Joint Surg Am. 2007;89(4):780–5. https://doi.org/10.2106/JBJS.F.00222.
2. Sloan M, Premkumar A, Sheth NP. Projected volume of primary Total Joint arthroplasty in the U.S., 2014 to 2030. J Bone Joint Surg Am. 2018;100(17):1455–60. https://doi.org/10.2106/JBJS.17.01617.
3. Kurtz SM, Ong KL, Lau E, Bozic KJ. Impact of the economic downturn on total joint replacement demand in the United States: updated projections to 2021. J Bone Joint Surg Am. 2014;96(8):624–30. https://doi.org/10.2106/JBJS.M.00285.
4. Pabinger C, Lothaller H, Geissler A. Utilization rates of knee-arthroplasty in OECD countries.

Osteoarthr Cartil. 2015;23(10):1664–73. https://doi.org/10.1016/j.joca.2015.05.008.

5. Krause A, Sayeed Z, El-Othmani M, Pallekonda V, Mihalko W, Saleh KJ. Outpatient Total knee arthroplasty: are we there yet? (part 1). Orthop Clin North Am. 2018;49(1):1–6. https://doi.org/10.1016/j.ocl.2017.08.002.

6. Huang A, Ryu JJ, Dervin G. Cost savings of outpatient versus standard inpatient total knee arthroplasty. Can J Surg. 2017;60(1):57–62. https://doi.org/10.1503/cjs.002516.

7. Centers for Medicare & Medicaid Services (CMS), HHS. Medicare program; Comprehensive Care for Joint Replacement Payment Model for acute care hospitals furnishing lower extremity Joint Replacement services. Final rule. Fed Regist. 2015;80(226):73273–554.

8. Barnett ML, Wilcock A, McWilliams JM, et al. Two-year evaluation of mandatory bundled payments for joint replacement. N Engl J Med. 2019;380(3):252–62. https://doi.org/10.1056/NEJMsa1809010.

9. DiGioia AM III, Greenhouse PK, Giarrusso ML, Kress JM. Determining the true cost to deliver Total hip and knee arthroplasty over the full cycle of care: preparing for bundling and reference-based pricing. J Arthroplast. 2016;31(1):1–6. https://doi.org/10.1016/j.arth.2015.07.013.

10. Sullivan R, Jarvis LD, O'Gara T, Langfitt M, Emory C. Bundled payments in total joint arthroplasty and spine surgery. Curr Rev Musculoskelet Med. 2017;10(2):218–23. https://doi.org/10.1007/s12178-017-9405-8.

11. Nwachukwu BU, Dy CJ, Burket JC, Padgett DE, Lyman S. Risk for complication after Total Joint arthroplasty at a Center of Excellence: the impact of patient travel distance. J Arthroplast. 2015;30(6):1058–61. https://doi.org/10.1016/j.arth.2015.01.015.

12. Wodowski AJ, Pelt CE, Erickson JA, Anderson MB, Gililland JM, Peters CL. 'Bundle busters': who is at risk of exceeding the target payment and can they be optimized? Bone Joint J. 2019;101-B(7_Supple_C):64–9. https://doi.org/10.1302/0301-620X.101B7.BJJ-2018-1522.R1.

13. Boyce L, Prasad A, Barrett M, et al. The outcomes of total knee arthroplasty in morbidly obese patients: a systematic review of the literature. Arch Orthop Trauma Surg. 2019;139(4):553–60. https://doi.org/10.1007/s00402-019-03127-5.

14. Puhto T, Puhto AP, Vielma M, Syrjälä H. Infection triples the cost of a primary joint arthroplasty. Infect Dis (Lond). 2019;51(5):348–55. https://doi.org/10.1080/23744235.2019.1572219.

15. Fisher R, Hamilton V, Reader S, Khatun F, Porteous M. Virtual arthroplasty follow-up: five-year data from a district general hospital. Ann R Coll Surg Engl. 2020;102(3):220–4. https://doi.org/10.1308/rcsann.2019.0139.

16. Ferdinandus S, Smith LK, Pandit H, Stone MH. Setting up an arthroplasty care practitioner-led virtual clinic for follow-up of orthopaedic patients.

Br J Nurs. 2019;28(20):1326–30. https://doi.org/10.12968/bjon.2019.28.20.1326.

17. Parkes RJ, Palmer J, Wingham J, Williams DH. Is virtual clinic follow-up of hip and knee joint replacement acceptable to patients and clinicians? A sequential mixed methods evaluation. BMJ Open Qual. 2019;8(1):e000502. Published 2019 Mar 1. https://doi.org/10.1136/bmjoq-2018-000502.

18. Ng VY, Lustenberger D, Hoang K, et al. Preoperative risk stratification and risk reduction for total joint reconstruction: AAOS exhibit selection. J Bone Joint Surg Am. 2013;95(4):e191–15.

19. Greene KA, Wilde AH, Stulberg BN. Preoperative nutritional status of total joint patients. Relationship to postoperative wound complications. J Arthroplast. 1991;6(4):321–5.

20. Jahic D, Omerovic D, Tanovic AT, Dzankovic F, Campara MT. The effect of Prehabilitation on postoperative outcome in patients following primary Total knee arthroplasty. Mediev Archaeol. 2018;72(6):439–43. https://doi.org/10.5455/medarh.2018.72.

21. Chen H, Li S, Ruan T, Liu L, Fang L. Is it necessary to perform prehabilitation exercise for patients undergoing total knee arthroplasty: meta-analysis of randomized controlled trials. [published correction appears in Phys Sportsmed. 2018 Sep;46(3):399–403]. Phys Sportsmed. 2018;46(1):36–43. https://doi.org/10.1080/00913847.2018.1403274.

22. Henderson KG, Wallis JA, Snowdon DA. Active physiotherapy interventions following total knee arthroplasty in the hospital and inpatient rehabilitation settings: a systematic review and meta-analysis. Physiotherapy. 2018;104(1):25–35. https://doi.org/10.1016/j.physio.2017.01.002.

23. Buhagiar MA, Naylor JM, Harris IA, et al. Effect of inpatient rehabilitation vs a monitored home-based program on mobility in patients with Total knee arthroplasty: the HIHO randomized clinical trial. JAMA. 2017;317(10):1037–46. https://doi.org/10.1001/jama.2017.1224.

24. Ko V, Naylor J, Harris I, et al. One-to-one therapy is not superior to group or home-based therapy after total knee arthroplasty: a randomized, superiority trial. J Bone Joint Surg Am. 2013;95(21):1942–9.

25. Shukla H, Nair SR, Thakker D. Role of telerehabilitation in patients following total knee arthroplasty: evidence from a systematic literature review and meta-analysis. J Telemed Telecare. 2017;23(2):339–46. https://doi.org/10.1177/1357633X16628996.

26. Soffin EM, Memtsoudis SG. Anesthesia and analgesia for total knee arthroplasty. Minerva Anestesiol. 2018;84(12):1406–12. https://doi.org/10.23736/S0375-9393.18.12383-2.

27. Cullom C, Weed JT. Anesthetic and analgesic Management for Outpatient Knee Arthroplasty. Curr Pain Headache Rep. 2017;21(5):23. https://doi.org/10.1007/s11916-017-0623-y.

28. Moucha CS, Weiser MC, Levin EJ. Current strategies in anesthesia and analgesia for Total knee arthro-

plasty. J Am Acad Orthop Surg. 2016;24(2):60–73. https://doi.org/10.5435/JAAOS-D-14-00259.

29. Molloy IB, Martin BI, Moschetti WE, Jevsevar DS. Effects of the length of stay on the cost of Total knee and Total hip arthroplasty from 2002 to 2013. J Bone Joint Surg Am. 2017;99(5):402–7. https://doi.org/10.2106/JBJS.16.00019.

30. Sukhonthamarn K, Grosso MJ, Sherman MB, Restrepo C, Parvizi J. Risk factors for unplanned admission to the intensive care unit after elective Total Joint arthroplasty. J Arthroplast. 2020;35(7):1937–40. https://doi.org/10.1016/j.arth.2020.03.003.

31. Kort NP, Bemelmans YF, van der Kuy PH, et al. Patient selection criteria for outpatient joint arthroplasty. Knee Surg Sports Traumatol Arthrosc. 2017;25(9):2668–75.

32. Edwards PK, Milles JL, Stambough JB, Barnes CL, Mears SC. Inpatient versus outpatient Total knee arthroplasty. J Knee Surg. 2019;32(8):730–5. https://doi.org/10.1055/s-0039-1683935.

33. Liu L, Liu H, Zhang H, Song J, Zhang L. Bilateral total knee arthroplasty: simultaneous or staged? A systematic review and meta-analysis. Medicine (Baltimore). 2019;98(22):e15931. https://doi.org/10.1097/MD.0000000000015931.

34. Wong E, Nguyen CL, Park S, Parker D. Simultaneous, same-anaesthetic bilateral total knee arthroplasty has low mortality and complication rates. Knee Surg Sports Traumatol Arthrosc. 2018;26(11):3395–402. https://doi.org/10.1007/s00167-018-4908-4.

35. Lindberg-Larsen M, Pitter FT, Husted H, Kehlet H, Jørgensen CC. Lundbeck Foundation Centre for fast-track hip and knee Replacement collaborative group. Simultaneous vs staged bilateral total knee arthroplasty: a propensity-matched case-control study from nine fast-track centres. Arch Orthop Trauma Surg. 2019;139(5):709–16. https://doi.org/10.1007/s00402-019-03157-z.

36. Davidson IU, Brigati DP, Faour M, UdoInyang IJ, Ibrahim M, Murray TG. Same-day bilateral Total knee arthroplasty candidacy criteria decrease length of stay and facility discharge. Orthopedics. 2018;41(5):293–8. https://doi.org/10.3928/01477447-20180815-02.

37. Sobh AH, Siljander MP, Mells AJ, Koueiter DM, Moore DD, Karadsheh MS. Cost analysis, complications, and discharge disposition associated with simultaneous vs staged bilateral Total knee arthroplasty. J Arthroplast. 2018;33(2):320–3. https://doi.org/10.1016/j.arth.2017.09.004.

38. Wyles CC, Robinson WA, Maradit-Kremers H, Houdek MT, Trousdale RT, Mabry TM. Cost and patient outcomes associated with bilateral Total knee arthroplasty performed by 2-surgeon teams vs a single surgeon. J Arthroplast. 2019;34(4):671–5. https://doi.org/10.1016/j.arth.2018.12.029.

39. Biazzo A, Masia F, Verde F. Bilateral unicompartmental knee arthroplasty: one stage or two stages? Musculoskelet Surg. 2019;103(3):231–6. https://doi.org/10.1007/s12306-018-0579-z.

40. Siedlecki C, Beaufils P, Lemaire B, Pujol N. Complications and cost of single-stage vs. two-stage bilateral unicompartmental knee arthroplasty: a case-control study. Orthop Traumatol Surg Res. 2018;104(7):949–53. https://doi.org/10.1016/j.otsr.2018.01.021.

41. Almaguer AM, Cichos KH, McGwin G Jr, Pearson JM, Wilson B, Ghanem ES. Combined total hip and knee arthroplasty during the same hospital admission: is it safe? Bone Joint J. 2019;101-B(5):573–81. https://doi.org/10.1302/0301-620X.101B5.BJJ-2018-1438.

42. Beard DJ, Davies LJ, Cook JA, et al. The clinical and cost-effectiveness of total versus partial knee replacement in patients with medial compartment osteoarthritis (TOPKAT): 5-year outcomes of a randomised controlled trial. Lancet. 2019;394(10200):746–56. https://doi.org/10.1016/S0140-6736(19)31281-4.

43. Cross MB, Berger R. Feasibility and safety of performing outpatient unicompartmental knee arthroplasty. Int Orthop. 2014;38(2):443–7.

44. Sabatini L, Giachino M, Risitano S, Atzori F. Bicompartmental knee arthroplasty. Ann Transl Med. 2016;4(1):5. https://doi.org/10.3978/j.issn.2305-5839.2015.12.24.

45. Parratte S, Pauly V, Aubaniac JM, Argenson JN. Survival of bicompartmental knee arthroplasty at 5 to 23 years. Clin Orthop Relat Res. 2010;468(1):64–72. https://doi.org/10.1007/s11999-009-1018-0.

46. Ma JX, He WW, Kuang MJ, et al. Efficacy of bicompartmental knee arthroplasty (BKA) for bicompartmental knee osteoarthritis: a meta analysis. Int J Surg. 2017;46:53–60. https://doi.org/10.1016/j.ijsu.2017.08.556.

47. Weinhardt C, Barisic M, Bergmann EG, et al. Early results of subvastus versus medial parapatellar approach in primary total knee arthroplasty. Arch Orthop Trauma Surg. 2004;124(6):401–3.

48. Alcelik I, Sukeik M, Pollock R, Misra A, Naguib A, Haddad FS. Comparing the mid-vastus and medial parapatellar approaches in total knee arthroplasty: a meta-analysis of short term outcomes. Knee. 2012;19(4):229–36. https://doi.org/10.1016/j.knee.2011.07.010.

49. Berger RA, Sanders S, Gerlinger T, et al. Outpatient total knee arthroplasty with a minimally invasive technique. J Arthroplast. 2005;20(7 Suppl 3):33–8.

50. Rivière C, Iranpour F, Auvinet E, et al. Alignment options for total knee arthroplasty: a systematic review. Orthop Traumatol Surg Res. 2017;103(7):1047–56. https://doi.org/10.1016/j.otsr.2017.07.010.

51. Haaker RG, Stockheim M, Kamp M, et al. Computer-assisted navigation increases precision of component placement in total knee arthroplasty. Clin Orthop Relat Res. 2005;433:152–9.

52. Beal MD, Delagramaticas D, Fitz D. Improving outcomes in total knee arthroplasty-do navigation or customized implants have a role? J Orthop Surg Res. 2016;11(1):60.

53. van der List JP, Chawla H, Joskowicz L, Pearle AD. Current state of computer navigation and robot-

ics in unicompartmental and total knee arthroplasty: a systematic review with meta-analysis. Knee Surg Sports Traumatol Arthrosc. 2016;24(11):3482–95. https://doi.org/10.1007/s00167-016-4305-9.

54. Khakha RS, Chowdhry M, Norris M, et al. Five-year follow-up of minimally invasive computer assisted total knee arthroplasty (MICATKA) versus conventional computer assisted total knee arthroplasty (CATKA) - a population matched study. Knee. 2014;21(5):944–8.

55. Chona D, Bala A, Huddleston JI III, Goodman SB, Maloney WJ, Amanatullah DF. Effect of computer navigation on complication rates following Unicompartmental knee arthroplasty. J Arthroplast. 2018;33(11):3437–3440.e1. https://doi.org/10.1016/j.arth.2018.06.030.

56. Matassi F, Cozzi Lepri A, Innocenti M, Zanna L, Civinini R, Innocenti M. Total knee arthroplasty in patients with extra-articular deformity: restoration of mechanical alignment using accelerometer-based navigation system. J Arthroplast. 2019;34(4):676–81. https://doi.org/10.1016/j.arth.2018.12.042.

57. Urish KL, Conditt M, Roche M, Rubash HE. Robotic Total knee arthroplasty: surgical assistant for a customized Normal kinematic knee. Orthopedics. 2016;39(5):e822–7. https://doi.org/10.3928/01477447-20160623-13.

58. Khlopas A, Sodhi N, Sultan AA, Chughtai M, Molloy RM, Mont MA. Robotic arm-assisted Total knee arthroplasty. J Arthroplast. 2018;33(7):2002–6. https://doi.org/10.1016/j.arth.2018.01.060.

59. Kayani B, Konan S, Tahmassebi J, Pietrzak JRT, Haddad FS. Robotic-arm assisted total knee arthroplasty is associated with improved early functional recovery and reduced time to hospital discharge compared with conventional jig-based total knee arthroplasty: a prospective cohort study. Bone Joint J. 2018;100-B(7):930–937:930. https://doi.org/10.1302/0301-620X.100B7.BJJ-2017-1449.R1.

60. Cotter EJ, Wang J, Illgen RL. Comparative cost analysis of robotic-assisted and jig-based manual primary total knee arthroplasty. [published online ahead of print, 2020 Jul 13]. J Knee Surg. 2020;35(2):176–84. https://doi.org/10.1055/s-0040-1713895.

61. Sodhi N, Khlopas A, Ehiorobo JO, et al. Robotic-assisted Total knee arthroplasty in the presence of extra-articular deformity. Surg Technol Int. 2019;34:497–502.

62. van der List JP, Chawla H, Pearle AD. Robotic-assisted knee arthroplasty: an overview. Am J Orthop (Belle Mead NJ). 2016;45(4):202–11.

63. Moschetti WE, Konopka JF, Rubash HE, Genuario JW. Can robot-assisted Unicompartmental knee arthroplasty be cost-effective? A markov decision analysis. J Arthroplast. 2016;31(4):759–65. https://doi.org/10.1016/j.arth.2015.10.018.

64. Fitz W. Unicompartmental knee arthroplasty with use of novel patient-specific resurfacing implants and per-sonalized jigs. J Bone Joint Surg Am. 2009;91(Suppl 1):69–76. https://doi.org/10.2106/JBJS.H.01448.

65. Thienpont E, Schwab PE, Fennema P. Efficacy of patient-specific instruments in Total knee arthroplasty: a systematic review and meta-analysis. J Bone Joint Surg Am. 2017;99(6):521–30. https://doi.org/10.2106/JBJS.16.00496.

66. Kizaki K, Shanmugaraj A, Yamashita F, et al. Total knee arthroplasty using patient-specific instrumentation for osteoarthritis of the knee: a meta-analysis. BMC Musculoskelet Disord. 2019;20(1):561. Published 2019 Nov 23. https://doi.org/10.1186/s12891-019-2940-2.

67. Alvand A, Khan T, Jenkins C, et al. The impact of patient-specific instrumentation on unicompartmental knee arthroplasty: a prospective randomised controlled study. Knee Surg Sports Traumatol Arthrosc. 2018;26(6):1662–70. https://doi.org/10.1007/s00167-017-4677-5.

68. Golladay GJ, Bradbury TL, Gordon AC, et al. Are patients more satisfied with a balanced Total knee arthroplasty? J Arthroplast. 2019;34(7S):S195–200. https://doi.org/10.1016/j.arth.2019.03.036.

69. Huang ZM, Ouyang GL, Xiao LB. Rotating-platform knee arthroplasty: a review and update. Orthop Surg. 2011;3(4):224–8. https://doi.org/10.1111/j.1757-7861.2011.00156.x.

70. Sabatini L, Risitano S, Parisi G, et al. Medial pivot in Total knee arthroplasty: literature review and our first experience. Clin Med Insights Arthritis Musculoskelet Disord. 2018;11:1179544117751431. Published 2018 Jan 4. https://doi.org/10.1177/1179544117751431.

71. Samy DA, Wolfstadt JI, Vaidee I, Backstein DJ. A retrospective comparison of a medial pivot and posterior-stabilized Total knee arthroplasty with respect to patient-reported and radiographic outcomes. J Arthroplast. 2018;33(5):1379–83. https://doi.org/10.1016/j.arth.2017.11.049.

72. Bozkurt M, Akkaya M, Tahta M, Gursoy S, Firat A. Tibial Base plate for Total knee arthroplasty: symmetric or asymmetric? Clin Orthop Surg. 2017;9(3):280–5. https://doi.org/10.4055/cios.2017.9.3.280.

73. Castellarin G, Pianigiani S, Innocenti B. Asymmetric polyethylene inserts promote favorable kinematics and better clinical outcome compared to symmetric inserts in a mobile-bearing total knee arthroplasty. Knee Surg Sports Traumatol Arthrosc. 2019;27(4):1096–105. https://doi.org/10.1007/s00167-018-5207-9.

74. Auvinet E, Maillot C, Uzoho C. Chapter 27: Augmented reality technology for joint replacement. In: Rivière C, Vendittoli PA, editors. Personalized hip and knee Joint Replacement. Cham (CH): Springer; 2020.

75. Tsukada S, Ogawa H, Nishino M, Kurosaka K, Hirasawa N. Augmented reality-based navigation system applied to tibial bone resection in total knee arthroplasty. J Exp Orthop. 2019;6(1):44. https://doi.org/10.1186/s40634-019-0212-6.

A Systematic Review of Kinematic Alignment and Implants in Total Knee Arthroplasties

19

Shrey Kapoor, Sandesh Rao, Safa Cyrus Fassihi, and Savyasachi C. Thakkar

Introduction and Native Knee Kinematics

Take Home Points

- The restoration of native kinematics of the knee is thought to potentially contribute to improved functional outcomes and patient satisfaction.
- Kinematic alignment uses a patient-specific approach since not all patients have the same native mechanical or anatomic axis.

TKA is the most commonly performed surgical procedure, with projections estimating over 3.5 million procedures in the United States done annually by 2030 [1]. There have been a variety of technological advances and innovation to TKA over the years centered around the optimal approach to final implant positioning in an attempt to recreate an individual's optimal knee mechanics. The purpose of this chapter is to explore the contemporary advancements in total knee arthroplasty, specifically with regards to kinematic alignment and implant options.

A review of normal knee kinematics and alignment will help us better understand the theory behind kinematically aligned and kinematically designed total knee arthroplasty. The knee is made up of the patellofemoral and the tibiofemoral joint, that have 6° of freedom of motion. There are three axes of translation: anterior–posterior, medial–lateral, and compression–distraction. There are three additional rotational axes: flexion–extension, varus–valgus, and internal–external rotation (Fig. 19.1).

The kinematics of the knee revolve around primarily two separate axes, the flexion–extension and the internal–external rotations. The osseous anatomy and the surrounding soft tissues facilitate this complex kinematic motion. The medial femoral condyle (MFC) is slightly larger and more uniformly circular with a similar radius of curvature and center of rotation for the distal and posterior aspect of the condyle than the lateral femoral condyle (LFC). This contributes to the medial femoral condyle remaining relatively stationary during flexion of the knee. The lateral femoral condyle conversely has a change in its center of rotation and a different radius of curvature between the distal femur and posterior femoral condyle that contributes to femoral rollback,

S. Kapoor (✉)
Research Assistant, Baltimore, MD, USA
e-mail: skapoo13@jhmi.edu

S. Rao
Adult Reconstruction Fellow, Chicago, IL, USA

Washington Orthopaedics & Sports Medicine, Washington, DC, USA

S. C. Fassihi
Adult Reconstruction Fellow, New York, NY, USA

S. C. Thakkar
Johns Hopkins Department of Orthopedic Surgery, Adult Reconstruction Division, Columbia, MD, USA
e-mail: savya@jhmi.edu

© The Author(s), under exclusive license to Springer Nature Switzerland AG 2023
A. J. Deshmukh et al. (eds.), *Surgical Management of Knee Arthritis*,
https://doi.org/10.1007/978-3-031-47929-8_19

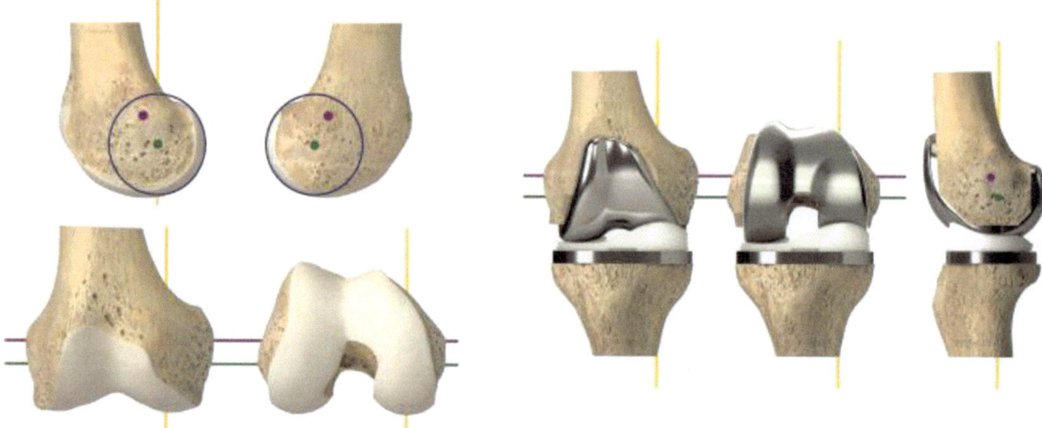

Fig. 19.1 The orange vertical lines demonstrate the longitudinal axis; the purple horizontal lines represent the transverse axis, about which the patella flexes and extends; and the green horizontal lines represent the transverse axis, about which the tibia flexes and extends [2]. (Reprinted with permission)

preventing impingement between the posterior tibia and femoral condyles, ultimately achieving maximal knee flexion. Because the MFC remains stationary while the LFC rolls back, this causes the distal femur to externally rotate in relation to an internally rotating tibia.

Another important kinematic mechanism that contributes to this pivoting motion in the native knee is known as the "screw home" mechanism. The medial tibial plateau is longer in the coronal plane and is concave than the lateral tibial plateau. As a result, during the last 20° of extension, the anterior lateral tibia glides further while the medial femoral condyle pivots on the medial tibial plateau, resulting in external rotation of the tibia. The restoration of these native kinematics of the knee is thought to potentially contribute to improved functional outcomes and patient satisfaction. Utilization of the above kinematic principles and kinematic alignment in total knee arthroplasty is thought to result in a prosthetic knee replacement that has a more natural motion.

Recreating the Native Knee

Three main strategies to create optimal knee function include employing a mechanical, anatomic, or kinematic approach to the final implant position. Recreating the mechanical axis through mechanical alignment has been the mainstay guide in total knee arthroplasty for several decades. The mechanical axis is determined by drawing a line from the center of the femoral head to the center of the ankle joint and is recreated by making cuts perpendicular to the mechanical axis of the femur and the tibia which ultimately results in neutral alignment of the final implant position [3, 4]. Anatomic alignment recreates the average anatomical axis of the distal femur and the proximal tibia. The femur, on average, is in 8–9° of valgus, while the tibia is in 2–3° of varus. This gives an overall alignment and final implant position of approximately 6° of valgus at the joint line during normal gait [3].

Kinematic alignment uses a patient-specific approach because not all patients have the same native mechanical or anatomic axis [5, 6] (Fig. 19.2).

Bellemans et al. conducted a study on adults without known knee pathology and found that 32% of males and 17% of females had a native mechanical alignment of >3° of varus. This has been referred to as constitutional varus, which has been present since skeletal maturity in these individuals [8]. By attempting to correct these patients to a neutral mechanical or an anatomic

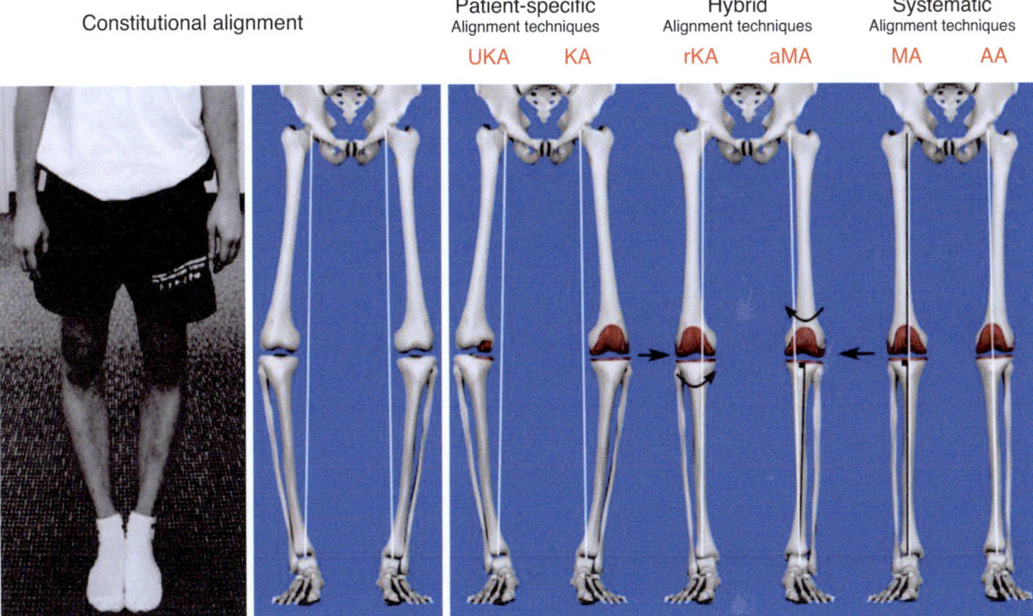

Fig. 19.2 Patient with varus deformity shown. *MA* mechanical alignment technique, *AA* anatomical alignment technique, *aMA* adjusted mechanical alignment technique; *rKA* restricted kinematic alignment technique, *UKA* unicompartmental knee arthroplasty [7]. (Reprinted with permission)

axis, these patients may have a total knee arthroplasty that functions dissimilarly to their native knee kinematics. Kinematic alignment provides an alternative option for such patients, and any patients that do not have "average" anatomic alignment. Utilization of kinematic alignment in total knee arthroplasty is thought to recreate native knee biomechanics and potentially result in improved functional outcomes and patient satisfaction [2]. The femoral and tibial cuts are made specifically to that individual patient's anatomic alignment. This may result in a femur that is in a few degrees more valgus and a tibia in a few degrees of varus [9, 10]. When done in the ideal patient, the bone resection achieved with kinematic alignment results in a perfectly balanced knee that does not require soft tissue balancing. The femoral and tibial components are often put in a more relatively internally rotated position when compared to mechanical alignment [10]. Proponents of kinematically aligned knees believe that this technique restores the anatomic joint line closer to the prearthritic knee [3]. The main concerns

that have risen with kinematic knees are the concern for higher tibial stress if an implant is placed in higher degrees of varus, depending on the patient's anatomy, and potential changes in patellofemoral contact stresses and patellar tracking due to internal rotation of the components.

Finally, how is implant survivorship affected by varying degrees of varus and valgus alignment through a myriad of component options? Implant survival has historically been a concern with regards to kinematically aligned total knee arthroplasty, with there being some degree of uncertainty surrounding the effect of kinematic, and potentially varus alignment, on implant longevity.

To evaluate the performance metrics of the various types of alignment and implant options, the following three questions were considered:

1. Is function restored?
2. Can patients forget they have a TKA?
3. How is implant and bone longevity affected by technique used to perform TKA?

Kinematic Alignment

Take Home Points

- Kinematic Alignment serves as a viable alternative to mechanical alignment to preserve normal knee kinematics and produce most likely comparable clinical outcomes undergoing TKA.
- Although kinematic alignment seems to indicate higher rates of restoring native knee kinematics, the jury is still out on whether function is superior to those with mechanical alignment implants in the long term.

In 2015, Ishikawa et al. conducted musculoskeletal computer simulations to determine the effects of mechanical and kinematically aligned TKAs [10]. Through the use of these simulations, they observed greater femoral rollback and more external rotation of the femoral component with kinematically aligned TKA than mechanically aligned TKA [10]. However, the patellofemoral and tibiofemoral contact stresses were increased in kinematically aligned TKA [10]. As a result, they concluded that KA preserves native kinematics more so than MA, but the long-term consequences of increased contact stresses were unclear. In 2019, these results were further corroborated by Koh et al., who found that KA TKA restores femoral rollback and laxity to the native condition better than MA TKA, thereby providing a more "normal" knee sensation [11].

Multiple meta-analyses have been recently performed to determine the restoration of kinematics with KA. In 2017, Courtney et al. did a systematic review of nine studies and found that similar or better clinical outcomes, as measured by the postoperative combined Knee Society Score, were produced by using a KA TKA at early-term follow-up. In 2019, Xu et al. analyzed eight studies and determined that by utilizing KA alignment to restore knee alignment, the original level of the knee joint line and surrounding soft tissue is preserved, resulting in comparative better range of motion. In 2020, Marinier et al. looked at five prospective randomized controlled trials published between 2014 and 2020 and

found no superiority of KA compared to MA technique for clinical and radiological outcomes, except in one study that showed a significant difference favoring KA between the two groups for all clinical scores, including the Knee Society Score, the Oxford Knee Score, the WOMAC score, and others [12].

In essence, the research suggests that KA serves as a viable alternative to MA to preserve normal knee kinematics and produces most likely comparable clinical outcomes undergoing TKA.

Ultimately, the question becomes: what impact does a kinematically aligned total knee arthroplasty have on long-term function and patient satisfaction?

In 2013, Howell et al. categorized patients as "in range," "varus outliers," or "valgus outliers" following their knee replacements. They found that regardless of alignment category, kinematically aligned TKA restores function without catastrophic failure at a mean follow-up of 38 months. Of note, 75% of patients in this study had their tibial components categorized as "varus outliers." This group was found to have high function and a zero incidence of catastrophic failure. Stemming from this, the authors concluded that kinematic alignment does not compromise function or implant longevity. In 2018, Howell again made a strong case for the long-term survival of the kinematically aligned knee, showing that treatment of patients with kinematically aligned TKA without restricting the preoperative deformity (varus/valgus outliers) did not adversely affect implant survival, yearly revision rate, or level of function at a mean follow-up of 10 years. Notably, this cohort was made up of 78% varus outliers.

Several studies continued to build on the notion that kinematic alignment represents a viable alternative to mechanical alignment in TKA. In 2016, Lee et al. reviewed nine studies and found that kinematically aligned TKA seemed to restore function without catastrophic failure regardless of preoperative alignment category. Lee's group found that similar or better clinical outcomes (as measured by clinical scores and radiological results) were produced by using a kinematically aligned TKA at early-term follow-up when compared to a mechanically aligned TKA. Xu et al. performed a systematic review of eight studies, concluding that kinematic alignment in TKA may produce better functional outcomes than mechanical alignment and have shorter operative times, with no difference in radiological outcomes and complication rates.

In a landmark randomized control trial published in 2016, Young et al. randomized 95 patients to either mechanically aligned or kinematically aligned TKA. They observed no difference in 2-year patient-reported outcome scores in TKAs implanted using the kinematic versus mechanical alignment technique. The theoretical advantages of improved pain and function in the case of kinematically aligned TKA were not observed. In another randomized control trial, also published in 2016, Waterson et al. randomized 71 patients to either mechanical or kinematic alignment. They concluded that kinematically aligned TKAs appeared to have comparable short-term results to mechanically aligned TKAs with no significant differences in function at 1-year postop.

Although kinematic alignment seems to indicate higher rates of restoring native knee kinematics, the jury is still out on whether function is superior to those with mechanical alignment implants in the long term. However, as recent studies have shown, there is at least somewhat comparable clinical and radiological outcomes for KA as MA, and this is an area that still needs to be further explored in the coming future.

In 2015, Howell et al. investigated the effect of varus alignment on implant survival and function at a mean follow-up of 6 years. His group found that varus alignment of the tibial component, knee, and limb did not adversely affect implant survival or function, providing support to the consideration of kinematic alignment as an alternative to mechanical alignment in TKA. Implant survivorship was 97.5% with a 0.40 rate of revision per 100 component years. In a 2017 meta-analysis of a total of 877 kinematic TKAs, Courtney et al. investigated early outcomes of kinematic alignment at a mean follow-up of 38 months, and found a 97.4% component survival rate, with the majority of revisions done

for patellar mal-tracking. In a retrospective review of 222 kinematically aligned TKAs published in 2018, Howell et al. found implant survivorship to be 97.5% for revision for any reason and 98.4% for aseptic failure at 10-year follow-up. They concluded that kinematic alignment of TKA did not have a negative impact on implant survival or significantly increase yearly revision rate. In a 2018 meta-analysis of six studies with a total of 561 patients, Li et al. demonstrated no significant difference in complication rate when comparing kinematically and mechanically aligned TKA. Revisiting Young's landmark randomized control trial from 2016, there was no significant difference in complications at 2-year follow-up between the kinematic and mechanically aligned groups. Additionally, implant survival in TKA has been investigated with regards to each kinematically designed implant type.

Mobile Bearing Knee

Take Home Points

- The Mobile-bearing (MB) knee design involves dual surface articulation, which mimics natural knee kinematics and theoretically decreases polyethylene wear and osteolysis by reducing rotational torque forces across the implant–bone interface.
- MB devices should be reserved for younger more active patients until more research is done on long term trends for older patients.

Mobile bearing devices attempt to reproduce medial pivot anatomy by allowing an additional ability to internally and externally rotate through the polyethylene insert on the tibia. The rotating tibial platform is designed to allow a partially fixed polyethylene insert to internally or externally rotate on the tibial base plate around a central axis about the medial plateau. The Meniscal Bearing polyethylene insert is not fixed to the tibial tray at all and is able to dynamically translate in a multitude of directions on the tibial insert through flexion and extension. The theoretical benefit of the Mobile-Bearing knee design is that

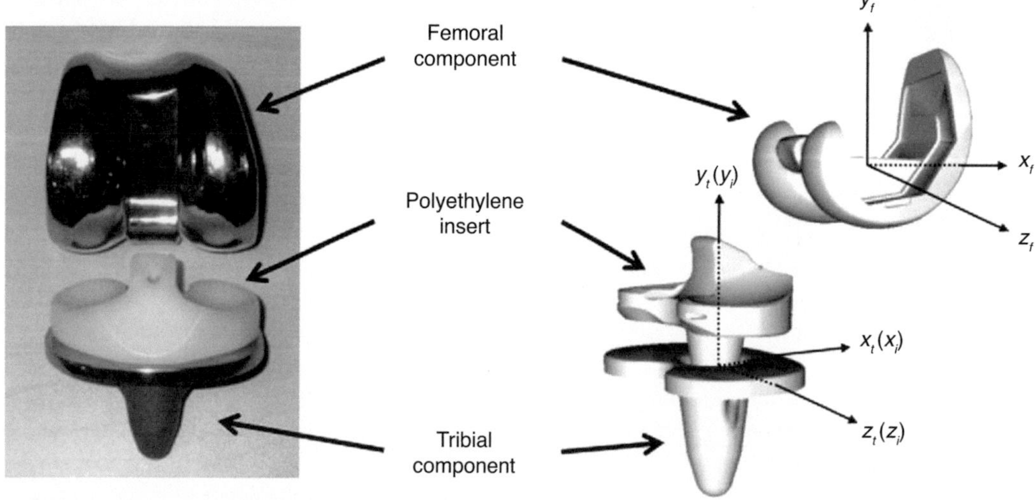

Fig. 19.3 Mobile-bearing TKA implant. The TKA implant consists of metallic femoral and tibial components and a polyethylene-bearing insert between them [14]. (Image taken from GEMINI SL at MedicalExpo.com)

a dual surface articulation, by mimicking natural knee kinematics, will decrease polyethylene wear and osteolysis by reducing rotational torque forces across the implant–bone interface [13] (Fig. 19.3).

With regard to complication rates, studies reveal similar outcomes compared to fixed-bearing total knee arthroplasty (TKA), with most complications involving early stiffness and postoperative thromboembolisms [15]. There are studies that detected higher rates of revision surgery in MB implants; however, these were ultimately attributed to the fact that MB implants were first originally used in younger patients who would ultimately place more stress and demand on the implants over a longer period of time. Once age of the patients was factored into this data, the trends were no longer significant [15, 16]. Other studies have shown equivocal rates of patellar component failure and hemarthrosis among all implants [15].

Looking at MB devices through mechanical lens, in vitro studies have shown less micromotion and reduced torque transfer across the bone–implant interface and this has been theorized to aid in long-term survival of MB implants [17]. Decreased polyethylene wear has also been shown which has led various authors to recommend MB implants for younger more active

patients and also for revision TKA in patients with poor bone quality [13, 18, 19]. Whether or not decreased wear contributes to lower rates of osteolysis requiring revision surgery is unclear at this point in general as studies have shown mixed results with differing rates of aseptic loosening and osteolysis [16, 19–21]. Overall longevity and durability have been shown to be comparable to other implants with no explicit benefit from one type of implant to another [13, 21, 22].

In terms of kinematics, given the increased freedom of motion in the MB implants, greater and more natural axial rotation is reported with their use [13]. Radiographic alignment has been reported to be better in MB implants compared to fixed-bearing knees; however, this was not shown to correlate with any changes in patient-reported range of motion of the joints and overall satisfaction [20]. Some studies have also suggested that decreased reported pain in patients can be attributed to the fact that even if components are malaligned, the rotating PE inserts are able to self-correct this and thus prevent unnatural kinematics at the knees [15].

From a patient-satisfaction and patient-reported outcomes perspective, there have been reported increases in difficulty with ADLS such as getting in and out of chairs. However, this was also attributed to MB implants being used in younger patients that had higher expectations of their ultimate outcomes [16]. Younger patients also tended to report more clicking, grinding, and popping with MB implants as compared to their fixed-bearing counterparts [23]. Stair climbing has so far been equivocal in RP and other implant types [24].

Overall, no major differences in clinical outcome and patient satisfaction have been found for the use of MB implants compared to fixed-bearing implants [18, 20, 23]. Even accounting for increased usage and higher expectations, most others do believe that in general MB devices should be reserved for younger more active patients until more research is done on long term trends for older patients [13].

Medial Pivot

Take Home Points

- The medial pivot implant has a tibial polyethylene insert, which creates a pivoting motion around the medial femoral condyle—to recreate the motion seen in native knee kinematics, including maintenance of posterior femoral rollback with deep flexion.
- The PCL has been shown to play an important role in the stability of the medial pivot design.
- Although the medial pivot design was created to better mimic native knee kinematics, some of the data suggest that it may lead to increased complications.

The medial pivot total knee arthroplasty was first developed in 1998 in an attempt to increase stability and recreate the kinematics of a native knee [25]. The native knee when ranged from −10 to 110° of flexion shows very limited medial compartment anterior–posterior movement, while the lateral compartment can translate between 0–15 mm. The stability of the medial compartment is created by the concavity of the medial tibial plateau combined with the similar center of rotation for the distal and posterior femur allowing for no femoral rollback with flexion. Additionally, the medial meniscus is fixed and

the medial collateral ligament is broad with no more than 3 mm of laxity [26].

There are several different designs that have been created to reproduce medial pivot anatomy. The medial pivot implant has a tibial polyethylene insert, which functions as a socket and limits anterior–posterior translation in the medial compartment, but allows for AP translation and medial lateral translation in the lateral component. Together this creates a pivoting motion around the medial femoral condyle—to recreate the motion seen in native knee kinematics, including maintenance of posterior femoral rollback with deep flexion [26]. Conventional posterior stabilized and posterior cruciate ligament-(PCL)retaining designs developed paradoxical anterior femoral translation in flexion. The medial pivot design was also hypothesized to lead to less postoperative patellofemoral pain secondary to the posterior location of contact points when the knee is in deep flexion. This design leads to less force from the quadriceps muscle on the patella and less contact pressure at the patellofemoral joint [27] (Fig. 19.4).

The stability of a medial pivot construct was assessed using a fluoroscopic motion study of 14 patients going through pivoting, kneeling, lunging, step-up and step-down motions. During all

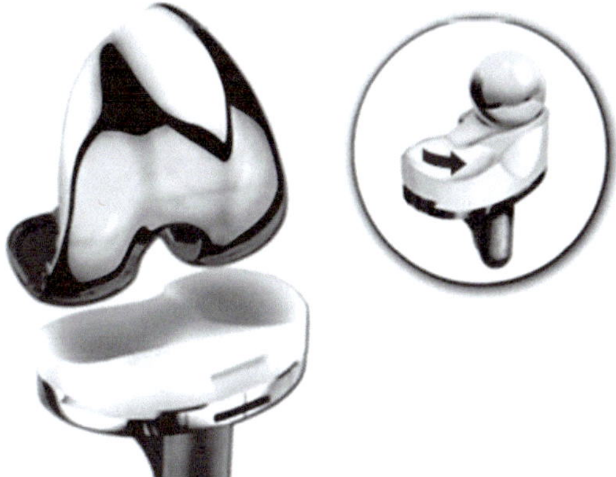

Fig. 19.4 Photograph of the medial pivot knee showing a deeper and more medial surface of the articular insert that articulates with a congruent medial femoral condyle and the anterior lip that provides stability in flexion and a less congruent lateral surface that allows free movement of lateral femoral condyle along an arcuate path [28]. (Reprinted with permission)

of these motions, Shimmin et al. found that there was no anterior femoral translation and that the medial femoral condyle remained stable while allowing the lateral femoral condyle to translate along the anterior–posterior axis recreating the native knee pivoting kinematic [29]. These results were confirmed using the dynamic finite element method by Shu L et al. to show no anterior femoral translation and improved kinematic behavior of the medial pivot design compared to cruciate retaining constructs [30].

Additionally, the PCL has been shown to play an important role in the stability of the medial pivot design. When the PCL was sacrificed intraoperatively, the femur is less constrained in flexion and may begin to translate anteriorly. In cruciate retaining and posterior stabilized approaches, the medial pivot design retains appropriate constraint throughout deep flexion. Fang et al. also showed that a posterior cam mechanism can also achieve appropriate constraint if the PCL is sacrificed in the medial pivot design [31]. In a comparison with other constrained designs, the medial pivot implant shows superior stability throughout the entire range of knee flexion [26]. In a comparison of speed of gait and length of stride, there was no difference between the medial pivot and posterior stabilized implant. These measures were used as an indirect marker for range of motion at the knee indicating that clinical outcomes were similar with each implant [26].

Bae et al. designed a strong study with a matched pair analysis between medial pivot and posterior stabilized total knee arthroplasties. The study recruited 125 patients and evaluated 150 knees for clinical outcomes and radiographs results. Both groups had significantly improved postoperative clinical scores, but there was no significant difference in the improvement. Radiographic analysis showed no difference in femorotibial angle or component positioning [27]. Additionally, the review by Shakespeare et al. found no difference in the mean flexion angle between medial pivot and posterior stabilized designs [32]. Together these findings suggest that neither implant design is superior

regardless of the improved stability seen in the medial pivot construct.

The native knee medial pivot mechanism can also be achieved with other implant designs. A retrospective review of primary total knee arthroplasties using cruciate retaining, cruciate sparing, and posterior stabilized constructs found that about 40% of constructs exhibited intraoperative medial pivot patterns. However, when clinical outcomes scores were compared at 1 year after surgery, there was no significant difference between patients that had intraoperative medial pivot patterns than those that did not. These findings suggest that achieving medial pivot kinematics may not be a keystone factor in clinical outcomes [33].

Although the medial pivot design was created to better mimic native knee kinematics, some of the data suggests that it may lead to increased complications. The Australian orthopedic association national joint replacement registry shows that medial pivot designed arthroplasties have a higher rate of revisions, most commonly from osteolysis and patellofemoral pain [27]. The increased rate of osteolysis may be related to the increased force along the interface between the cement and tibial component [25]. The dynamic finite element method study designed by Shu L et al. showed an increase in femoral internal rotation during gait and while going up and down stairs. This rotational movement may be a source of the anterolateral and patellofemoral pain seen in medial pivot constructs [30].

Asymmetric vs. Symmetric Tibial Components

Take Home Points

- Asymmetric components have been designed to theoretically more accurately represent native anatomy and allow for greater tibial coverage while decreasing rates of internal rotation and preventing overhang.
- Patients receiving asymmetric components had better performance with physical routines,

no pain in the anterior lateral portion of the knee, and lower tibial bone stress—but more research is needed to determine the long-term effects.

The three most important factors in positioning of tibial plateau components are proper rotational alignment, maximal coverage of the cut tibia, and minimal overhang. Mal-rotation may cause patellar mal-tracking and poor kinematics [34–36], reduced bone coverage may lead to periprosthetic fractures and loosening [37]; and overhang can lead to a reduction in range of motion, increased pain and increased inflammation of the soft tissues [38]. Historically, production and use of symmetric tibial components have been the standard of care. However, due to the difference in size and shape of the native lateral and medial plateaus, wherein the medial plateau is often larger, it can be difficult to optimize tibial bone coverage and maintain proper rotation. It can be easier to allow for symmetric fit while incorporating external rotation of the implant [39]. Asymmetric components have been designed to theoretically more accurately represent native anatomy and allow for greater tibial coverage while decreasing rates of internal rotation and preventing overhang [39] (Fig. 19.5).

There have been conflicting reports on outcomes of bone coverage with asymmetric and symmetric components. Some authors have found greater tibial bone coverage and cortical support for asymmetric designs [39], while others have shown better outcomes with coverage and rotational alignment with symmetric designs [40–42]. Recent work has shown that this may be due to not matching components to their optimized rotational axis, causing variability in coverage throughout all component types. In Meier et al., it was shown that surgeons must select the proper rotational axis for each specific component. By doing so, they found there was no difference in the optimized tibial coverage for both asymmetric and symmetric components [42].

As asymmetric tibial components are new to the field of orthopedics, larger studies with longer follow-ups will be needed prior to the ortho-

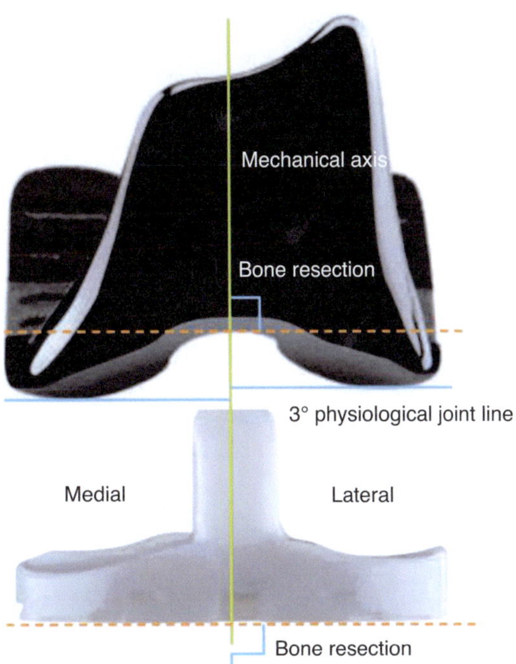

Fig. 19.5 Asymmetry can be in femoral and/or tibial components and the Polyethylene asymmetry tries to match native tibia. (Image taken from the JOURNEY II Bi-Cruciate Stabilized Knee System)

pedic community coming to a consensus. A recent 303-patient retrospective study with 1-year follow-up looking at outcomes and finite element analysis for different shape polyethylene inserts in mobile bearing total knees noted multiple positive outcomes for asymmetric components. Patients receiving asymmetric components had better performance with physical routines, no pain in the anterior lateral portion of the knee, and lower tibial bone stress [43].

Bicruciate-Retaining Total Knee Arthroplasty

Take Home Points

- The Bicruciate-Retaining (BCR)-TKA was designed with the idea that, with less soft tissue disruption during TKA, there would be more normal kinematics and stability, less

Fig. 19.6 Shows the prepared femur and tibia, including the retained tibial eminence and both cruciate ligaments. The femoral and two-piece tibial component is shown with the prepared slot in the tibia for the keel and pilot holes for the spikes of the tibial component [45]. (Reprinted with permission)

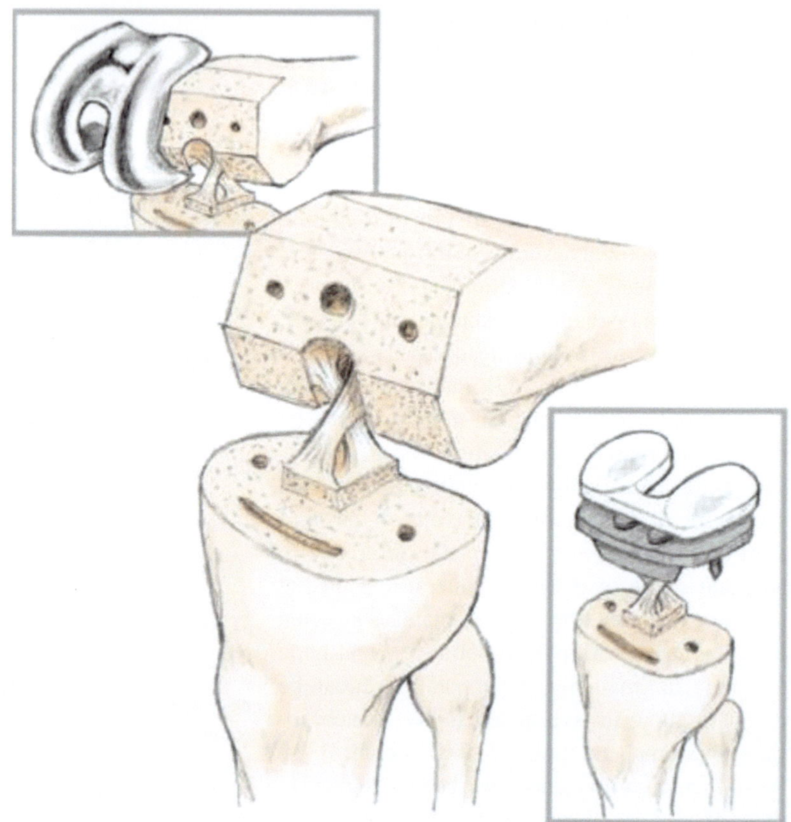

patient awareness of their TKA and better proprioception with retention of the densely innervated ACL.

- The primary disadvantage that is cited by studies is that it is more technically challenging to implant than ACL sacrificing implants.
- BCR-TKA is an excellent choice of implant for both patient satisfaction and longevity.

The ligaments that connect the knee are especially important for native knee kinematics. The ACL prevents the tibia from anterior displacement during hyperextension of the knee. The PCL prevents it from posterior displacement and stabilizes the knee during flexion. During typical total knee arthroplasty, before the tibia is resurfaced, the ACL and sometimes the PCL is sacrificed. Bicruciate-retaining total knee arthroplasty (BCR-TKA) has been attempted for decades, but with inconsistent results [44]. Recently, with the advent of more sophisticated operative planning tools and patient-specific cutting guides, there

has been a resurgence of BCR- TKAs. Studies into these techniques have found many advantages of BCR-TKA, primarily regarding kinematics and patient-reported outcomes. However, there are several notable disadvantages, challenges, and concerning gaps in knowledge concerning these implants (Fig. 19.6).

The BCR-TKA was designed with the idea that, with less soft tissue disruption during TKA, there would be more normal kinematics and stability, less patient awareness of their TKA and better proprioception with retention of the densely innervated ACL. These findings have been largely borne out in studies. Stiehl et al. performed fluoroscopic testing of posterior cruciate-retaining total knee arthroplasties (PCR-TKA) and BCR-TKAs during weightbearing knee flexion and extension, finding that, while BCR-TKA did not perfectly mirror the kinematics of normal knees, it was much more similar than PCR-TKAs [46]. Several cadaveric studies have also shown that, when comparing native knees to BCR-TKAs and traditional

TKAs, the stability profile of the BCR-TKA is much more similar to the native knee [47–49]. In a study comparing BCR-TKA to PCR-TKA during level and downhill walking tasks, Simon et al. found significantly less muscle activity required to stabilize the BCR-TKA, suggesting a more stable construct due to preserved soft tissues [50]. The restoration of normal knee kinematics and stability is not perfect, however. Hamada et al. found in a cadaveric study that BCR-TKA was more similar to PCR-TKA than a native knee with respect to rotational stability, especially in early flexion. They also found that BCR-TKA lacked the "screw home" mechanism of the normal knee. Interestingly, the changes in rotational stability were only present after tibial resurfacing and were not present after meniscectomy or femoral resurfacing [51]. In addition, Kono et al. compared BCR-TKA to native knees and unicompartmental arthroplasty (UKA) in a fluoroscopic study, and found that, while the kinematics of UKA closely mirrored that of native knees, BCR-TKA kinematics were significantly different during a deep squatting motion [52]. Regarding patient awareness of their BCR-TKA, Baumann et al. compared BCR-TKA, UKA, and posterior-stabilized TKA (PS-TKA) and found patients were equally aware of their BCR-TKA and UKA during activities of daily living, but that they were significantly more aware of their PS-TKA [53]. Another study by Baumann et al. looked at proprioception in BCR-TKA, UKA, and PS-TKA during a single-legged standing task with eyes open and closed, and found again that UKA and BCR-TKA performed similarly, and performed significantly better than PS-TKA [54]. Corroborating the advantages provided by BCR-TKA with regards to kinematics, stability, joint awareness, and proprioception, 440 patients with bilateral TKAs of different types (BCR-TKA, medial pivot TKA, PCR-TKA, PS-TKA, and mobile-bearing TKA) were surveyed to determine which knee they preferred. The study showed that patients preferred BCR-TKA to all other implant types other than medial pivot, with no difference in preference between BCR-TKA and medial pivot [55].

The BCR-TKA implant is not without its disadvantages. The primary disadvantage that is cited by studies is that it is more technically challenging to implant than ACL sacrificing implants [56, 57]. Other challenges with BCR-TKA that were cited were the unique challenges regarding both coronal and sagittal balancing, as well as reports of avulsion fractures of the tibial spine and a case report of three knees that developed the cyclops lesion (anterior arthrofibrotic lesion traditionally associated with ACL reconstruction) after BCR-TKA [58, 59].

BCR-TKA is a promising alternative to cruciate-sacrificing TKA. The preservation of the ACL and the minimal soft tissue releases inherent to this technique lead to more normal joint kinematics and stability, less joint awareness, better proprioception, and better patient outcomes. Survivorship studies of BCR-TKA with follow-up for as long as 23 years show no significant issues with implant survivorship, especially with the advent of more highly cross-linked polyethylene inserts, as many of the revisions were for polyethylene wear [56]. Due to the technical challenges of BCR-TKA, however, there is a need for larger, multisurgeon studies that will determine the prudence of encouraging the widescale use of this type of implant. Still, the current literature suggests that BCR-TKA is an excellent choice of implant for both patient satisfaction and longevity.

Conclusion

In conclusion, the native kinematics of the knee are complex, and this is a very active area of study as orthopedic surgeons strive to better understand the kinematics of the native knee. Along with that comes the complex challenge of trying to recreate and restore native kinematics with a kinematically aligned total knee arthroplasty. Despite the seemingly logical thought process that restoring native kinematics would be best for the patient, KA TKA does not always correlate with better outcomes. There is still an ongoing debate as to whether mechanically or kinematically aligned TKA is superior.

This is further complicated by the wide range of available implant designs, of which there is no clear-cut superior design based on the available literature. Many current implant designs add to the "kinematic" dynamics of the knee. The jury is still out on whether combining kinematic alignment and kinematic implant designs leads to better patient outcomes. However, these implants by themselves have shown to be powerful designs that drastically improve patient function scores. Nonetheless, kinematic alignment and kinematic implant designs all seem like an excellent new frontier for research and development in improving all spectra of total knee arthroplasties.

References

1. Feng JE, Novikov D, Anoushiravani AA, Schwarzkopf R. Total knee arthroplasty: improving outcomes with a multidisciplinary approach. J Multidiscip Healthc. 2018;11:63–73. https://doi.org/10.2147/JMDH.S140550.
2. Nisar S, Palan J, Rivière C, Emerton M, Pandit H. Kinematic alignment in total knee arthroplasty. EFORT Open Rev. 2020;5(7):380–90. https://doi.org/10.1302/2058-5241.5.200010.
3. Cherian JJ, Kapadia BH, Banerjee S, Jauregui JJ, Issa K, Mont MA. Mechanical, anatomical, and kinematic Axis in TKA: concepts and practical applications. Curr Rev Musculoskelet Med. 2014;7(2):89–95. https://doi.org/10.1007/s12178-014-9218-y.
4. An VVG, Twiggs J, Leie M, Fritsch BA. Kinematic alignment is bone and soft tissue preserving compared to mechanical alignment in total knee arthroplasty. Knee. 2019;26(2):466–76. https://doi.org/10.1016/j.knee.2019.01.002.
5. Jaffe WL, Dundon JM, Camus T. Alignment and balance methods in Total knee arthroplasty. J Am Acad Orthop Surg. 2018;26(20):709–16. https://doi.org/10.5435/JAAOS-D-16-00428.
6. Fahlman L, Sangeorzan E, Chheda N, Lambright D. Older adults without radiographic knee osteoarthritis: knee alignment and knee range of motion. Clin Med Insights Arthritis Musculoskelet Disord. 2014;7:1–11. https://doi.org/10.4137/CMAMD.S13009.
7. Rivière C, Iranpour F, Auvinet E, et al. Alignment options for total knee arthroplasty: a systematic review. Orthop Traumatol Surg Res. 2017;103(7):1047–56. https://doi.org/10.1016/j.otsr.2017.07.010.
8. Bellemans J, Colyn W, Vandenneucker H, Victor J. The Chitranjan Ranawat award: is neutral mechanical alignment normal for all patients? The concept of constitutional varus. Clin Orthop. 2012;470(1):45–53. https://doi.org/10.1007/s11999-011-1936-5.
9. Theodore W, Twiggs J, Kolos E, et al. Variability in static alignment and kinematics for kinematically aligned TKA. Knee. 2017;24(4):733–44. https://doi.org/10.1016/j.knee.2017.04.002.
10. Ishikawa M, Kuriyama S, Ito H, Furu M, Nakamura S, Matsuda S. Kinematic alignment produces near-normal knee motion but increases contact stress after total knee arthroplasty: a case study on a single implant design. Knee. 2015;22(3):206–12. https://doi.org/10.1016/j.knee.2015.02.019.
11. Koh IJ, Lin CC, Patel NA, et al. Kinematically aligned total knee arthroplasty reproduces more native roll-back and laxity than mechanically aligned total knee arthroplasty: a matched pair cadaveric study. Orthop Traumatol Surg Res. 2019;105(4):605–11. https://doi.org/10.1016/j.otsr.2019.03.011.
12. Sappey-Marinier E, Pauvert A, Batailler C, et al. Kinematic versus mechanical alignment for primary total knee arthroplasty with minimum 2 years follow-up: a systematic review. SICOT-J. 2020;6:18. https://doi.org/10.1051/sicotj/2020014.
13. White PB, Ranawat AS, Ranawat CS. Fixed bearings versus rotating platforms in Total knee arthroplasty. J Knee Surg. 2015;28(5):358–62. https://doi.org/10.1055/s-0035-1550338.
14. Yamazaki T, Futai K, Tomita T, et al. 3D kinematics of mobile-bearing total knee arthroplasty using X-ray fluoroscopy. Int J Comput Assist Radiol Surg. 2015;10(4):487–95. https://doi.org/10.1007/s11548-014-1093-x.
15. Scholes C, Ebrahimi M, Ektas N, Ireland J. Efficacy of a second-generation rotating bearing Tibial platform in Total knee arthroplasty: a prospective observational cohort study with registry analysis. J Knee Surg. 2020;33(5):513–24. https://doi.org/10.1055/s-0039-1678679.
16. Martin JR, Beahrs TR, Fehring KA, Trousdale RT. Rotating platform versus fixed bearing total knee arthroplasty at mid-term follow-up. Knee. 2016;23(6):1055–8. https://doi.org/10.1016/j.knee.2016.06.004.
17. Small SR, Rogge RD, Malinzak RA, et al. Micromotion at the tibial plateau in primary and revision total knee arthroplasty: fixed versus rotating platform designs. Bone Joint Res. 2016;5(4):122–9. https://doi.org/10.1302/2046-3758.54.2000481.
18. McEwen HMJ, Barnett PI, Bell CJ, et al. The influence of design, materials and kinematics on the in vitro wear of total knee replacements. J Biomech. 2005;38(2):357–65. https://doi.org/10.1016/j.jbiomech.2004.02.015.
19. Fisher J, McEwen H, Tipper J, et al. Wear-simulation analysis of rotating-platform mobile-bearing knees. Orthopedics. 2006;29(9 Suppl):S36–41.
20. Hernigou P, Huys M, Pariat J, Roubineau F, Flouzat Lachaniette CH, Dubory A. Comparison of fixed-bearing and mobile-bearing total knee arthroplasty after high tibial osteotomy. Int Orthop. 2018;42(2):317–22. https://doi.org/10.1007/s00264-017-3540-0.
21. Gothesen O, Lygre SHL, Lorimer M, Graves S, Furnes O. Increased risk of aseptic loosening for 43,525

rotating-platform vs. fixed-bearing total knee replacements. Acta Orthop. 2017;88(6):649–56. https://doi.org/10.1080/17453674.2017.1378533.

22. Argenson J-NA, Parratte S, Ashour A, Saintmard B, Aubaniac J-M. The outcome of rotating-platform total knee arthroplasty with cement at a minimum of ten years of follow-up. J Bone Joint Surg Am. 2012;94(7):638–44. https://doi.org/10.2106/JBJS.K.00263.

23. Nunley RM, Nam D, Berend KR, et al. New total knee arthroplasty designs: do young patients notice? Clin Orthop. 2015;473(1):101–8. https://doi.org/10.1007/s11999-014-3713-8.

24. Murakami K, Hamai S, Okazaki K, et al. Kinematic analysis of stair climbing in rotating platform cruciate-retaining and posterior-stabilized mobile-bearing total knee arthroplasties. Arch Orthop Trauma Surg. 2017;137(5):701–11. https://doi.org/10.1007/s00402-017-2662-6.

25. Kim Y-H, Park J-W, Kim J-S. Clinical outcome of medial pivot compared with press-fit condylar sigma cruciate-retaining Mobile-bearing Total knee arthroplasty. J Arthroplast. 2017;32(10):3016–23. https://doi.org/10.1016/j.arth.2017.05.022.

26. Benjamin B, Pietrzak JRT, Tahmassebi J, Haddad FS. A functional comparison of medial pivot and condylar knee designs based on patient outcomes and parameters of gait. Bone Joint J. 2018;100-B(1 Supple A):76–82. https://doi.org/10.1302/0301-620X.100B1.BJJ-2017-0605.R1.

27. Bae DK, Cho SD, Im SK, Song SJ. Comparison of midterm clinical and radiographic results between Total knee arthroplasties using medial pivot and posterior-stabilized prosthesis-a matched pair analysis. J Arthroplast. 2016;31(2):419–24. https://doi.org/10.1016/j.arth.2015.09.038.

28. Kulshrestha V, Sood M, Kanade S, Kumar S, Datta B, Mittal G. Early outcomes of medial pivot Total knee arthroplasty compared to posterior-stabilized design: a randomized controlled trial. Clin Orthop Surg. 2020;12(2):178–86. https://doi.org/10.4055/cios19141.

29. Shimmin A, Martinez-Martos S, Owens J, Iorgulescu AD, Banks S. Fluoroscopic motion study confirming the stability of a medial pivot design total knee arthroplasty. Knee. 2015;22(6):522–6. https://doi.org/10.1016/j.knee.2014.11.011.

30. Shu L, Yamamoto K, Kai S, Inagaki J, Sugita N. Symmetrical cruciate-retaining versus medial pivot prostheses: the effect of intercondylar sagittal conformity on knee kinematics and contact mechanics. Comput Biol Med. 2019;108:101–10. https://doi.org/10.1016/j.compbiomed.2019.03.005.

31. Fang C-H, Chang C-M, Lai Y-S, et al. Is the posterior cruciate ligament necessary for medial pivot knee prostheses with regard to postoperative kinematics? Knee Surg Sports Traumatol Arthrosc. 2015;23(11):3375–82. https://doi.org/10.1007/s00167-014-3249-1.

32. Shakespeare D, Ledger M, Kinzel V. Flexion after total knee replacement. A comparison between the medial pivot knee and a posterior stabilised implant. Knee. 2006;13(5):371–3. https://doi.org/10.1016/j.knee.2006.05.007.

33. Warth LC, Ishmael MK, Deckard ER, Ziemba-Davis M, Meneghini RM. Do medial pivot kinematics correlate with patient-reported outcomes after Total knee arthroplasty? J Arthroplast. 2017;32(8):2411–6. https://doi.org/10.1016/j.arth.2017.03.019.

34. Fitz W, Bliss R, Losina E. Current fit of medial and lateral unicompartmental knee arthroplasty. Acta Orthop Belg. 2013;79(2):191–6.

35. Martin S, Saurez A, Ismaily S, Ashfaq K, Noble P, Incavo SJ. Maximizing tibial coverage is detrimental to proper rotational alignment. Clin Orthop. 2014;472(1):121–5. https://doi.org/10.1007/s11999-013-3047-y.

36. Keshmiri A, Maderbacher G, Baier C, Zeman F, Grifka J, Springorum HR. Significant influence of rotational limb alignment parameters on patellar kinematics: an in vitro study. Knee Surg Sports Traumatol Arthrosc. 2016;24(8):2407–14. https://doi.org/10.1007/s00167-014-3434-2.

37. Abram SGF, Marsh AG, Brydone AS, Nicol F, Mohammed A, Spencer SJ. The effect of tibial component sizing on patient reported outcome measures following uncemented total knee replacement. Knee. 2014;21(5):955–9. https://doi.org/10.1016/j.knee.2014.05.010.

38. Mahoney OM, Kinsey T. Overhang of the femoral component in total knee arthroplasty: risk factors and clinical consequences. J Bone Joint Surg Am. 2010;92(5):1115–21. https://doi.org/10.2106/JBJS.H.00434.

39. Dai Y, Scuderi GR, Bischoff JE, Bertin K, Tarabichi S, Rajgopal A. Anatomic tibial component design can increase tibial coverage and rotational alignment accuracy: a comparison of six contemporary designs. Knee Surg Sports Traumatol Arthrosc. 2014;22(12):2911–23. https://doi.org/10.1007/s00167-014-3282-0.

40. Clary C, Aram L, Deffenbaugh D, Heldreth M. Tibial base design and patient morphology affecting tibial coverage and rotational alignment after total knee arthroplasty. Knee Surg Sports Traumatol Arthrosc. 2014;22(12):3012–8. https://doi.org/10.1007/s00167-014-3402-x.

41. Bozkurt M, Akkaya M, Tahta M, Gursoy S, Firat A. Tibial Base plate for Total knee arthroplasty: symmetric or asymmetric? Clin Orthop Surg. 2017;9(3):280–5. https://doi.org/10.4055/cios.2017.9.3.280.

42. Meier M, Webb J, Collins JE, Beckmann J, Fitz W. Do modern total knee replacements improve tibial coverage? Knee Surg Sports Traumatol Arthrosc. 2018;26(11):3219–29. https://doi.org/10.1007/s00167-018-4836-3.

43. Castellarin G, Pianigiani S, Innocenti B. Asymmetric polyethylene inserts promote favorable kinematics and better clinical outcome compared to symmetric inserts in a mobile bearing total knee arthro-

plasty. Knee Surg Sports Traumatol Arthrosc. 2019;27(4):1096–105. https://doi.org/10.1007/s00167-018-5207-9.

44. Alnachoukati OK, Emerson RH, Diaz E, Ruchaud E, Ennin KA. Modern day Bicruciate-retaining Total knee arthroplasty: a short-term review of 146 knees. J Arthroplast. 2018;33(8):2485–90. https://doi.org/10.1016/j.arth.2018.03.026.

45. Pritchett JW. Bicruciate-retaining Total knee replacement provides satisfactory function and implant survivorship at 23 years. Clin Orthop Relat Res. 2015;473(7):2327–33. https://doi.org/10.1007/s11999-015-4219-8.

46. Parcells BW, Tria AJ. The cruciate ligaments in Total knee arthroplasty. Am J Orthop Belle Mead NJ. 2016;45(4):E153–60.

47. Halewood C, Traynor A, Bellemans J, Victor J, Amis AA. Anteroposterior laxity after Bicruciate-retaining Total knee arthroplasty is closer to the native knee than ACL-resecting TKA: a biomechanical cadaver study. J Arthroplast. 2015;30(12):2315–9. https://doi.org/10.1016/j.arth.2015.06.021.

48. Lo J, Müller O, Dilger T, Wülker N, Wünschel M. Translational and rotational knee joint stability in anterior and posterior cruciate-retaining knee arthroplasty. Knee. 2011;18(6):491–5. https://doi.org/10.1016/j.knee.2010.10.009.

49. Arnout N, Victor J, Vermue H, Pringels L, Bellemans J, Verstraete MA. Knee joint laxity is restored in a bi-cruciate retaining TKA-design. Knee Surg Sports Traumatol Arthrosc. 2020;28(9):2863–71. https://doi.org/10.1007/s00167-019-05639-4.

50. Simon JC, Della Valle CJ, Wimmer MA. Level and downhill walking to assess implant functionality in Bicruciate- and posterior cruciate-retaining Total knee arthroplasty. J Arthroplast. 2018;33(9):2884–9. https://doi.org/10.1016/j.arth.2018.05.010.

51. Hamada D, Wada K, Takasago T, et al. Native rotational knee kinematics are lost in bicruciate-retaining total knee arthroplasty when the tibial component is replaced. Knee Surg Sports Traumatol Arthrosc. 2018;26(11):3249–56. https://doi.org/10.1007/s00167-018-4842-5.

52. Kono K, Inui H, Tomita T, Yamazaki T, Taketomi S, Tanaka S. Bicruciate-retaining total knee arthroplasty reproduces in vivo kinematics of normal knees to a lower extent than unicompartmental knee arthroplasty. Knee Surg Sports Traumatol Arthrosc. 2020;28(9):3007–15. https://doi.org/10.1007/s00167-019-05754-2.

53. Baumann F, Krutsch W, Worlicek M, et al. Reduced joint-awareness in bicruciate-retaining total knee arthroplasty compared to cruciate-sacrificing total knee arthroplasty. Arch Orthop Trauma Surg. 2018;138(2):273–9. https://doi.org/10.1007/s00402-017-2839-z.

54. Baumann F, Bahadin Ö, Krutsch W, et al. Proprioception after bicruciate-retaining total knee arthroplasty is comparable to unicompartmental knee arthroplasty. Knee Surg Sports Traumatol Arthrosc. 2017;25(6):1697–704. https://doi.org/10.1007/s00167-016-4121-2.

55. Pritchett JW. Patients prefer a bicruciate-retaining or the medial pivot total knee prosthesis. J Arthroplast. 2011;26(2):224–8. https://doi.org/10.1016/j.arth.2010.02.012.

56. Baumann F. Bicruciate-retaining total knee arthroplasty compared to cruciate-sacrificing TKA: what are the advantages and disadvantages? Expert Rev Med Devices. 2018;15(9):615–7. https://doi.org/10.1080/17434440.2018.1514256.

57. Osmani FA, Thakkar SC, Collins K, Schwarzkopf R. The utility of bicruciate-retaining total knee arthroplasty. Arthroplast Today. 2017;3(1):61–6. https://doi.org/10.1016/j.artd.2016.11.004.

58. Barrett TJ, Shi L, Parsley BS. Bicruciate-retaining total knee arthroplasty, a promising technology, that's not quite there. Ann Transl Med. 2017;5(Suppl 1):S17. https://doi.org/10.21037/atm.2017.03.77.

59. Klaassen MA, Aikins JL. The cyclops lesion after bicruciate-retaining total knee replacement. Arthroplast Today. 2017;3(4):242–6. https://doi.org/10.1016/j.artd.2017.06.002.

Knee Distraction for Managing Knee Osteoarthritis

Beth Lineham, Paul Harwood, and Hemant G. Pandit

Introduction

Osteoarthritis (OA) is a common and disabling musculoskeletal condition, affecting 3.8% of the world's population [1]. The knee is the most commonly affected joint, with treatment sought by 1 in 6 people over the age of 55 in the UK every year [2]. This number is increasing, with rates of primary total knee arthroplasty (TKA) tripling in the UK since the early 1990s [3]; this increase appears likely to continue due to rising obesity rates and an aging population [4, 5]. There is currently no definitive treatment that arrests the progression of, or cures, OA. Initial management at the knee is symptomatic, with lifestyle modification, analgesia and physiotherapy [6]. Some patients may benefit from a realignment osteotomy to correct mechanical axis malalignment [7]. The gold standard treatment for end stage knee OA with failure of symptomatic treatment is total knee arthroplasty. This is proven and effective, with more than 790,000 procedures carried out in the USA per year, this rate is projected to increase in the future [8].

There are, however, limitations to knee arthroplasty surgery, 10–20% of patients remain dissatisfied with the results and 30–50% have residual symptoms [9–11]. Knee arthroplasty prostheses have a finite life span, with survival without revision ranging from 70–96% at 20 years [12, 13]. Rates of revision surgery are increasing and predicted to present a significant economic burden in the future [5].

Demand for TKA in younger patients is predicted to increase over time [14], currently 13% of patients are under 55 years of age [15]. Managing younger patients with knee OA presents specific difficulties. Though TKA results in good initial clinical outcomes in these patients [16], higher rates of complication and increased early failure rates have been reported [17]. Revision surgery is more costly than primary TKA [18], more prone to complications [19] and has a higher early failure rate [20]. There is therefore a need to develop alternative treatments for young patients in particular.

Joint distraction has been proposed as a potential treatment for osteoarthritis at various sites. In this technique, an external fixator is placed to apply temporary distraction across the joint, unloading the cartilage. This was first described in 1978 using a hinged apparatus applied following various surgical procedures, including arthrolysis, to allow motion whilst maintaining joint space. Formation of fibrous tissue was observed following such a procedure undertaken

B. Lineham (✉) · H. C. Pandit
Leeds Institute of Rheumatic and Musculoskeletal Medicine (LIRMM), University of Leeds, Leeds, UK
e-mail: Beth.lineham@nhs.net; h.pandit@leeds.ac.uk

P. Harwood
Department of Trauma and Orthopaedic Surgery, Leeds Teaching Hospitals, Leeds, UK
e-mail: Paulharwood@nhs.net

at the ankle [21]. A subsequent case series reported results of ankle joint distraction (AJD) for post-traumatic OA using an Ilizarov device in 11 patients [22]. The initial rationale for the joint distraction was to correct foot position; however, improvements in pain and mobility were observed alongside a radiological increase in joint space. The authors postulated the effects were due to a combination of reduced mechanical stress and intermittent intra-articular hydrostatic pressures changes produced during distraction and loading. Intermittent hydrostatic pressure on osteoarthritic cartilage has been shown to produce an improvement in cartilage quality in vitro with synthesis of proteoglycans increased by more than 50% [23].

Outcomes of joint distraction at various sites have been reported in a number of case series. Though relatively small numbers of patients have been involved, results are encouraging in at least providing temporary symptom relief. At the ankle, improvements in reported symptoms were seen in 73–91% of patients at mean follow-up time of 1–12 years. [22, 24, 25] Conversion to final ankle arthrodesis or total ankle arthroplasty ranged between 6.2% and 44% with failure of 44% in the longest follow up. Thirty seven percent of patients underwent further surgery within the first 5 years, with women having a higher rate of failure [26].

AJD has also been compared to ankle joint debridement in a randomised controlled trial (RCT) of 17 patients. Superior clinical outcomes were reported in the AJD patients at 1 year of follow up. The same group also followed 57 patients with AJD prospectively, with three quarters demonstrating significant clinical benefit [24]. Joint distraction has also been demonstrated to give good clinical outcomes in first carpometacarpal joint osteoarthritis, albeit in a very limited number of patients. Patients were followed up for 1 year and had improved functional scores compared to baseline [27]. It has also been utilised in combination with trapeziectomy for OA as an alternative to trapeziectomy and ligament interposition with good outcomes reported at 6 years [28, 29].

Knee joint distraction is therefore a potential management option for osteoarthritis, particularly in younger patients. Early reported outcomes appear encouraging and this information is outlined hereafter in this chapter. If this technique is proven to be clinically effective, it would potentially offer significant financial benefits, by delaying TKA and reducing need for subsequent revisions [30].

Mechanism of Action of Joint Distraction

It had been traditionally accepted that articular cartilage has low regenerative potential; however, the cartilage offloading seen in HTO has been observed to produce cartilage repair. Total coverage with newly regenerated fibrocartilage or hyaline-like cartilage has been reported, indicating an endogenous repair mechanism exists [31]. Full thickness hyaline repair has also been demonstrated following microfracture treatment [32]. Though there remains no proven mechanism of action to explain the clinical improvements seen in more severe OA in KJD, various theories have been proposed. Changes are seen in the mechanical and biological environment as discussed previously, but it is unclear as to whether these changes demonstrate a cause or effect. Offloading of the joint during joint distraction is postulated to allow regeneration by temporarily preventing mechanical stress on the cartilage. However, complete abolition of movement or weight bearing at a joint leads to reduced bone quality and can potentiate osteoarthritic changes [33, 34]. However, low levels of intermittent fluid pressure in an offloaded joint has been shown to decrease IL-1 and TNF-alpha in osteoarthritic synovial fluid mononuclear cells [35] and to increase proteoglycan synthesis [23] which is implicated in endogenous cartilage repair mechanisms. Low levels of intermittent fluid pressure have been shown to be achieved in even static joint distraction on weightbearing, with changes in mean hydrostatic pressure ranging from 3.0 ± 0.5 kPa during relaxation to 10.3 ± 0.6 kPa during loading [22]. Mesenchymal stem cells in synovial fluid adhere better to damaged cartilage in OA synovial fluid in certain concentrations of hyaluronic acid (HA). A dense HA layer appears to inhibit adherence of MSCs to cartilage defects. Therefore, the modulation of SF-HA provided by KJD may ensure a more favourable environment for cartilage regeneration [36].

Methods of Joint Distraction

Hinged Distractors

Ankle joint distraction was first described using a circular external fixator; these devices remain the most commonly employed. Circular frames, particularly where employing tensioned fine wires, lead to axial micromotion on compressive loading, whilst providing a stable environment for distraction [37]. Intra-articular pressure fluctuations have been demonstrated during both static and hinged distraction and this is theorised to contribute to cartilage regeneration [22]. Static and hinged joint distractors have been assessed with most AJD being undertaken using a hinge to allow motion at the ankle joint. Joint motion during AJD appears to correlate with superior results, with improved outcome scores compared to fixed distraction [38]. Weight bearing is typically allowed immediately post-operatively as tolerated, with the hinge unlocked for range of movement exercises initially and then progression to unlocked weight bearing when comfortable [39].

Hinged distractors have also been utilised in KJD, allowing range of motion at the knee during distraction with improved clinical outcomes in a small group of patients, although have not been directly compared to static distractors. [40]

Spring-Loaded Distractor

The majority of studies investigating KJD for OA employ the use of non-hinged fixators. Earlier studies utilised Ilizarov or biplanar tubular devices; these techniques were usually combined with other procedures such as arthroscopic lavage and drilling of cartilage defects [40, 41]. More recently, specifically designed spring-loaded dis-

tractors have been developed in an attempt to simplify the procedure. These consist of two tubular fixators with internal coil springs, one placed on either side of the limb in parallel, spanning the knee joint. Fixation to the distal femur and proximal tibia is achieved by a number of half-pins. The joint is distracted either at the time of surgery, or gradually over a few days post-operatively. These fixators do not allow for flexion at the knee joint and fixation in extension is usually maintained for the entire treatment period. [30, 42, 43] Periodic motion during distraction using a continuous passive movement machine has also been described which required temporary removal of the tubular fixators periodically throughout the distraction period [44]. It is unclear whether this improves range of motion post-operatively as this has not been directly compared.

Current evidence demonstrates significant improvement in patient-reported outcomes following KJD distraction using different devices. There are currently no comparative studies of hinged versus fixed or spring-loaded versus static KJD devices and therefore no conclusions can be drawn in this regard.

Operative Technique

Operative techniques will vary dependent on what device is employed. We describe here the authors' preferred technique using Ilizarov equipment. This is versatile in its nature and alternative constructs can be utilised which would achieve similar biomechanical results. A static distractor is described here. It is also possible to apply a hinged distractor using this equipment. It is important that the centre of rotation of the knee is carefully identified to allow proper orientation and positioning of the hinges. The technique for this is also described at the end of the section below.

Figure 20.1 demonstrates preoperative imaging in a patient with predominantly medial compartment osteoarthritis with a relatively symmetrical mechanical axis.

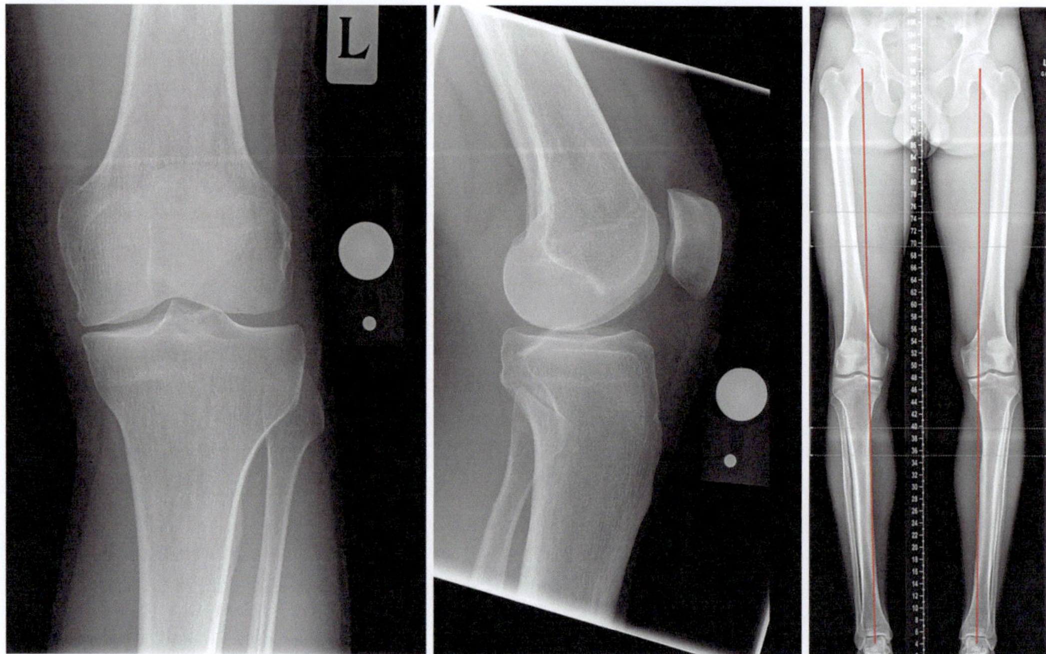

Fig. 20.1 Knee joint distraction case pre-op radiographs. 48-year-old patient with significantly symptomatic predominantly medial compartment osteoarthritis. Full thickness cartilage loss on MRI scan. Note relatively symmetrical mechanical axis

Static Distraction Frame

Preoperatively, a definitive external fixation construct should be planned which enables controlled linear distraction across the knee joint. Distraction at the joint measured radiographically at 5 mm is recommended. The construct should consist of at least 4 fixation elements at 2 levels in both the tibia and femur in a near-far arrangement. Appropriate antibiotic prophylaxis and interventions to reduce the risk of thromboembolism should be utilised. The patient will be supine on a radiolucent table, it is important that this allows imaging of the whole femur as well as the tibia. Typically, a tourniquet is not used, but some surgeons may choose to apply one but leave uninflated in case of unexpected serious vascular injury. This must allow access proximally for proper placement of femoral fixation. Following prepping and draping according to local protocols, the limb should be positioned in neutral rotation and elevated to allow free access medially and laterally (Fig. 20.2).

The exact surgical steps depend on surgeon preference and the type of external fixation utilised. However, generally anatomic landmarks should be marked radiographically at the start of the procedure and fixation planned. A 'reference' wire or pin should be placed perpendicular to the mechanical axis of the limb to facilitate correct alignment of the fixator (Fig. 20.3).

When placing the fixation elements, an awareness of relevant cross-sectional anatomy is required to avoid injury to critical neurovascular structures. Care should be taken to avoid breach of the knee joint to avoid serious septic complication. Therefore, in the tibia, pins should be placed at least 13–15 mm distal to the joint surface, below the physeal scar (Fig. 20.4). In the femur, medial and lateral pins should be placed above the superior pole of the patella or with reference to the complex anatomy of the joint capsule, if more distal. If anterior pins are utilised, they must be above the supra-patellar pouch.

When inserting pins, care must be taken to minimise the risk of complications. For half pins, a small incision should be made in the

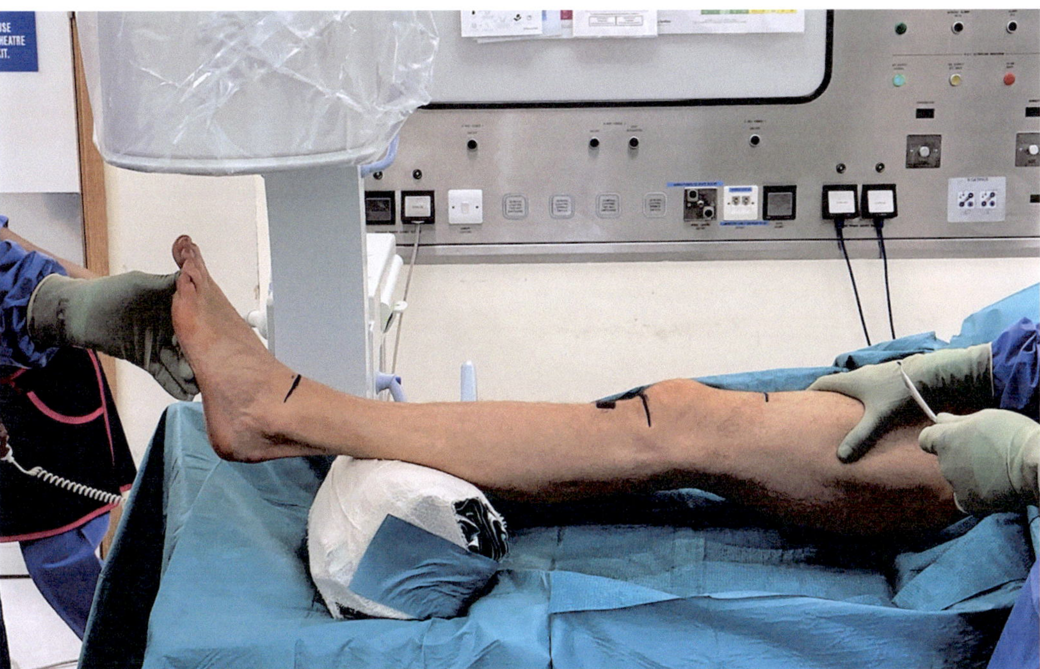

Fig. 20.2 Patient has been prepared and draped for procedure. Note that the ankle, tibial tuberosity and knee joints have been identified and marked. A further line has been marked approximately 10 cm proximal to the patella estimating the extent of the suprapatellar pouch

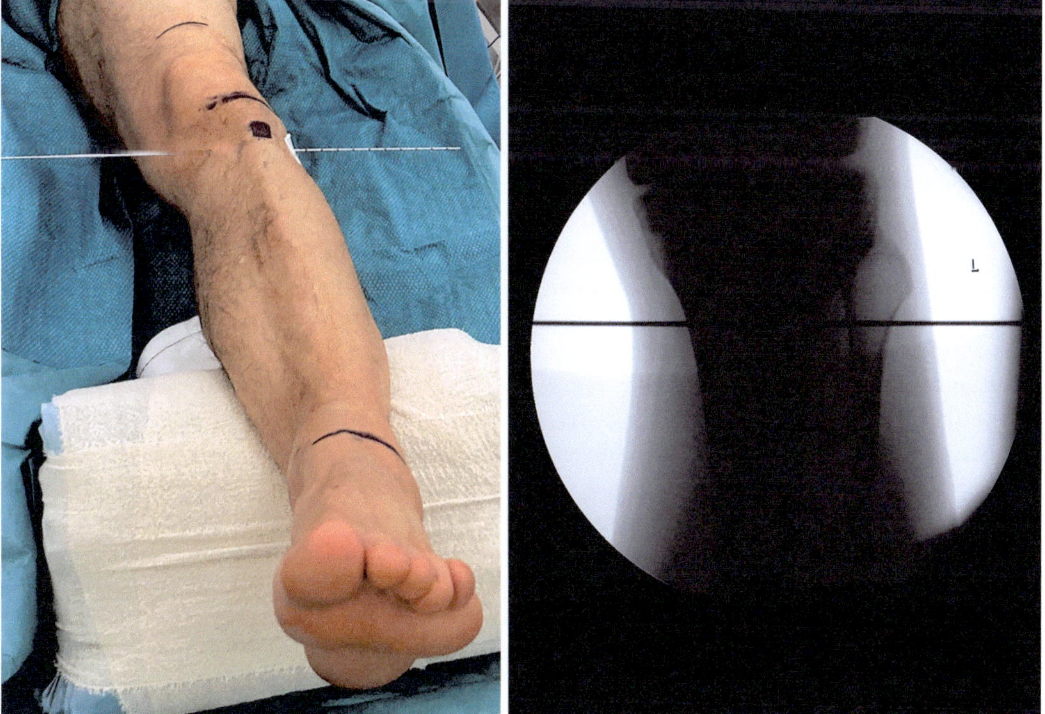

Fig. 20.3 A proximal tibial reference wire has been placed at right angles to the mechanical axis as planned from the preoperative standing alignment radiographs. This will be used to align the frame on both segments

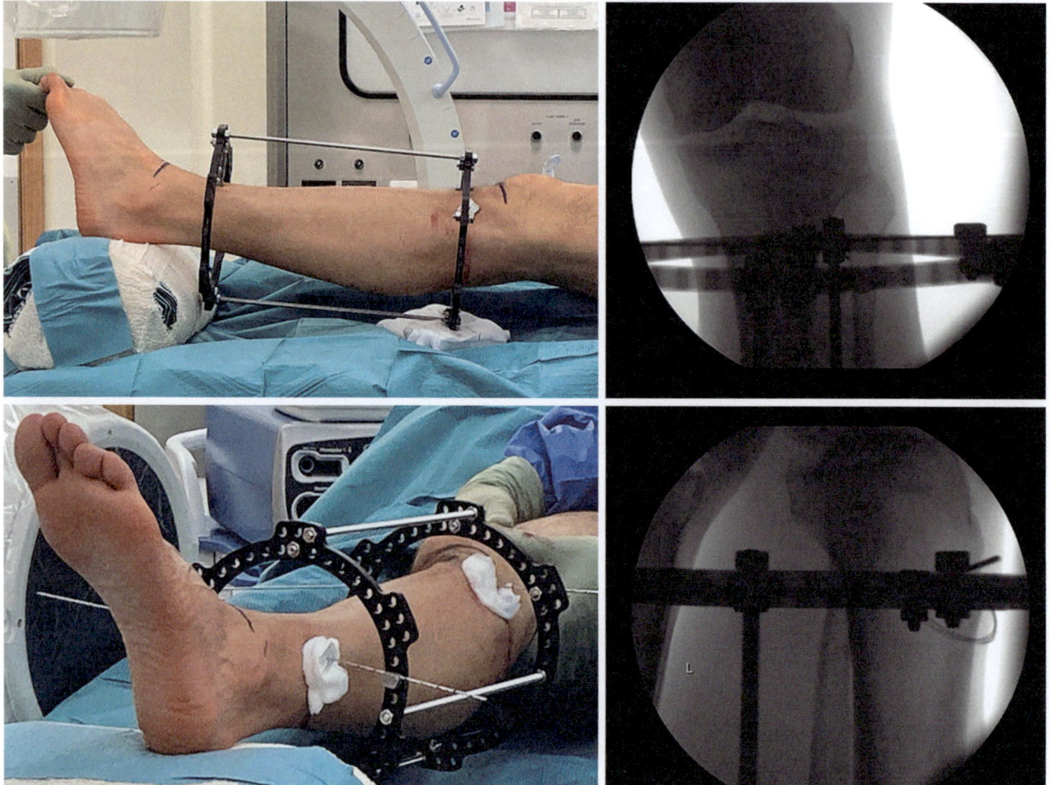

Fig. 20.4 The preliminary tibial construct has been applied on 2 wires. Fluoroscopic images are taken to ensure that the frame is aligned with the mechanical axis in the coronal and sagittal planes

appropriate incision, oriented to allow soft tissue release if required, with blunt dissection continued to bone. A pilot hole should be made using an appropriately sized drill with soft tissue protection. The drill should be pulsed and can be irrigated to avoid excessive heat generation and thermal necrosis. The pins should be placed in an equatorial position in the bone where possible to achieve bicortical purchase and optimise stability. This will reduce the risk of bone damage, pin loosening and iatrogenic fracture. Half pins are then placed by hand. For fine wires, a similar technique can be employed in anatomically critical areas. Otherwise, wires may be placed percutaneously and drilled until the far cortex is breached. The drill should be pulsed, and again wires placed in an equatorial

position in relation to their trajectory where possible. To reduce thermal osseous injury and damage to soft tissue structures on the far side of the bone, the wire can be hammered into position once the far cortex is breached. Wires can then be attached to the external fixator assembly and tensioned as required by the construct utilised (Fig. 20.5).

The external fixator construct can then be applied aligned with the mechanical axis of the limb in the coronal and sagittal planes to allow consistent linear distraction across the knee joint (Figs. 20.6 and 20.7).

Following assembly, initial axial distraction should be applied across the knee joint with radiological confirmation (Figs. 20.8 and 20.9). Some surgeons will apply all 5 mm of this intra-

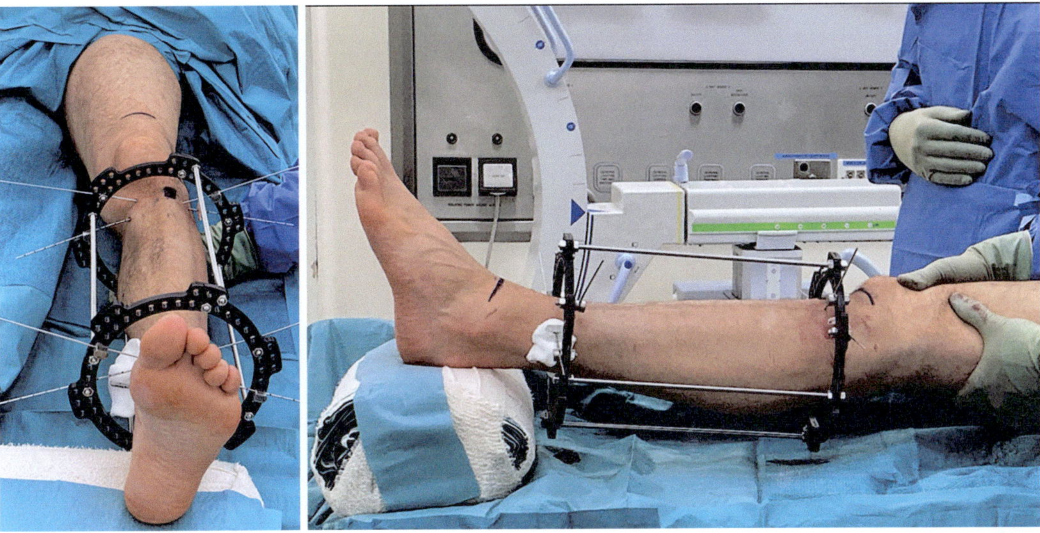

Fig. 20.5 The tibial construct is completed, and the wires tensioned. Further images are taken at this stage to ensure the alignment has been maintained. Additional fixation will be added to this segment once the femoral fixation has been completed

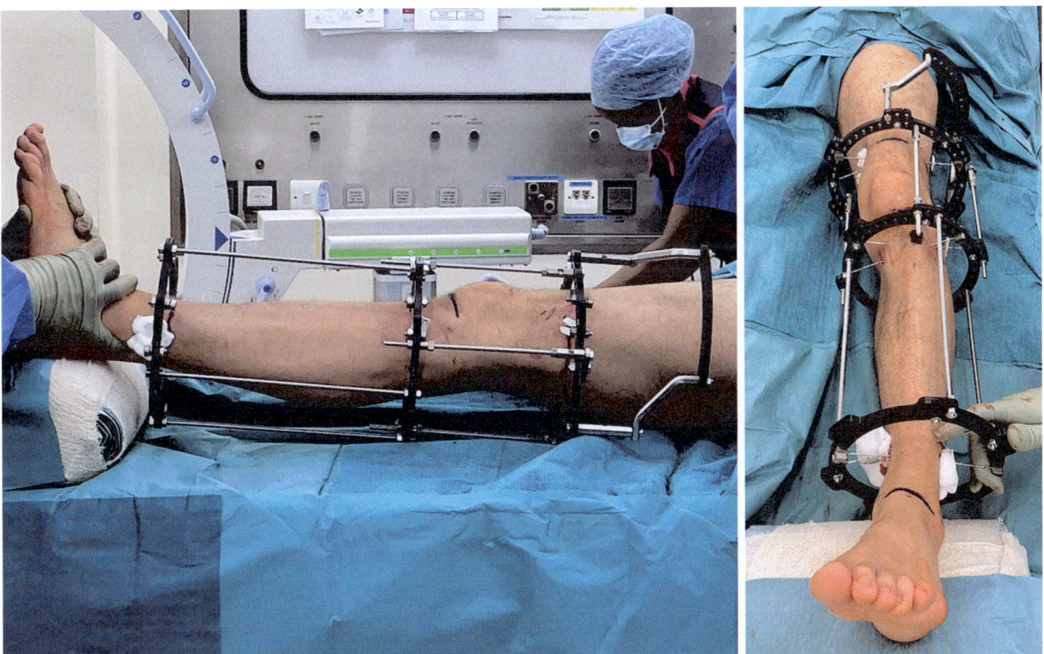

Fig. 20.6 The frame is extended to the femur, maintaining the current axis. Note that the distal femoral ring has been offset medially to accommodate the limb contour and that at femoral arch has been used proximally. Wires have been added from this on the distal ring, taking care not to penetrate the supra-patellar pouch. Counter nuts have been placed on the distal end of the rods spanning the knee so that controlled distraction can be applied

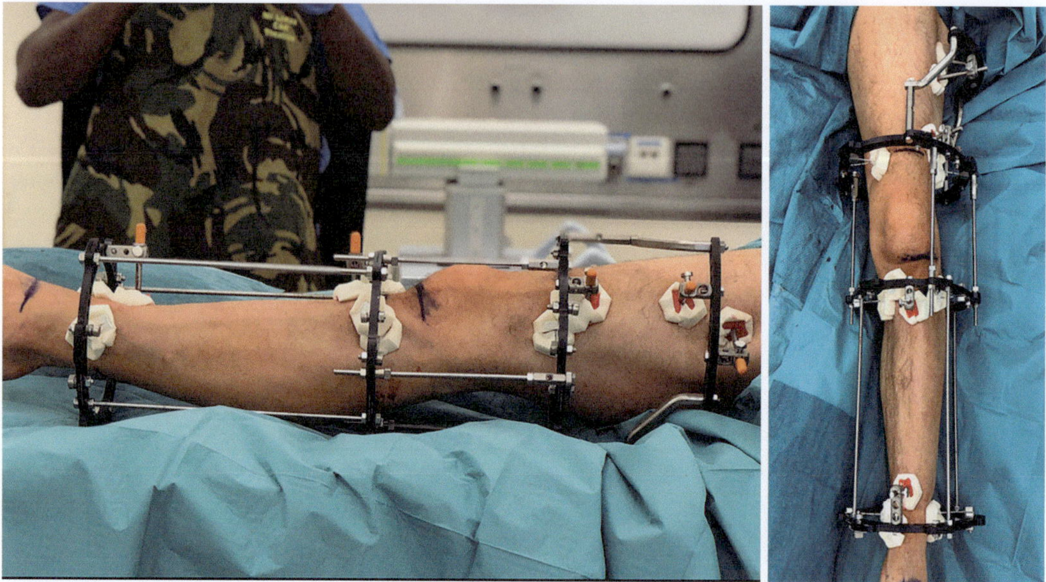

Fig. 20.7 Fixation has been completed by adding half-pins throughout. Note that only half pins are used for proximal femoral fixation

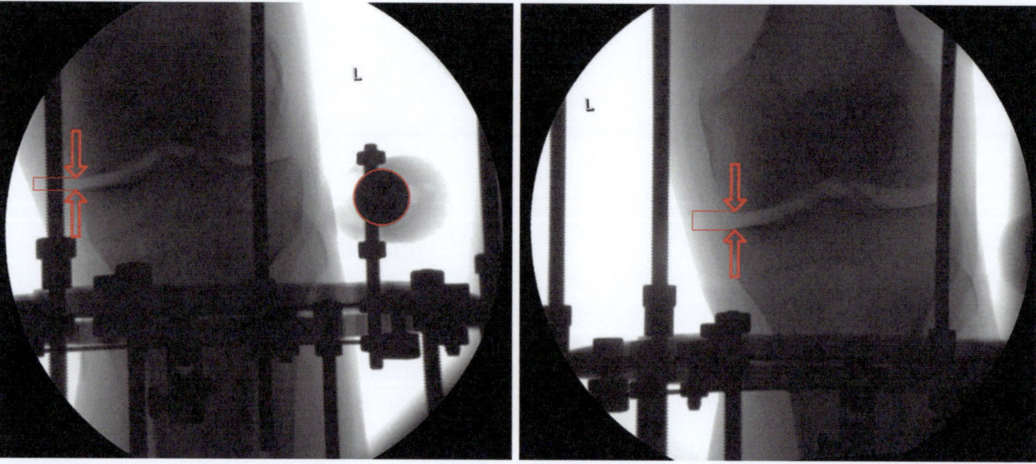

Fig. 20.8 Fluoroscopic images have been taken at the end of the procedure with a calibration ball in place to allow accurate measurements to be taken. The image on the left is before distraction and that on the right after. Approximately 3 mm has been achieved medially

operatively. This may result in increased post-operative pain, and it may be preferable to partially distract the knee and then complete the distraction in the early post-operative period. If this approach is chosen, then proper distraction should be confirmed radiographically.

A final check should be made for soft tissue releases required and pin sites dressed with an

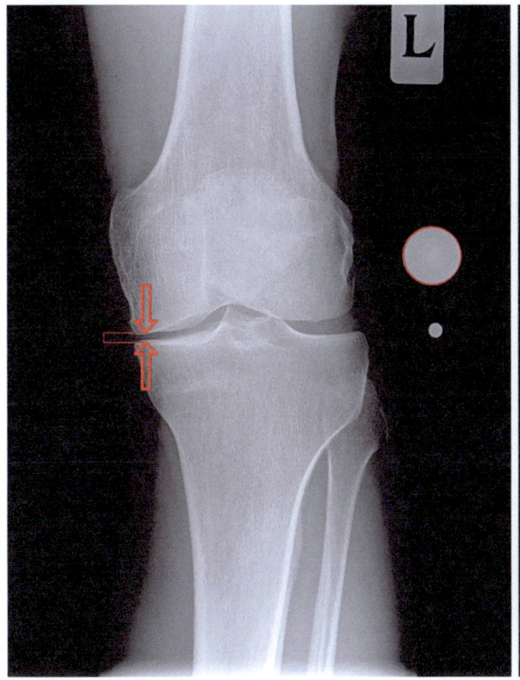

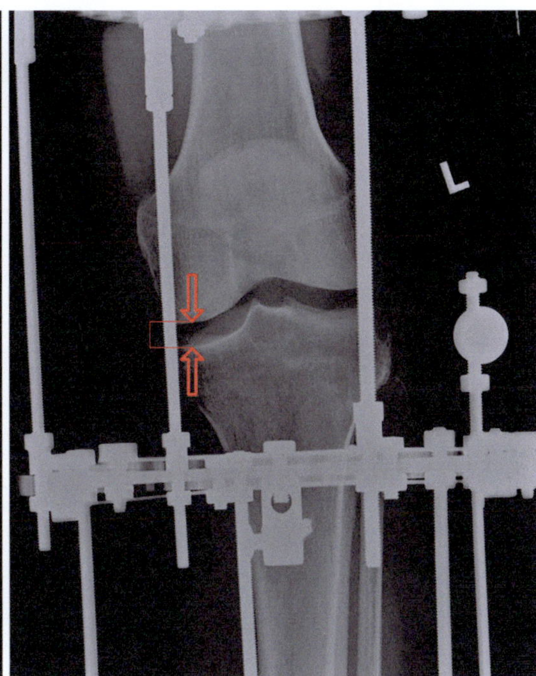

Fig. 20.9 Radiographs comparing pre- and post-operative joint space. The post-operative radiographs were taken the day after surgery. Ongoing distraction has occurred at the joint due to creep of the soft tissues. Using the calibration ball, it is calculated that just over 6 mm of distraction has been achieved compared to the joint space on the preoperative radiographs. This is therefore accepted, and no further distraction applied. Had less than 5 mm of distraction been measured, further distraction would have been applied until this was achieved

absorbent non-shedding dressing. Post-operatively, patients can fully weight bear on the first day post-op under physio supervision as pain allows (Fig. 20.10). If delayed distraction has been planned, a further 1 mm of distraction should be applied per day until a total of 5 mm articular distraction is achieved. Maintenance of distraction should be confirmed at 1 week post-op both on the fixator and radiographically.

Technique for Applying Hinged Distraction

Where hinged distraction is planned, it is important that the hinges are positioned and aligned along the axis of knee rotation, at the isometric point of the femur. This can be estimated radiographically and is demonstrated in Fig. 20.6. A true lateral radiograph of the knee should be obtained. The C-arm is positioned and the limb moved to achieve this view. Once a projection along the joint is obtained, the limb is rotated so that the posterior condyles of the femur perfectly overlap. The correct axis in this rotation is found at the intersection between a line drawn along the posterior femoral and the Blumensaat line. The author prefers to place a wire carefully along this line to secure the position and then place the hinges along this. The knee should be cycled with the hinges in place to ensure they are properly aligned. Otherwise, construct application is as described above.

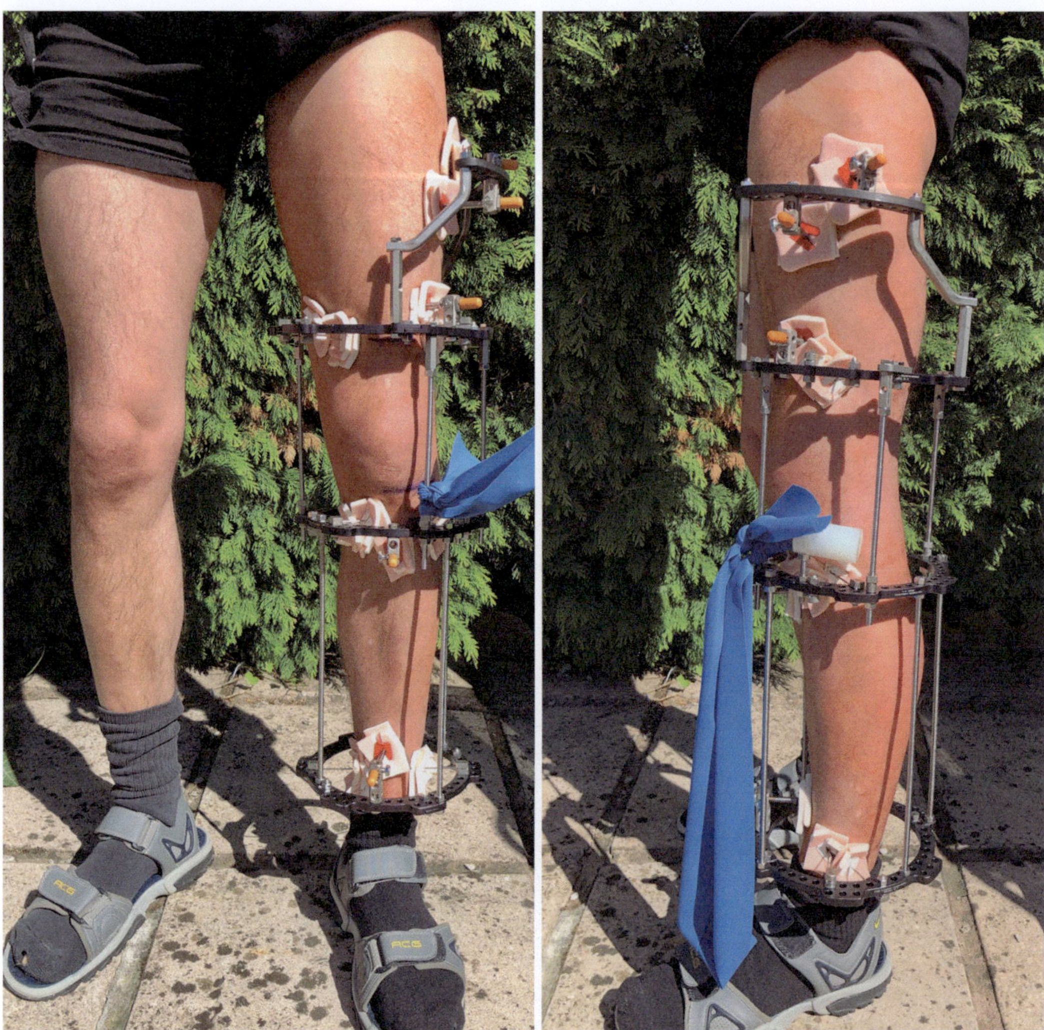

Fig. 20.10 Patient weight bearing in their frame following discharge from hospital

Results of Knee Joint Distraction

Animal Studies

Markers of cartilage repair or breakdown have been utilised to estimate response to KJD in animal models. Articular tissue from an animal model of OA in dogs has been assessed [22]. Prior to distraction, changes in biomarkers typical of OA were observed with significant increases in proteoglycan (PG) synthesis and the percentage of PG released alongside a decrease in PG content compared to control knees. Immediately following KJD, PG synthesis and release returned to equivalent levels to those measured in control joints. This effect was, however, only observed in the joint treated by articulating distraction. In non-articulating distraction, PG synthesis was significantly reduced, and PG release significantly increased, compared to controls. The reduction observed in PG content was particularly striking in the non-articulating distraction group. This was lower than in the untreated OA joints with almost complete PG depletion. There was no significant difference in histologic analysis of the articular cartilage between specimens from different groups. The implications of this for clinical practice remain unclear. The authors note that their methods modelled early OA in young animals rather than severe OA in older humans with the samples taken immediately following distraction, highlighting that changes in cartilage metabolism may require normal joint use to go on to tissue repair. This observation remains worthy of further investigation. A further study in a canine animal OA model assessed cartilage samples at 6 months post distraction. In the treated group, less histologic and macroscopic evidence of articular damage was observed with increased proteoglycan content and better retention of newly formed proteoglycans when compared to controls. These improvements were also seen to a degree in the group managed with a fixator without distraction, though to a lesser extent. This study again used a hinged distraction fixator [45]. A similar study in a rat OA model observed significantly reduced levels of IL-1B, less evidence of histologic damage, and a lower percentage of MMP13 or Col X positive chondrocytes following distraction compared with controls [46]. Raised levels of IL-1B have been reported in cartilage and synovial fluid from joint affected by OA; MMP13 appears to be involved in the progression of OA and is being investigated as a therapeutic target [47, 48].

Clinical Outcomes

Pain and Function Scores

The literature regarding KJD is difficult to assess due to the heterogeneity of devices and methods used. A recent literature review included three studies, one cohort study and two randomised controlled trials, all of which came from the same research group, including a total of 62 patients (Table 20.1) [51]. These studies all utilised a spring-loaded static distractor. All of the studies

Table 20.1 Review of included studies

	Number of patients	Fixator used	Additional procedures	Outcomes	Complications
Deie (2007) [40]	$n = 6$	Articulated device 7–12 weeks	Arthroscopy ± partial meniscectomy	Mean 3 years Significant improvement in Japan orthopaedic association score (JOA) ($p < 0.001$) Mean JSW increased from 0.4 mm preoperatively to 1.5 mm at final follow up	Superficial skin infection (17%)
Aly (2011) [41]	$n = 19$	Ilizarov 3 months	Debridement and abrasioplasty of large ulcers of femoral and tibial condyles	3–5 years Significant improvement of pain ($p < 0.004$) and walking capacity ($p < 0.001$) compared to no significant improvement in debridement only group Mean JSW increased from 2.5 mm preoperatively to 4.5 mm at final follow up ($p < 0.000$)	Pin tract infection (18%) DVT (11%)
Intema (2011) [44]	$n = 20$	2 monotubes with internal coil springs 2 months	Nil	1 year follow-up Significant improvement in WOMAC score ($p < 0.001$) Mean JSW increased from 2.7 to 3.6 mm ($p < 0.05$) MRI showed increase in cartilage thickness (2.4 to 3.0 mm; $p < 0.001$)	Pin tract infection (85%) PE (10%)

(continued)

Table 20.1 (continued)

	Number of patients	Fixator used	Additional procedures	Outcomes	Complications
Weigant (2013) [45]	$n = 20$ Same population as Intema 2011	2 monotubes with internal coil springs 2 months	Nil	2 years Significant improvement WOMAC score ($p < 0.001$) Mean JSW increased by 21%, a fall from 24% at 1 year MRI showed increase in cartilage thickness (2.4 to 2.78 mm; $p = 0.03$)	Pin tract infection (85%)
Besselink (2018) [49]	$n = 20$ Same population as Intema 2011 Compared to HTO $n = 20$	2 monotubes with internal coil springs 2 months	Nil	2 years MRI analysis— Overall average dGEMRIC change nonsignificant ($p = 0.260$) HTO dGEMRIC showed worsening in medial dGEMRIC indices and improvement on the lateral side, KJD showed changes over 2 years not significant	Conversion to HTO (15%)
van der Woude (2017) [42]	$n = 20$ Same population as Intema 2011	2 monotubes with internal coil springs 2 months	Nil	5 years Significant improvement in WOMAC score ($p = 0.002$) Mean JSW on X-ray and mean cartilage thickness no longer statistically different from baseline ($p = 0.177$)	3 patients converted to TKA at 3.8, 4.4 and 4.8 years
Jansen (2020) [50]	$n = 84$ in open prospective study of regular care (OPS) $n = 62$ in clinical trials (RCT)	2 monotubes with internal coil springs 6 weeks OPS 8 weeks RCT	Nil	1 year Significant improvement in WOMAC score ($p < 0.001$)	Pin tract infection (85% OPS; 57% RCT) Osteomyelitis (4%) Flexion limitation requiring MUA (2%) DVT (1%) PE (2%) Compartment syndrome (0.68%)

reported Western Ontario and McMaster Universities Osteoarthritis Index (WOMAC) scores at baseline and at 1 year post KJD, with significant improvements observed [30, 42, 43]. WOMAC score improvements were significantly greater than conservatively managed osteoarthritis [42], and not inferior to TKA [30], or HTO [43]. Two of these studies [30, 43] also reported Knee Injury and Osteoarthritis Outcome Score (KOOS), Intermittent and Constant Osteoarthritis Pain (ICOAP) score, EuroQol 5 Dimensions (EQ-5D) and Short form (SF)-36 with significant improvements between baseline and 1-year scores seen in all scores except for the SF-36 mental component score. There was no significant difference in these improvements compared to TKA or HTO. Pain score assessed on a pain visual analogue scale 0 to 100 was also reported in the two studies and showed improvements at 1 year with no significant difference between KJD and HTO or TKA.

Further studies were not included in the review due to the incorporation of other procedures such as arthroscopic debridement or microfracture alongside joint distraction, although significant clinical improvements have been demonstrated [40, 41].

Radiographic Outcomes

Radiographic assessment of the physical joint structure has been undertaken in various studies, with imaging at the time of distraction or follow-up. These have demonstrated increased joint space compared to pre-treatment measurements, which appear to be sustained following removal of the distraction device. In one study, mean joint space width measure using standardised digital techniques increased from 2.7 mm at baseline to 3.6 mm at 12 months post fixator removal [44]. Three further studies by the same group with a total of 62 patients appear to confirm this finding. Radiographic minimum joint space width was shown to increase by an average of 0.8 mm at 12 months compared to baseline [30, 42, 43]. This group also utilised MRI to assessing structural recovery. The mean cartilage thickness was shown to increase on both the tibial and femoral sides. The percentage of the joint surface appearing as denuded subchondral bone also decreased [51].

Other groups have used alternate MRI techniques. Delayed gadolinium-enhanced magnetic resonance imaging of cartilage can assess the quality of cartilaginous tissue [52]. A study using this approach found no difference in relevant indices obtained by this technique following either HTO or KJD, despite radiographic and clinical improvements [49].

Biomarker Outcomes

Changes in relevant biomarkers have also been used to estimate response to KJD for OA in humans [44]. Ongoing increases in the synthesis of type II collagen along with lower rates of breakdown have been observed 1 year after static distraction therapy. Similarly, cartilage collagen synthesis and breakdown has been estimated by measuring the serum N-propeptide of type IIA procollagen and urinary C-telopeptide of type II collagen. During distraction, these biomarkers were raised, returning to baseline levels 1 month after distraction was removed. Over the next 6–12 months, an increased ratio of type II collagen synthesis over breakdown was demonstrated which persisted at 2 years follow-up [45].

Complications

The most frequently reported complication in KJD patients is pin site infection. Rates approaching 70% have been reported, whilst the majority responded to oral antibiotics, almost 20% of patients affected required intravenous therapy. [51] In the series of 62 patients described above, 2 required surgical intervention for pin-site infection during distraction, with a further case of osteomyelitis requiring surgery following fixator removal [30, 42, 43]. These rates of infection are somewhat at odds with those reported in patients treated by definitive external fixation for other reasons. Pin-site infection rates of around 40% are found fairly consistently, even where fixators are in place for much longer, the reasons for this are unclear [53]. Whilst transient pin-site infection seldom has long-term implications, it is unpleasant for the patient and may impair rehabilitation. Deep infections may be much more worrisome, especially considering the expected progression of osteoarthritis following distraction potentially requiring eventual arthroplasty. TKA following significant osteomyelitis is significantly more complex and has a risk of further infection even when infection is considered eradicated [54]. The current literature around KJD does not provide sufficient evidence to estimate serious infection rates following conversion to TKA. In one ankle distraction study with a minimum of 5 years of follow up, there was no infection seen in the 5 patients who had conversion to total ankle arthroplasty [25].

Loss of knee range of movement immediately following distraction therapy is consistently reported. This has been observed to improve to approximately baseline around 1 year, with a small number of patients undergoing joint manipulation under anaesthetic to achieve this [30, 50]

Uncertainties

As to be expected with an emerging management technique, and alluded to earlier in this chapter, multiple uncertainties remain regarding KJD which require further investigation.

Device Choice

As described earlier, there is no evidence on the superiority of one device or mode of fixation over another. It is unclear if joint movement is required to create the optimum environment for cartilage regeneration or if holding the joint static whilst allowing weight bearing generates sufficient pressure changes within the joint to initiate and maintain cartilage regeneration. There is no consensus on benefit of spring-loaded devices compared to conventional monolateral, biplanar or ring fixators or the benefits of half pin or fine wire constructs. This is further complicated by the fact that the mechanism of action and therefore optimal mechanical environment for arthro-distraction have yet to be determined. Further research in this area is warranted.

Duration and Timing of Treatment

The time period required for a device to be in situ varies between studies, with a span of 6–8 weeks most commonly utilised [30, 42, 43]. In an observational study comparing 6–8 weeks distraction, there was no significant difference in WOMAC scores and radiographic outcomes at 3, 6 and 12 months [55]. Arthro-distraction of other joints for OA has used time periods of up to 22 weeks [22]. Although it might be anticipated that prolonged immobilisation would result in decreased ROM post fixator removal, this has not been definitively demonstrated [41]. The optimal tim-

ing of distraction has also not been determined. Some parties advocate applying the distraction at the time of frame positioning, with others applying this gradually over days or weeks. The consequences of these different approaches have not been directly compared. Most studies allow weight bearing from the time of fixation unless it is combined with other procedures that require a period of non-weight bearing [40, 41].

Gender Differences

Gender difference in outcome following TKA has been widely documented; females are more likely to have significant loss of knee flexion and lower knee scores preoperatively, but consistently achieve greater improvement in social and physical functioning scores post-operatively. [56, 57] Reasons for this gender disparity appear to be multi-factorial with physiological and social factors postulated, including differences in willingness to undergo surgery, pain responses, treatment preferences, and provider, system and research level issues [57]. A gender difference is apparent following KJD also, with women more likely to require earlier conversion to TKA following KJD [42]. The reasons for this are unclear and require further investigation.

Length of Improvement

Probably the most significant uncertainty regarding KJD relates to long-term outcome. Ankle distraction is somewhat more established and therefore has better long-term data available, though still in relatively small numbers of patients. In one study, conversion to arthrodesis or arthroplasty had been undertaken in 17% of patients within 2 years, 37% within 5 years and 44% at 12 years [25]. For KJD, only intermediate term outcomes have been reported, with 70% of patients still not requiring revision to the previously planned TKA at 5 years [42]. The effectiveness of repeat procedures has not been investigated. Even when average time to failure is more well known, there will need to be further evaluation of the risk benefit balance and cost-effectiveness of using KJD to delay the need for the likely eventuality of an arthroplasty procedure versus early arthroplasty procedures.

Conclusion

This is an exciting emerging technique with potential for great clinical benefit in this common and disabling condition. Despite the well-established management options available for OA, joint preservation remains desirable, particularly in younger patients. As a less invasive procedure, KJD may provide a solution with subsequent improvements in clinical outcomes and eventual reduction in arthroplasty revision burden. Early outcomes are promising with a low incidence of significant complications. However, numbers of patients in current studies are small and follow-up periods are short, therefore there are multiple areas requiring further investigation. Concerns remain surrounding the uncertainty of long-term outcomes and potential infection following conversion to TKA. Clinical and economic effectiveness, when compared to more established treatments, particularly joint arthroplasty, have not been determined. Randomised controlled trials with larger numbers of patients and more extensive follow-up are required to address these concerns.

References

1. Cross M, Smith E, Hoy D, et al. The global burden of hip and knee osteoarthritis: estimates from the global burden of disease 2010 study. Ann Rheum Dis. 2014;73(7):1323–30.
2. Peat G, McCarney R, Croft P. Knee pain and osteoarthritis in older adults: a review of community burden and current use of primary health care. Ann Rheum Dis. 2001;60(2):91–7.
3. Culliford DJ, Maskell J, Beard DJ, Murray DW, Price AJ, Arden NK. Temporal trends in hip and knee replacement in the United Kingdom: 1991 to 2006. J Bone Joint Surg (Br). 2010;92(1):130–5.
4. Zhang Y, Jordan JM. Epidemiology of osteoarthritis. Clin Geriatr Med. 2010;26(3):355–69.
5. Patel A, Pavlou G, Mújica-Mota RE, Toms AD. The epidemiology of revision total knee and hip arthroplasty in England and Wales: a comparative analysis with projections for the United States. A study using the National Joint Registry dataset. Bone Joint J. 2015;97-B(8):1076–81.
6. Excellence NIfHaC. Osteoarthritis: care and management Clinical Guideline [CG177]. 2014.
7. Surgeons AAoO. Treatment of Osteoarthritis of the Knee. 2013.
8. Kurtz S, Ong K, Lau E, Mowat F, Halpern M. Projections of primary and revision hip and knee arthroplasty in the United States from 2005 to 2030. J Bone Joint Surg Am. 2007;89(4):780–5.
9. Nam D, Nunley RM, Barrack RL. Patient dissatisfaction following total knee replacement: a growing concern? Bone Joint J. 2014;96-B(11 Supple A):96–100.
10. Parvizi J, Nunley RM, Berend KR, et al. High level of residual symptoms in young patients after total knee arthroplasty. Clin Orthop Relat Res. 2014;472(1):133–7.
11. Kahlenberg CA, Nwachukwu BU, McLawhorn AS, Cross MB, Cornell CN, Padgett DE. Patient satisfaction after Total knee replacement: a systematic review. HSS J. 2018;14(2):192–201.
12. Evans JT, Walker RW, Evans JP, Blom AW, Sayers A, Whitehouse MR. How long does a knee replacement last? A systematic review and meta-analysis of case series and national registry reports with more than 15 years of follow-up. Lancet. 2019;393(10172):655–63.
13. Bae DK, Song SJ, Park MJ, Eoh JH, Song JH, Park CH. Twenty-year survival analysis in total knee arthroplasty by a single surgeon. J Arthroplast. 2012;27(7):1297–1304.e1291.
14. Culliford D, Maskell J, Judge A, et al. Future projections of total hip and knee arthroplasty in the UK: results from the UK clinical practice research datalink. Osteoarthr Cartil. 2015;23(4):594–600.
15. Kurtz SM, Lau E, Ong K, Zhao K, Kelly M, Bozic KJ. Future young patient demand for primary and revision joint replacement: national projections from 2010 to 2030. Clin Orthop Relat Res. 2009;467(10):2606–12.
16. Keeney JA, Eunice S, Pashos G, Wright RW, Clohisy JC. What is the evidence for total knee arthroplasty in young patients?: a systematic review of the literature. Clin Orthop Relat Res. 2011;469(2):574–83.
17. Bayliss LE, Culliford D, Monk AP, et al. The effect of patient age at intervention on risk of implant revision after total replacement of the hip or knee: a population-based cohort study. Lancet. 2017;389(10077):1424–30.
18. Bhandari M, Smith J, Miller LE, Block JE. Clinical and economic burden of revision knee arthroplasty. Clin Med Insights Arthritis Musculoskelet Disord. 2012;5:89–94.
19. Lee DH, Lee SH, Song EK, Seon JK, Lim HA, Yang HY. Causes and clinical outcomes of revision Total knee arthroplasty. Knee Surg Relat Res. 2017;29(2):104–9.
20. Ong KL, Lau E, Suggs J, Kurtz SM, Manley MT. Risk of subsequent revision after primary and revi-

sion total joint arthroplasty. Clin Orthop Relat Res. 2010;468(11):3070–6.

21. Judet R, Judet T. The use of a hinge distraction apparatus after arthrolysis and arthroplasty (author's transl). Rev Chir Orthop Reparatrice Appar Mot. 1978;64(5):353–65.

22. van Valburg AA, van Roermund PM, Lammens J, et al. Can Ilizarov joint distraction delay the need for an arthrodesis of the ankle? A preliminary report. J Bone Joint Surg (Br). 1995;77(5):720–5.

23. Lafeber F, Veldhuijzen JP, Vanroy JL, Huber-Bruning O, Bijlsma JW. Intermittent hydrostatic compressive force stimulates exclusively the proteoglycan synthesis of osteoarthritic human cartilage. Br J Rheumatol. 1992;31(7):437–42.

24. Marijnissen AC, Van Roermund PM, Van Melkebeek J, et al. Clinical benefit of joint distraction in the treatment of severe osteoarthritis of the ankle: proof of concept in an open prospective study and in a randomized controlled study. Arthritis Rheum. 2002;46(11):2893–902.

25. Nguyen MP, Pedersen DR, Gao Y, Saltzman CL, Amendola A. Intermediate-term follow-up after ankle distraction for treatment of end-stage osteoarthritis. J Bone Joint Surg Am. 2015;97(7):590–6.

26. Rodriguez-Merchan EC. Joint distraction in advanced osteoarthritis of the ankle. Arch Bone Jt Surg. 2017;5(4):208–12.

27. Spaans AJ, Minnen LPV, Braakenburg A, Mink van der Molen AB. Joint distraction for thumb carpometacarpal osteoarthritis: a feasibility study with 1-year follow-up. J Plast Surg Hand Surg. 2017;51(4):254–8.

28. Sandvall BK, Cameron TE, Netscher DT, Epstein MJ, Staines KG, Petersen NJ. Basal joint osteoarthritis of the thumb: ligament reconstruction and tendon interposition versus hematoma distraction arthroplasty. J Hand Surg [Am]. 2010;35(12):1968–75.

29. Gray KV, Meals RA. Hematoma and distraction arthroplasty for thumb basal joint osteoarthritis: minimum 6.5-year follow-up evaluation. J Hand Surg [Am]. 2007;32(1):23–9.

30. van der Woude JA, Nair SC, Custers RJ, et al. Knee joint distraction compared to Total knee arthroplasty for treatment of end stage osteoarthritis: simulating long-term outcomes and cost-effectiveness. PLoS One. 2016;11(5):e0155524.

31. Koshino T, Wada S, Ara Y, Saito T. Regeneration of degenerated articular cartilage after high tibial valgus osteotomy for medial compartmental osteoarthritis of the knee. Knee. 2003;10(3):229–36.

32. Hoemann CD, Tran-Khanh N, Chevrier A, et al. Chondroinduction is the Main cartilage repair response to microfracture and microfracture with BST-CarGel: results as shown by ICRS-II histological scoring and a novel zonal collagen type scoring method of human clinical biopsy specimens. Am J Sports Med. 2015;43(10):2469–80.

33. Brandt KD. Response of joint structures to inactivity and to reloading after immobilization. Arthritis Rheum. 2003;49(2):267–71.

34. Vanwanseele B, Lucchinetti E, Stüssi E. The effects of immobilization on the characteristics of articular cartilage: current concepts and future directions. Osteoarthr Cartil. 2002;10(5):408–19.

35. van Valburg AA, van Roy HL, Lafeber FP, Bijlsma JW. Beneficial effects of intermittent fluid pressure of low physiological magnitude on cartilage and inflammation in osteoarthritis. An in vitro study. J Rheumatol. 1998;25(3):515–20.

36. Baboolal TG, Mastbergen SC, Jones E, Calder SJ, Lafeber FP, McGonagle D. Synovial fluid hyaluronan mediates MSC attachment to cartilage, a potential novel mechanism contributing to cartilage repair in osteoarthritis using knee joint distraction. Ann Rheum Dis. 2016;75(5):908–15.

37. Gessmann J, Baecker H, Jettkant B, Muhr G, Seybold D. Direct and indirect loading of the Ilizarov external fixator: the effect on the interfragmentary movements and compressive loads. Strategies Trauma Limb Reconstr. 2011;6(1):27–31.

38. Saltzman CL, Hillis SL, Stolley MP, Anderson DD, Amendola A. Motion versus fixed distraction of the joint in the treatment of ankle osteoarthritis: a prospective randomized controlled trial. J Bone Joint Surg Am. 2012;94(11):961–70.

39. Bernstein M, Reidler J, Fragomen A, Rozbruch SR. Ankle distraction arthroplasty: indications, technique, and outcomes. J Am Acad Orthop Surg. 2017;25(2):89–99.

40. Deie M, Ochi M, Adachi N, Kajiwara R, Kanaya A. A new articulated distraction arthroplasty device for treatment of the osteoarthritic knee joint: a preliminary report. Arthroscopy. 2007;23(8):833–8.

41. Aly TA, Hafez K, Amin O. Arthrodiatasis for management of knee osteoarthritis. Orthopedics. 2011;34(8):e338–43.

42. van der Woude JAD, Wiegant K, van Roermund PM, et al. Five-year follow-up of knee joint distraction: clinical benefit and cartilaginous tissue repair in an open uncontrolled prospective study. Cartilage. 2017;8(3):263–71.

43. van der Woude JAD, Wiegant K, van Heerwaarden RJ, et al. Knee joint distraction compared with high tibial osteotomy: a randomized controlled trial. Knee Surg Sports Traumatol Arthrosc. 2017;25(3):876–86.

44. Intema F, Van Roermund PM, Marijnissen AC, et al. Tissue structure modification in knee osteoarthritis by use of joint distraction: an open 1-year pilot study. Ann Rheum Dis. 2011;70(8):1441–6.

45. Wiegant K, van Roermund PM, Intema F, et al. Sustained clinical and structural benefit after joint distraction in the treatment of severe knee osteoarthritis. Osteoarthr Cartil. 2013;21(11):1660–7.

46. Chen Y, Sun Y, Pan X, Ho K, Li G. Joint distraction attenuates osteoarthritis by reducing secondary inflammation, cartilage degeneration and subchondral bone aberrant change. Osteoarthr Cartil. 2015;23(10):1728–35.

47. Vincent TL. IL-1 in osteoarthritis: time for a critical review of the literature. F1000Res. 2019:8.

48. Wang M, Sampson ER, Jin H, et al. MMP13 is a critical target gene during the progression of osteoarthritis. Arthritis Res Ther. 2013;15(1):R5.
49. Besselink NJ, Vincken KL, Bartels LW, et al. Cartilage quality (dGEMRIC index) following knee joint distraction or high Tibial osteotomy. Cartilage. 2020;11(1):19–31.
50. Jansen MP, Mastbergen SC, van Heerwaarden RJ, et al. Knee joint distraction in regular care for treatment of knee osteoarthritis: a comparison with clinical trial data. PLoS One. 2020;15(1):e0227975.
51. Takahashi T, Baboolal TG, Lamb J, Hamilton TW, Pandit HG. Is knee joint distraction a viable treatment option for knee OA?-a literature review and meta-analysis. J Knee Surg. 2019;32(8):788–95.
52. Rutgers M, Bartels LW, Tsuchida AI, et al. dGEMRIC as a tool for measuring changes in cartilage quality following high tibial osteotomy: a feasibility study. Osteoarthr Cartil. 2012;20(10):1134–41.
53. Ferguson D, Harwood P, Allgar V, et al. The PINS trial: a prospective randomized clinical trial comparing a traditional versus an emollient skincare regimen for the care of pin-sites in patients with circular frames. Bone Joint J. 2021;103-B(2):279–85.
54. Williams RL, Khan W, Roberts-Huntleigh N, Morgan-Jones R. Total knee arthroplasty in patients with prior adjacent multi-organism osteomyelitis. Acta Orthop Belg. 2018;84(2):184–91.
55. van der Woude JA, van Heerwaarden RJ, Spruijt S, et al. Six weeks of continuous joint distraction appears sufficient for clinical benefit and cartilaginous tissue repair in the treatment of knee osteoarthritis. Knee. 2016;23(5):785–91.
56. Lim JB, Chi CH, Lo LE, et al. Gender difference in outcome after total knee replacement. J Orthop Surg (Hong Kong). 2015;23(2):194–7.
57. Novicoff WM, Saleh KJ. Examining sex and gender disparities in total joint arthroplasty. Clin Orthop Relat Res. 2011;469(7):1824–8.

Lateral Unicompartmental Knee Replacement Surgery for Lateral Knee Osteoarthritis

Irene Yang, Bernard H. van Duren, and Hemant G. Pandit

The Lateral Compartment of the Knee: Anatomy and Physiology

The lateral compartment of the knee differs from the medial compartment to the knee with distinct geometry and biomechanics [1, 2]. Compared with the medial, the lateral tibial condyle is smaller [3] and convex in the sagittal plane [3, 4].

The lateral meniscus is a semi-lunar or crescent-shaped fibro-cartilaginous disc which primarily functions to facilitate load transmission [5]. Secondary functions include stabilisation of the knee [6], to provide lubrication [6] and nutrition [6], aid proprioception [6], and shock absorption [7] in the knee joint. It is smaller than the medial meniscus [3] and has been shown to be more mobile with up to 20 mm posterior translation of the lateral meniscus following flexion compared with 8 mm medially—though the extent of meniscal movement depends on the loading conditions [8]. While the medial com-

partment is stabilised by the Medial Collateral Ligament (MCL) providing stability throughout the range of motion [4], the lateral knee is predominantly stabilised by the popliteus and the iliotibial tract during dynamic motion of the knee [9]. The Lateral Collateral Ligament (LCL) is only tight in extension, providing limited support in flexion; with maximum laxity occurring when the knee is in 90° of flexion [10]. In a Magnetic Resonance Imaging (MRI) study, Tokuhara et al. have shown that the lateral compartment of the knee can distract on average 6.7 ± 1.9 mm (as compared to 2.1 ± 1.1 mm medially) following application of a varus stress to a knee joint in 90° of knee flexion [11]. In addition to a larger distraction possible in the lateral knee, during high flexion, the lateral femoral condyle translates posteriorly, until eventually, it lies posterior to the lateral tibial plateau in high flexion (~160° of knee flexion) [12].

These anatomical and biomechanical differences between the medial and lateral compartments of the knee have a direct effect on knee replacement surgery and the associated implants.

Lateral Knee Osteoarthritis: Aetiology and Prevalence

Osteoarthritis (OA) is the most common joint disorder worldwide [13]. It is a debilitating musculoskeletal disorder characterised by deteriora-

I. Yang
Nuffield Department of Orthopaedics, Rheumatology and Musculoskeletal Sciences, University of Oxford, Oxford, UK
e-mail: irene.yang@ndorms.ox.ac.uk

B. H. van Duren · H. G. Pandit (✉)
Leeds Orthopaedic Trauma Sciences, Leeds Institute of Rheumatology and Musculoskeletal Medicine, University of Leeds, Leeds, UK
e-mail: B.H.vanDuren@leeds.ac.uk;
H.Pandit@leeds.ac.uk

© The Author(s), under exclusive license to Springer Nature Switzerland AG 2023
A. J. Deshmukh et al. (eds.), *Surgical Management of Knee Arthritis*,
https://doi.org/10.1007/978-3-031-47929-8_21

Table 21.1 Aetiology of lateral knee OA

Aetiology	Reference
Primary lateral compartment OA	[16–23]
Rheumatoid arthritis	[24, 25]
Secondary lateral compartment OA	
Post traumatic	[16, 18, 25–27]
Valgus deformity	[28, 29]
Tibial plateau fracture	[19, 30]
Osteonecrosis	[18, 22, 25–27]
Avascular necrosis of lateral femoral condyle	[21, 23]
Meniscectomy	[21, 31]

tion of the articular cartilage lining the contact surfaces of bones and subchondral bone, causing bone-on-bone articulation leading to pain, compromised function, and ultimately joint destruction [13]. Half of knee OA cases involve a single compartment, with the prevalence of isolated lateral tibiofemoral OA being 5% [14].

The main aetiologies of lateral knee OA are primary osteoarthritis and secondary to trauma. The wear in lateral compartment osteoarthritis, is frequently located more posteriorly on the tibial plateau [15]. These findings were supported by a study in 2009 analysing full thickness cartilage lesions in 20 knees with lateral knee OA which showed that the femoral lesions were located on average at 40° of knee flexion (as compared to at 11° knee flexion medially). The aetiology of lateral compartment OA is summarised in Table 21.1.

Diagnosis

Lateral knee OA is comparatively well tolerated by the patient for a longer time than medial OA [16], in part, due to preserved movement and, in part, due to delayed diagnosis. Weight-bearing AP and lateral radiographs of the knee underplay the extent of OA and for accurate diagnosis of lateral knee OA, patients should undergo stress views (at 40° of knee flexion) or Rosenberg views.

Treatments

Treatment options depend on disease severity [32, 33], patient age [32], and the clinician's expertise and opinion [32].

Conservative

Treatment typically begins with managing symptoms conservatively through weight reduction, physical therapy (muscle strengthening), knee bracing, exercise (aerobic, water-based), walking aids, knee bracing, footwear and insoles, thermal treatments, transcutaneous electrical nerve stimulation, and acupuncture [34]. A study on unloading knee braces found to improve pain and functional ability [35]; however, unloading does not prevent disease progression [36] and is less effective in obese patients [37]. Nevertheless, knee bracing may delay the need for surgery [38].

A systematic review of guidelines for knee OA found that the optimal treatment involves combining non-pharmacological with pharmacological treatments [39]. Central to the management of knee OA, is education and self-management alongside land-based exercise, irrespective of dietary management [40]. Indeed in the literature, exercise has been shown to be an effective and critical component in the conservative management of knee OA [41]. Further, topical non-steroidal anti-inflammatory drugs (NSAIDs) were recommended [40]. In addition, the National Institute for Health and Care Excellence (NICE) recommends intra-articular therapies such as corticosteroid injections, which are recommended for use as an adjunct to core treatments [42]. According to the Osteoarthritis Research Society international guidelines on OA management [40], additional treatment recommendations were dependent on specific patient comorbidities, e.g. intra-articular hyaluronic acid injections are regarded as relatively safe and based on evidence showing improvement of symptoms beyond 12 weeks, is now conditionally recommended for longer term treatment.

Oral and transdermal opioids were strongly not recommended due to high risk of chemical dependency. Finally, intra-articular stem cell therapy and intra-articular platelet-rich plasma were also not recommended due to low quality evidence and the formulations being non-standardised.

Non-Conservative

With disease progression and conservative treatment options exhausted, end stage lateral knee OA can be treated surgically. Surgical options include arthroscopic debridement [18, 32], interpositional arthroplasty [43], osteotomy—high tibial osteotomy or distal femoral osteotomy [44], knee replacement surgery—either UKR or TKR. Distal femoral osteotomy (DFO) or high tibial osteotomy (HTO) may be performed to realign the mechanical axis of the lower limb and have the benefit of retaining the native knee joint structures. Osteotomies have been reported as an effective strategy to reduced knee osteoarthritis pain, particularly in younger and more active patients [45–47], delaying the need for knee replacement surgery. In addition to osteotomies, TKR surgery is where the entire knee joint is replaced with an artificial knee system. TKR is the most common knee-replacement surgery, accounting for 83% of knee-replacement surgeries in the UK [48]. While osteotomies, UKRs, and TKRs are all viable surgical treatment options for end-stage lateral knee OA, this chapter will focus on the UKR procedure as the remaining treatments fall outside the scope of this chapter.

Lateral UKR Surgical Technique

Most surgeons perform the lateral UKR through a lateral approach [49]. The original anterolateral approach for the Oxford implant (Biomet, Bridgend, UK) was first described by the designer group [50] and involved a lateral parapatellar incision with patellar tendon dislocation to enable direct access to the lateral compartment of the knee. This technique was later modified [4, 51] and the full surgical technique involved placing the knee in a leg holder which enables the knee to hang freely in 100°–110° flexion.

A short lateral parapatellar skin incision is made over the junction of the central and lateral third of the patella and begins at the level of superior pole of the patella extending down to and just lateral to the tibial tubercle. The retinacular incision is made around the lateral side of the patella and down beside the patellar tendon. The anterolateral portion of the proximal tibia is exposed and Gerdy's tubercle and attachment of Iliotibial tract identified. Generous excision of fat pad is often needed. The functional integrity of the ACL and medial compartment is confirmed. Osteophytes from around the lateral condyle, intercondylar notch, lateral patella facet anterior tibia, and those in front of the ACL are removed. The patella is not dislocated, instead a transpatellar tendon approach is adopted whereby an internally rotated vertical tibial cut is made through the centre of the patellar tendon. The horizontal tibial cut is made with 7° posterior slope, just below the top of Gerdy's tubercle, usually 2 to 3 mm below the defect. In general, more bone is removed from the lateral tibial plateau than during medial Oxford UKR as the domed tibial component is thicker than the flat.

An assessment is made to ensure that an adequate resection has been undertaken by inserting an appropriate tibial template and a 3 mm feeler gauge. The knee is brought into full extension to check for ligament tension. Appropriate bearing thickness is chosen with the knee in extension so that the gap in full extension with the tibial template in place is an estimate of the final bearing thickness.

Femoral preparation is fundamentally different to the medial Oxford UKR philosophy. Ligament balance on the lateral side is impossible to judge as the LCL is slack in flexion. Therefore, the aim is to place the femoral component anatomically. The femoral cartilage in lateral OA is relatively preserved at 0° and 90° flexion. The technique therefore aims to position the implant flush to the condyle surfaces at 0° and 90° flexion. This is achieved by using the standard femoral jig, referencing from the posterior cartilage for AP position and by milling with a 4 mm spigot for distal positioning. Rest of the preparation of femoral and tibial condyles is similar to that of medial UKR (including checking for and dealing with potential causes of bearing impingement) except for the use of anterior mill, as this may remove too much bone and the patella can jam in the defect. It is important to ensure that the bearing does not jam against the wall in full extension. Both the two-peg femoral and tibial components are fixed with polymethylmethacrylate (PMMA) bone cement. Definitive bearing assessment is now undertaken. A bearing that is just gripped in full extension is ideal and it will be loose in flexion. It is difficult to insert the bearing from the front at times and it may be inserted antero-laterally. Routine closure is undertaken.

In view of high dislocation rates, the Oxford group recommends use of fixed-bearing components at least for the first few cases. The Fixed Lateral Oxford (FLO) prosthesis can be used with the same instruments and the same surgical technique.

Lateral UKR Implants

LUKR is less common than medial UKR owing to the lower disease prevalence and accounts for about 1% of all prosthetic procedures [32] and 5–10% of all UKRs [15, 18, 48]. For patients with end-stage isolated lateral compartment OA, Lateral UKR (LUKR) surgery is an effective alternative to TKR [32] as it retains the medial compartment, minimises bone resection, retains the native knee ligaments, especially the anterior and posterior cruciate ligaments essential for normal knee function [43, 52, 53]. Furthermore, compared with TKR, UKR patients have more natural knee kinematics [19], better proprioception, improved range of motion [43], and superior pain relief that is more predictable [43, 54]. The operative time is shorter, recovery faster, with

patients able to return to daily activities quicker [54], and it is more cost-effective [55]. A propensity score-matched cohort analysis comparing UKR to TKR found UKR to have better long-term outcomes and quality of life [56]. Although there are many potential reasons for better function with UKR as compared to TKR, one key determinant is the preservation of normal knee kinematics and normal patella tendon length with UKR as compared to TKR. TKR has been shown to cause shortening of the patella tendon, which is associated with subsequent joint stiffness and eventually onset of patellofemoral arthrosis [57].

Due to the unique anatomy and kinematics in the lateral knee, achieving correct ligament balance is more challenging than the medial UKR, making LUKR a more technically challenging procedure [44]. However, with more experience and greater appreciation for the unique lateral knee anatomy and biomechanics, the results for LUKR saw improvement [52]. Developments in implant design and instrumentation alongside better patient selection has led to recent studies reporting excellent patient outcomes, improved satisfaction and excellent early implant survivorship [20–23, 58–60]. In addition, surgeon experience [61, 62] has been linked to improved patient outcomes with some studies demonstrating a protracted learning curve for less experienced surgeons/low volume surgeons [32] and better outcomes reported for high volume surgeons [19].

Since the introduction of resurfacing implants in the 1950s, among which the McIntosh surface arthroplasty [50] and the McKeever implant [63], the first modern UKR was the Marmor modular knee in the early 1970s [64]. Since then, many UKR implants have been developed; however, few have been designed specifically with the lateral compartment as the primary focus [32]. Table 21.2 lists LUKR implants reported in the literature and in active registries around the world reflecting the implants in clinical use for comparison. Table 21.3 summarises the reported outcomes in literature, and Table 21.4 provides the relevant demographic data. Table 21.5 lists existing arthroplasty registries, and Table 21.6 lists excluded UKR implants in this review along with the reasoning behind the exclusion.

Table 21.2 LUKR implants reported in literature and/or registries

Implant	Manufacturer	Bearing type	Medial/lateral	Literature reference	Registry
Allegretto	Sulzer orthopedics	Fixed	Medial or lateral	N/A	Switzerland [65], Australia [66], Italy [67]
Alpina	Biomet, France, valence	Fixed	Medial or lateral	[26, 27, 68, 69]	Switzerland [65]
AMC unicompartmental knee	Alphanorm, Quiershied, Germany	Mobile	Medial or lateral	[2]	N/A
AMC Uniglide prosthesis	Corin PLC, Cirencester, UK	Fixed	Medial or lateral	[17]	Australia [66], UK [48]
Balansys Uni system	Mathys European orthopedics	Fixed	Medial or lateral	N/A	Switzerland [65], Australia [66], Italy [67]
Brigham prosthesis	NS	Fixed	Medial or lateral	[70]	N/A
Duracon UKA	Howmedica, Rutherford, NJ	Fixed	Not found	[24, 71]	N/A
Endo-model sled	Link	Fixed	Medial or lateral	N/A	Australia [66], Italy [67]
Genesis Unicondylar implant/Accuris system	Smith & Nephew, Memphis, TN	Fixed	Medial or lateral	[61]	Australia [66], Italy [67], Norway [72], Sweden [73]
GKS	Permedica	Fixed		N/A	Italy [67]
GMK Uni	Medacta international	Fixed	Medial or lateral	N/A	Switzerland [65]
HLS Uni evolution	Tornier, Inc., Grenoble, France	Fixed	Medial or lateral	[26, 30, 74].	Portugal [75], Italy [67]
iBalance Uni	Arthrex	Fixed	Medial or lateral	N/A	Switzerland [65]
Journey Uni	Smith & nephew	Fixed	Medial or lateral	N/A	Slovenia [76], Switzerland [65], USA [77], New Zealand [78], Germany [79], Australia [66], UK [48], Belgium [80], Italy [67], Norway [72], Netherlands [81]
KAPS® uni knee arthroplasty system	X.NOV (Héricourt, France)	Mobile or fixed	Medial or lateral	[82]	N/A
Link sled	Link	Fixed	Medial or lateral	N/A	New Zealand [78], Germany [79], Norway [72], Sweden [73]
Marmor, Marmor II	Smith & nephew Richards, Orthez, France	Fixed	Medial or lateral	[30, 83, 84]	N/A
Miller-Galante	Zimmer, Warsaw, Indiana	Fixed	Medial or lateral	[30, 84, 85]	Australia [66], UK [48], Italy [67], Norway [72], Sweden [73]
New Jersey low contact stress knee	DePuy international, Leeds, UK	Mobile	Medial or lateral	[44, 63, 83]	N/A
Optetrak uni	Exactec	Fixed (all-poly tibial)	Medial or lateral	N/A	Italy [67]

(continued)

Table 21.2 (continued)

Implant	Manufacturer	Bearing type	Medial/lateral	Literature reference	Registry
Oxford domed lateral implant	Zimmer Biomet, Bridgend, UK	Mobile	Lateral	[86, 87]	*:Germany [79], Australia [66], UK [48], USA [77], Italy [67], Netherlands [81], New Zealand [78], Norway [72], Portugal [75], Slovenia [76], Sweden [73], Switzerland [65]
Oxford fixed bearing implant	Biomet Inc., Warsaw, IN, USA	Fixed	Lateral	[23]	Germany [79]
Physica ZUK	Lima corporate, Udine, Italy	Fixed	Medial or lateral	[58]	Slovenia [76], Switzerland [65], Germany [79], UK [48], Belgium [80], Italy [67], Netherlands [81]
Porous coated anatomic UKA	Howmedica, Rutherford, NJ	Fixed	Medial or lateral	[88]	N/A
Preservation UKA	DePuy Orthopaedics Inc., USA	Fixed or Mobile	Medial or lateral	[25, 44, 89]	Portugal [75], Australia [66], Italy [67], Norway [72]
Repicci II®	Biomet, Inc., Warsaw, IN	Fixed	Medial or lateral	[90]	Australia [66]
Restoris MCK	Stryker	Fixed	Medial or lateral	N/A	USA [77], New Zealand [78], Australia [66], Italy [67]
Sigma HP ®	DePuy Synthes	Fixed	Medial or lateral	[26]	Switzerland [65], USA [77], New Zealand [78], Germany [79], Australia [66], UK [48], Italy [67], Norway [72], Sweden [72]
St Georg sled prosthesis	Waldemar, Link, Hamburg, Germany	Fixed	Medial or lateral	[52, 91]	N/A
Triathlon PKR	Stryker	Fixed	Medial or lateral	N/A	Switzerland [65], USA [77], New Zealand, Germany [79], Australia [66], UK [48], Belgium [80], Norway [72], Sweden [72], Netherlands [81]
UC plus solution	Smith & Nephew	Fixed	Medial or lateral	N/A	Italy [67]
Uni score®	Amplitude	Fixed	Medial or lateral	[26]	Slovenia [76]
Unix UKR	Stryker orthopedics, Mahwah, NJ	Fixed	Medial or lateral	[68, 92]	Australia [66]
Vanguard M™	Biomet, Inc., Warsaw, IN	Fixed	Medial or lateral	[90]	N/A
Zimmer unicompartmental high flex knee system (ZUK)	Zimmer, Indiana	Fixed	Medial or lateral	[18, 93]	Australia [66], Norway [72], Sweden [73]
Zimmer natural-knee UKA	Zimmer Biomet, Warsaw, IN	Fixed	Medial or lateral	[68]	N/A
ZUK	Smith & nephew	Fixed	Medial or lateral	[27, 74]	N/A

Table 21.3 LUKR implants reported outcomes and implant survival rates

Author	Year	Implant	Bearing type	Functional outcomes	Implant survival
Gunther [1]	1996	Flat lateral Oxford (phase I and II)	Mobile	In activity pain: 71% no pain, 24% mild pain, 0% moderate pain, 5% severe At rest: 79% no pain, 17% mild pain, 0% moderate pain, 5% severe	(a) All re-operations: 5 years: 82% ± 15.4% (95% CI) (b) All aseptic re-operations (infection excluded): 5 years: 86% ± 14.1% (95% CI)© re-operations for aseptic loosening: 5 years: 98% ± 6.7% (95% CI)
Ohdera [24]	2001	Marmor Oxford PCA Omnifit	Both	JOAKS: 64.2 ± 13.2 points -- > 85.3 ± 9.9 points	NS
Ashraf [91]	2002	St Georg sled prosthesis	Fixed	BKS: 88 pre-op, 55 2 years, 44 5 years and 23 10 years	Revision for any cause—Cumulative survival rate: 83% at 10 years (excl. Pain), with 74.5% knees still at risk at 15 years
Pennington [85]	2006	Miller Galante	Fixed	HSS: Average pre-op 60 (42–79), post-op 93 (82–100), excellent (100–85 points), good (84–70 points), fair (69–60 points), or poor (b60 points)	100
Forster [44]	2007	Preservation UKA	Fixed	AKSS knee: Pre-op 41, 95 at 1 year, 95 at 2 years AKSS function: Pre-op 50, 100 at 1 year, 95 at 2 years OKS: Pre-op 40, 16 at 1 year, 15 at 2 years	NS
			Mobile	AKSS knee: Pre-op 48, 95 at 1 year, 95 at 2 years AKSS function: Pre-op 60, 100 at 1 year, 100 at 2 years OKS: Pre-op 41, 19 at 1 year, 13 at 2 years	NS
Sah [94]	2007	Brigham unicondylar prosthesis	Fixed	AKSS knee: Pre-op 39, 89 post-op AKSS function: Pre-op 45, post-op 80	5 years 100
		Press fit condylar (PFC) prosthesis	NS		
		PFC sigma prosthesis	NS		
		Preservation Unicompartmental knee	Fixed or mobile		

(continued)

Table 21.3 (continued)

Author	Year	Implant	Bearing type	Functional outcomes	Implant survival
Volpi [32]	2007	Miller Galante	Fixed	HSS: Average pre-op 52.9 (48–68), post-op 88.04 (71–95)	NS
Argenson [27]	2008	Marmor-like	Fixed	KSS-KS: Pre-op 57 ± 10 (35–75 SD), post-op 88 ± 5 (40–100 SD) KSS-FS: Pre-op 46 ± 5 (10–89 SD), post-op 78 ± 3 (20–100 SD)	Revision for any reason: 92% at 10 years (95% CI: 0.79–0.99), 84% at 16 years (95% CI: 0.71–0.97)
		Alpina	Fixed		
		Miller Galante	Fixed		
		ZUK	Fixed		
Pandit [51]	2010	Flat lateral Oxford phase III	Mobile	86%: No pain/mild pain at rest and on activity. Mean flexion improved from 111° pre-op to 117° post-op. OKS improved from 24–36	NS
John [95]	2011	Miller Galante	Fixed	Average total BKS at follow-up was 43.61 (range: 28–50). The mean functional score was 16.3 (9–20) Patient satisfaction: 88% of patients had good or excellent total score and 73% patients had good or excellent functional score. Fifteen patients had a fair/poor functional score while only eight had their total score in the fair/poor The mean range of movement at follow-up was 110.6° (80–130°). Overall, 25 (45%) of the knees had no pain, 24 (43%) mild or occasional pain and 7 (12%) moderate pain All patients stated that they had improved after the procedure	97% at 5 years, it dropped to 41% at 8 years
Lustig [96]	2011	Cemented all-polyethylene tibial component	N/A	IKS knee average: 68.2 (range 35–92) pre-op to 94.9 points (range 70–100 points) Mean range of flexion of 132.6° (range, 115°–150°) Mean IKS function score: 68.9 (range 0–100) pre-op to 81.8 points (range 25–100 points) post-op	Prosthesis removal endpoint: 98.08% (94.38%–100%) at 10 years
Scievine Panni [97]	2011	ZUK metal backed tibial tray	Fixed	IKS knee 46 pre-op to 80 post-op IKS function 54 pre-op to 94 post-op	100%
Berend [33]	2012	Repicci II	Fixed	Average KSS: – Pain: From 8 (range, 0–45) pre-op to 46 (range, 10–50) post-op for pain – Total clinical: 49 (range, 10–95) pre-op to 94 (range, 10–95) post-op – Function: 47 (range, 0–90) pre-op to 89 (range, 40–100) post-op Average ROM: 115° (range, 70°–125°) pre-op to 124° (range, 95°–45°) post-op	NS
		Vanguard M ™	Fixed		

Table 21.3 (continued)

Author	Year	Implant	Bearing type	Functional outcomes	Implant survival
Heyse [61]	2012	Genesis Unicondylar implant/Accuris system—Full poly	Fixed	Average KS-KS: – All-poly: 97.0 ± 2.4 male, 96.8 ± 2.9 female Average KS-FS: – All-poly: 98.6 ± 2.5 male, 96.5 ± 4.2 female	Overall LUKR: 91.8% at 10 and 15 years All poly: 93.3% at 10 and 15 years Metal backed cemented: 88.7% at 10 years and 82.4% at 15 years Metal backed uncemented: 97.3% at 10 years and 74.9% at 15 years
		Genesis Unicondylar implant/Accuris system—Metal-backed cemented		Average KS-KS: Metal backed and cemented: 93.5 ± 0.7 male, 95.5 ± 4.8 female Average KS-FS: Metal backed and cemented: 95.0 ± 0.0 male, 91.2 ± 7.5 female	
		Genesis Unicondylar implant/Accuris system—Metal-backed uncemented		Average KS-KS: – Metal backed and uncemented: 93.8 ± 2.8 male, 90.4 ± 3.6 female Average knee society function scores: – Metal backed and uncemented: 98.8 ± 2.5 male, 93.6 ± 3.8 female	
Lustig [30]	2012	HLS Uni evolution	Fixed	Mean IKS knee scores improved from 51 points (range, 29–75 points) pre-op to 88 points (range, 65–100 points) post-op Mean IKS knee function scores improved from 51 points (range, 10–89 points) pre-op to 87 points (range, 35–100 points) post-op	Revision for any reason as the end point, the implant survivorship rates were 100% at 5 and 10 years and 80% at 15 years
		Marmor II	Fixed		
		Miller-Galante unicompartmental knee system	Fixed		
Liebs [25]	2013	Preservation (R) mobile bearing prosthesis	Mobile	WOMAC(TM) function score (points): 33.6 ± 29.5 WOMAC(TM) pain score (points): 33.7 ± 31.3 WOMAC(TM) stiffness score (points): 22.8 ± 27.1 SF-36 PCS (points): 38.0 ± 11.4 SF-36 MCS (points): 48.1 ± 12.2 Lequesne knee score (points): 7.9 ± 4.1	Implant survival was 91.8% at 5 years and 83% at 9 years
Schelfaut [28]	2013	Domed lateral Oxford UKR	Mobile	General patient satisfaction at the latest follow-up was excellent in 84%, good in 12% and fair in 4% The OKS improved significantly (p < 0.0001) from a pre-op mean of 23.3 (range 8–40, SD 8.4) to 42.1 (range 23–48, SD 6.7) post-op The mean post-op flexion was 127° (range 110°–155°, SD 10.5°)	NS
Lustig [98]	2014	HLS Uni evolution	Fixed	Mean KSS knee score was 95.1 points and mean KSS function score was 82.2 points. The mean ROM was 132.6° (range, 115–150°)	Implant survival was 94.4% at 10 years and 91.4% at 15 years

(continued)

Table 21.3 (continued)

Author	Year	Implant	Bearing type	Functional outcomes	Implant survival
Marson [93]	2014	Domed lateral Oxford UKR	Mobile	Average Oxford knee scores was 36.6 (95% CI 29.0–44.2)	100% at 2 years
		Zimmer unicompartmental high flex knee system	Fixed	Average Oxford knee scores was 28.6 (19.8–37.5) for the Zimmer fixed-bearing prosthesis ($p = 0.15$)	90% at 2 years
Smith [17]	2014	AMC Uniglide prosthesis	Fixed	The mean total AKSS increased from 100 (30–182) pre-op to 159 (69–200) at 5 years ($p < 0.001$). Mean OKS was 20 (5–45) pre-op and 37 (9–48) at 5 years ($p < 0.001$). WOMAC scores were 36 (15–53) pre-op, and 22 (12–48) at 5 years ($p < 0.001$)	All 101 UKRs were included in survivorship calculations Taking removal of prosthesis as the end-point, implant survival was 98.7% at 2 and 95.5% at 5 years
Walker [99]	2014	Domed lateral Oxford UKR	Mobile	Mean postoperative OKS and ROM: Mean OKS was 43 [standard deviation (SD) 4] ROM was 127° (SD 13)	Revision for any reason as the endpoint was 96% [95% confidence interval (CI) 72–99] at 2 years
Kim [18]	2016	Zimmer unicompartmental high-flex knee (ZUK) prosthesis	Fixed	The mean KS knee score increased from 63.2 points (range, 48 to 70 points) pre-op to 86.0 points (range, 74 to 95 points) at the final follow-up ($p < 0.001$) The mean KS knee function score increased from 68.6 points (range, 35 to 80 points) pre-op to 92.4 points (range, 60 to 100 points) at the final follow-up ($p < 0.001$)	NS
Masud [100]	2018	Domed lateral Oxford UKR	Mobile	Pre-op OKS 20, post-op OKS 37	96.30%
Newman [19]	2017	Domed lateral Oxford UKR	Mobile	Median OKS was 26 (range nine to 36) pre-op and 42 (10–48) at final follow-up	Re-operation plots a cumulative survival of 0.80 at 119 months
Edmiston [59]	2018	Before 2004: Miller-Galante Unicompartmental Knee Thereafter: cemented Zimmer Unicompartmental Knee	Fixed	Mean KSS pre-op (SD) 124.8 (23.4) and 144.7 (30.8) post-op Mean KSS pre-op was 126.6 (25.1 SD) and 155.2 (36.1 SD) post-op	Overall survivorship was 94% at a mean of 82 months
Fornell [21]	2018	Domed lateral Oxford UKR	Mobile	At latest follow-up: The VAS score mean pre-op of 9.3 (range: 8–10) to post-op of 1.25 (range: 0–6) The mean pre-op OKS was 26 (20–36) and the mean post-op score was 44 (38–48)	Survival, with revision for any reason as the endpoint, was 97.5% at 5 years and 86.4% at 6 years

Table 21.3 (continued)

Author	Year	Implant	Bearing type	Functional outcomes	Implant survival
Saragaglia [82]	2018	KAPS® prosthesis	Fixed Mobile	The mean post-op OKS was 18 ± 5 (13–30)	NS for lateral only
Walker [20]	2018	Domed lateral Oxford UKR	Mobile	Mean OKS of 40.3 (95% CI 39.4 to 41.2), a mean Tegner activity score of 3.2 (95% CI 3.1 to 3.3) and a mean University of California, Los Angeles score of 5.7 (95% CI 5.5 to 5.9)	Survival rate of 90.1% at 3 years (95% CI: 86.1 to 93.1; number at risk: 155) and 85.0% at 5 years (95% CI 77.9 to 89.9; number at risk: 43)
Deroche [74]	2019	HLS Uni evolution	Fixed	The mean functional IKS score was 66.5 ± 26.8, with a mean objective score of 84.4 points ± 13.2	Cumulative survival rate was 82.1% at 15 years and 79.4% at 20 years
Gill [58]	2019	Physica ZUK	Fixed	KS-KS and KS-FS pre-op was 46.4 and 48.7, and 91.3 and 93.1, respectively post-op ($p = 0.0001$)	100%
Burger [60]	2020	Metal-backed tibial onlay components	NS	Of 152 knees: Mean post-op KOOS score (SD) 85.6 (14.3) 150/162 (92.6%) of patients were either very satisfied or satisfied with their knee function	Five-year survivorship was 97.7% (95% CI 94.9 to 100)
Burger [101]	2020	NS Domed lateral Oxford UKR	Fixed Mobile	NS NS	Five-year crude cumulative revision rate using the Kaplan-Meier Analysis was 12.9% (95% confidence interval [CI] 6.6–16.2) Risk analysis: 12.6% (95% CI 9.7–16.4)
Deroche [26]	2020	HLS Uni evolution Alpina Uni® ZUK® Sigma HP® Uni score®	Fixed Fixed Fixed Fixed Fixed	At last follow-up: Mean IKS knees score was 87.0 ± 10.9 (range, 45–100) and mean function score 80.2 ± 14.3 (range, 30–100). Mean maximum flexion was 125 ± 11° (range, 85°–140°). 94.3% of patients were satisfied or very satisfied	All-cause revision surgery was 85.4% at 10 years and 79.4% at 20 years.
Kagan [68]	2020	Zimmer natural-knee UKA	Fixed	KOOS, JR was 101.3 (94.5 to 108.02) Satisfaction was 92% (28/30) in the lateral UKAs ($p = 0.309$)	The cumulative incidence of revision TKA at 10 years was approximately 5% for the lateral UKAs (SHR, 0.67; 95% confidence interval, 0.22–20.2, $p = 0.476$) when including death as a competing risk

(continued)

Table 21.3 (continued)

Author	Year	Implant	Bearing type	Functional outcomes	Implant survival
Kennedy [22]	2020	Domed lateral Oxford UKR	Mobile	Median OKS was 43 (interquartile range (IQR) 37 to 47), with 260 (80%) achieving a good or excellent score (OKS > 34)	Ten-year survival was 85% (95% confidence interval (CI) 79 to 90, at risk 72)
Walker [23]	2020	Oxford fixed lateral prosthesis	Fixed	OKS pre-op was 26.4 ± 6.9 (12–41) and 39.7 ± 8.4 (15–48) post-op AKSS-O pre-op was 54.3 ± 15.3 (18–90) and 82.2 ± 15.6 (40–100) post-op AKS-FS was 56.4 ± 21.3 (10–100) pre-op and 83.1 ± 20.2 (five to 100) post-op ROM was 123.5 ± 13.5 (90–140) pre-op and 134 ± 10.3 (95–150) post-op	Survivorship was 100% at 2 years for revision for any reason (exchange any component) as the end point. Survivorship was 94.2% (95% confidence interval (CI): 83.2–98.1%) with the endpoint 'any reoperation'
Mohammad [102]	2021	Domed lateral Oxford UKR	Mobile	NS	The 5- and 10-year cumulative implant survival rates were 92.4% (CI: 90.3–94.1) and 88.6% (CI: 85.3–91.2), respectively.
Murray [103]	2021	St Georg sled UKA	Fixed	Mean BKS, mean OKS and WOMAC: Pre-op: 52.7, N/A, N/A 10 years: 84.5, 35.3, 23.2 15 years: 76.6, 27.3, 30.3 20 years: 74, 21, 34 25 years: 90, 37.7, 18.75	Survivorship was 72% at 15 years, and 68% at 20 and 25 years
Xue [104]	2021	St Georg sled UKA	Fixed	At last follow-up, the HSS score was 52.1 (range, 38–80) pre-op and 85.6 (range, 61–98) post-op The OKS improved from 22.8 (range, 16–32) pre-op to 42.7 (range, 30–47) post-op	The 5 year survival was 99.5%

Fixed vs. Mobile Bearing Lateral UKR

LUKR implants are available as either a fixed bearing or a mobile bearing. Mobile bearing designs have theoretical advantages over fixed bearing designs, including more normal knee kinematics and reduced bearing wear. In a cadaveric knee study by Goodfellow et al., knees implanted with the Oxford Knee implant showed obligatory sliding of the mobile bearing on the tibial component surface [52]. As a result, mobile bearing designs eliminate the artificial constraint on the bearing, thereby restoring nearly normal knee motion [83] and subsequently reducing bearing wear. This is particularly important in the lateral knee, which exhibits larger meniscal excursion in the natural knee [8]. Mobile bearing designs have been shown to reflect this phenomenon where bearings implanted laterally moved 2.25 mm more than medial bearings across an 80° knee flexion range [52].

Despite theoretical advantages of mobile-bearing implants over fixed-bearing implants, a recent study with a minimum 10-year follow up found no difference in implant survival or functional outcomes when comparing the mobile-bearing Phase III Oxford Knee implant with the fixed-bearing implants (Miller-Galante and the Zimmer Unicompartmental High Flex Knee

System) [105], with other studies similarly reporting little difference between fixed- and mobile-bearing designs [106–108].

Of the 25 devices listed in Table 21.2, 20 (80%) are fixed-bearing implants and three (12%) are mobile-bearing designs. Two implants (8%) are semi-constrained designs: the Preservation UKA (DePuy) and the New Jersey Low contact Stress Uni (DePuy International, Leeds, UK). Both implants feature a curved groove/track in the tibial component to partially restrain the bearing movement: enabling AP movement but not mediolateral movement [44, 63]. While initial results were promising [63], the Preservation Uni was recalled in 2009, due to poor implant performance and similarly, early failure of the LCS mobile-bearing prosthesis has been reported with over-constraint of the mobile bearing cited as the cause [109].

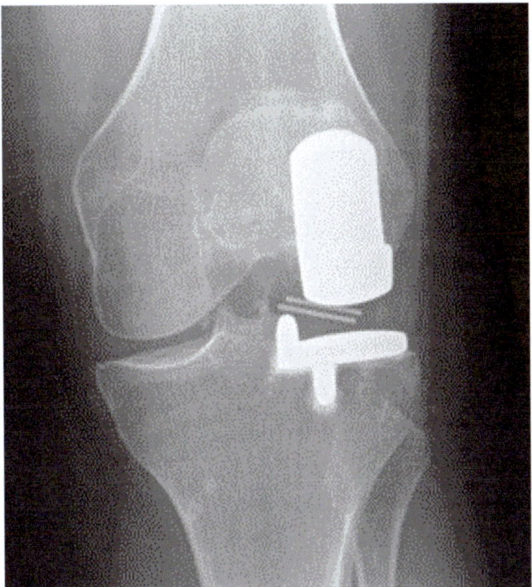

Fig. 21.1 X-ray shows mobile bearing dislocation medially into the knee joint. Bearing position is seen by the radio-opaque lines showing bearing lodged on top of the tibial component wall

Why Do LUKRs Fail?

The most common failure mode for LUKR implants is OA progression followed by aseptic loosening [110]. However, for mobile-bearing designs, the most common failure mode is dislocation of the mobile bearing [2, 51, 87]. As dislocations tend to occur early (most within 12 months post-operatively [1], average 16 months post-operatively [111]), this is likely the cause for poor early survivorship seen in mobile bearing designs. Revision surgery often involves conversion to TKR; however, some authors have advocated for conversion to bi-compartmental UKR for progression of arthritis or use of supplementary screws (in the intercondylar notch) to treat subluxed/dislocated mobile bearing [112].

The choice of implant has an impact on the reasons for failure. For instance, prior to its recall, Liebs & Herzberg reported that the most common reason for revision of the Preservation Knee (DePuy Orthopaedics Inc., USA) was aseptic loosening followed by disease progression [25]. For the HLS Uni Evolution prosthesis (Tornier, Inc., Grenoble, France), it was reversed, with disease progression exceeding the cases of aseptic

loosening [74]. In contrast, the Oxford Domed Lateral UKR implant (Zimmer Biomet, Bridgend, UK) predominantly fails as a result of dislocation of the mobile bearing [102] (see Fig. 21.1).

Discussion/Further Work

LUKR is an established and effective treatment for end-stage osteoarthritis isolated to the lateral compartment of the knee. Other surgical treatment options include osteotomies (HTO or DFO) or TKR. Compared with HTO, mobile-bearing UKR had superior short-term clinical outcomes for advanced unicompartmental knee OA of the medial knee [113]. Similarly, another study found that while HTO and UKR showed similar long-term survival between the two procedures to 12 years, beyond 12 years, UKR was found to have superior post-operative survival [114]. Whilst TKR is also a viable treatment option for lateral knee OA, UKR has also been shown to be superior to TKR as it replaces just the damaged tissues, retaining the native knee ligaments, resulting in more natural knee kinematics [19] with better long-term outcomes and better quality of life [56]. Further, compared with UKR, TKRs are more sensitive to minor misalignment, which may cause component loosening or joint instability [52] and UKR consistently outperforms TKR with better functional outcomes, shorter hospital stays, lower mortality, and lower early reoperation for any reason [115].

UKR replaces just the damaged tissues in the knee, allows for the retention of native knee ligaments, preservation of bone stock, and involves a minimally invasive procedure. Over five decades of research have led to improvements in patient selection, surgical technique, implant design and surgeon experience, all of which have contributed to the improvement of patient-functional outcomes and therefore greater confidence in this procedure. However, the use of LUKR globally remains limited due to increased technical difficulty of the procedure (and therefore a protracted learning curve for less experienced surgeons), particularly with ligament balancing of LCL laxity in flexion, and less familiarity with the lateral knee likely as a result of the lower disease prevalence [14]. The learning curve associated with medial UKRs has been studied, with satisfactory outcomes achieved following 25 operations per year [116].

Few devices have been designed specifically for use in the lateral knee, with most implants being designed for the medial knee and used laterally. The Oxford Domed Lateral (ODL) implant and the Fixed Lateral Oxford (FLO) implant [23] are uniquely designed for the lateral knee for implantation through a minimally invasive procedure. The ODL implant features a spherical femoral component, a tibial component with a domed tibial surface, and a biconcave mobile bearing [52]. The design maximises the bearing entrapment, in order to reduce the risk of bearing dislocation [117]. Following ongoing dislocation of the mobile bearing in the ODL implant, it is now recommended that surgeons use the FLO interchangeably if the bearing is deemed unstable intra-operatively [22] (see Fig. 21.2).

Patient-specific implants for the lateral knee have also been trialled, namely, the iUni (ConforMIS, Burlington, Massachusetts, USA) [118]. Compared with the Miller_Galante Unicompartmental System (Zimmer Warsaw, Indiana, USA), iUni showed better tibial coverage and excellent short-term clinical results (mean post-op KSS 94 ± 7.6 SD with minimum 24 months follow up, survivorship of iUni was 97% at 37 months follow up) [118]. The impetus

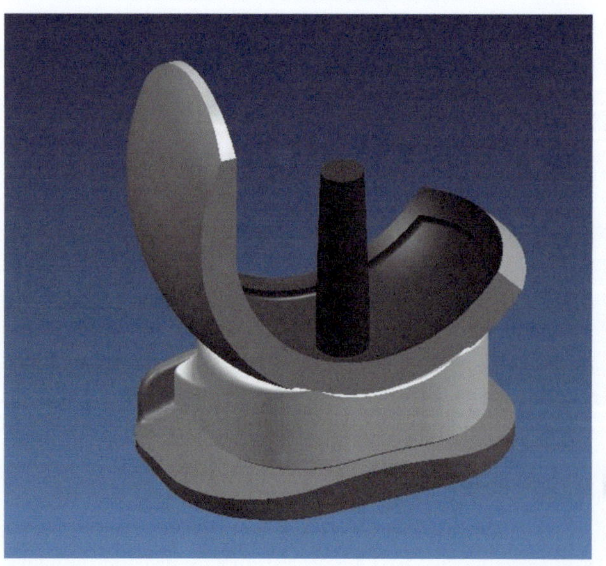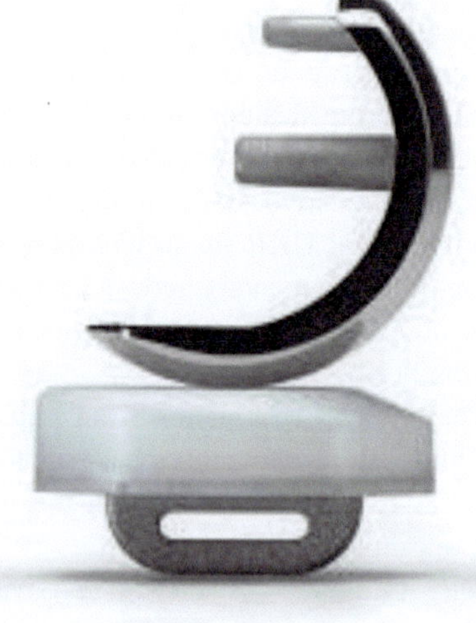

Fig. 21.2 Mobile bearing Oxford Domed Lateral implant (left) and the Fixed bearing Lateral Oxford implant (right)

for lateral-specific implants is clear due to the unique anatomy and kinematics of the lateral knee; however, the long-term success of patient-specific implants over conventional ones remains unknown.

Approximately 85% of implants available on the market are fixed-bearing constructs, which do not predispose to bearing dislocation. However, the importance of mobile-bearing constructs, which allow for more normal knee kinematics [119], reduced bearing wear [52], and therefore longer implant survival, may become more prominent with a greater demand for implants with greater longevity as a result of an ageing population and a greater demand for treatments for younger and more active patients. Key to the development of mobile-bearing constructs is solving the problem of bearing dislocation [2, 51], which occurs more frequently in the lateral knee (ODL implant: 3.7% laterally [111] versus 0.5% medially [120]). The most popular and well researched mobile-bearing design in the literature is the ODL implant [22], so the remaining discussion will focus predominantly on bearing dislocation specific to the ODL implant. Many attempts have been made to address the problem of mobile bearing dislocation, including careful patient selection [2], changes to the surgical technique (including introduction of lateral parapatellar approach [1, 50], internally rotating the tibial cut [51], dividing the popliteus tendon to avoid bow-string [1], inserting screws into the tibial eminence to augment the tibial component wall height [121] (see Fig. 21.3) and avoiding lateral tibial joint line elevation [86, 122]), modifying the implant design (increasing tibial component wall height [52], introduction of lateral specific meniscus [1], improved instrumentation [1] and introduction of the ODL with increased bearing entrapment [117]), and increased surgeon experience [123].

A recent systematic review on the ODL implant found that changing the design of the tibial component from a flat tibial surface to a domed tibial surface reduced the bearing dislocation rate from 17% to 3.7% [111]. While the authors attributed the reduction in dislocation rate to changing the tibial component from a flat

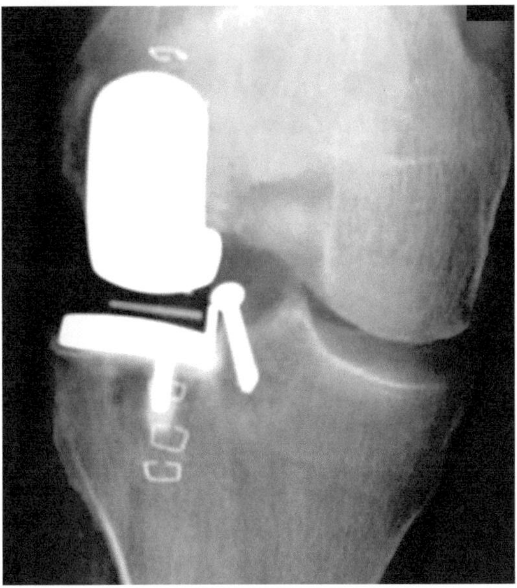

Fig. 21.3 Screws inserted into the tibial eminence to augment the tibial component wall height in an attempt to reduce dislocation of the mobile bearing medially

to a domed tibial surface design, concurrent changes overtime to the patient selection, instrumentation, surgeon experience, surgical technique were not accounted for. Nevertheless, the dislocation rate has reduced over time, with most recent studies reporting a similar dislocation rate of 2–4% [19, 21, 22, 28, 51, 102]. Despite similar implant survivorship shown for fixed-bearing versus mobile-bearing implants, resolving the complication of bearing dislocation may see mobile-bearing constructs outperforming fixed-bearing designs, given that bearing dislocations tend to occur early (average 16 months post-op [111]), potentially masking the long-term benefits of mobile-bearing designs.

Conversely, with continuing improvements in bearing materials resulting in more failure resistant and durable Ultra-High Molecular Weight Polyethylene (UHMWPEs), the need for a mobile bearing may become less pressing. Nanocomposite materials have been developed which focus on reinforcing pure UHMWPEs to improve material physicochemical properties. One study showed that compared with pure UHMWPEs, UHMWPE reinforced with functionalised single-walled carbon nanotubes (f-SWCNTs) has been shown to increase Young's Modulus by 12% [124]. Other improvements in the manufacturing technique have been developed which improve the polyethylene wear rates [125]. High-dose radiation cross-linking with treatment using potent antioxidants such as vitamin E for oxidation have been shown to improve the strength, toughness, oxidation resistance, and wear rate [126]. These developments may reduce the bearing wear rate; however, the kinematic similarity of mobile-bearing implants to native knees remains a benefit of mobile-bearing designs over fixed-bearing implants.

One less understood and discussed effect of LUKR with the ODL implant is its effect on the patellar tendon length. LUKR has been found to cause lengthening of the patellar tendon length [57, 127] at similar rates whether using a flat or domed tibial component design [127]. Further research regarding the cause of patellar tendon lengthening as well as its effects on clinical outcomes are required.

Conclusion

Ongoing research and development of the LUKR procedure has led to LUKR being the preferred treatment option for patients suffering from end-stage isolated lateral knee osteoarthritis. Many implants exist on the market for LUKR treatment; however, few are specifically designed for the lateral compartment and with most being fixed-bearing designs. With an ageing population and greater demand for implants for younger and more active patients, further research to address the problem of mobile bearing dislocation may allow more patients to benefit from the advantages of mobile-bearing designs over fixed-bearing designs of reduced bearing wear and more normal knee kinematics.

Appendix A: Demographic Information for Studies

See Table 21.4.

Table 21.4 Demographic information of LUKR studies

Author	Year	Country of study	Implant	Bearing type	Manufacturing company	Total no. of knees	Total no. of patients	Male	Female	Mean age	Age range	Study start date	Study end date	No. of patients followed up	No. of knees followed up	Mean follow up duration (months)	Follow up range (months)
Gunther [1]	1996	United Kingdom	Flat lateral Oxford (phase I and II)	Mobile Both	Biomet, Bridgend, UK	53	51	4	47	68	40–88	Apr-83	Dec-91	NS	53	62	24–119
							14									40	20–72
Ohdera [24]	2001	Japan	Marmor Oxford PCA Omnifit	Fixed		38	37	8	29	65.1		Aug-77	Dec-99	17	18	99	60–189
Ashraf [91]	2002	United Kingdom	St Georg sled prosthesis	Fixed	Waldemar Link, Hamburg, Germany	83	75	NS	NS	69	35–81	Jan-78	Dec-99	71	NS	9	2–21
Pennington [85]	2006	USA	Miller Galante	Fixed	Zimmer, Warsaw, Indiana	29	24					Aug-88	Jan-01		29	149	37.2–187.2
Forster [44]	2007	Australia	Preservation UKA	Mobile	DePuy, Warsaw, Indiana	17	NS	5	11	75	55–93	May-01	May-03				
				Fixed		13	NS	7	5	55	36–87						
Sah [94]	2007	USA	Brigham unicondylar prosthesis	NS	Johnson and Johnson Orthopaedics, Raynham, Massachusetts	48				61	37–84	1981	1991			62.4	24–180
			Press fit condylar (PFC) prosthesis	NS									1990s				
			PFC sigma prosthesis	Fixed or mobile									2001				
			Preservation Uni	Fixed	DePuy, Warsaw, Indiana							2002	2004				
Volpi [32]	2007	Italy	Miller Galante	Fixed	Zimmer, Warsaw, Indiana	28	27	2	25	73	65–82			24	25	NS	12–60
Argenson [27]	2008	France	Marmor-like	Fixed	Zimmer, Warsaw, Indiana	15		15	24	61 ± 7 years	34–79	Feb-82	Dec-04	37			
			Alpina	Fixed	Biomet, Bridgend, UK	1											
			Miller Galante	Fixed		20											
			ZUK	Mobile	Zimmer	4											

(continued)

Table 21.4 (continued)

Author	Year	Country of study	Implant	Bearing type	Manufacturing company	Total no. of knees	Total no. of patients	Male	Female	Mean age	Age range	Study start date	Study end date	No. of patients followed up	No. of knees followed up	Mean follow up duration (months)	Follow up range (months)
Pandit [51]	2010	UK	Flat lateral Oxford phase III	Fixed	Biomet UK limited, Swindon, UK	65	64	28	36	53	39–83	Apr-98	Oct-04	NS	65	56	36–108
John [95]	2011	UK	Miller Galante	N/A		66				67		1989	2006			129.6	24–192
Lustig [96]	2011	France	Cemented all-polyethylene tibial component	Fixed	N/A	54	52			72.2 ± 3	25–88			47	49	101	64–189
Scievine Panni [97]	2011	Italy	ZUK metal backed tibial tray	Fixed		9	NS			69		Feb-05	Dec-07			60	
Berend [33]	2012	USA	Repicci II	Fixed	Biomet, Inc., Warsaw, IN	42	125	38	89	68		Apr-04	Dec-08	93	100	39	24–81
			Vanguard M ™	Fixed		90											
Heyse [61]	2012	Germany	Genesis Unicondylar implant/Accuris system—Full poly	Fixed Fixed	Smith & Nephew, Memphis< TN	23						1993	2005				
			Genesis Unicondylar implant/Accuris system—Metal-backed cemented			7											
			Genesis Unicondylar implant/Accuris system—Metal-backed uncemented			20											
Lustig [30]	2012	France	HLS Uni evolution	Fixed	Tornier, Inc., Grenoble, France		6	6	7	50							
			Marmor II	Fixed	Richards Orthopaedics, Memphis, TN		2										
			Miller-Galante uni knee system	Mobile	Zimmer, Inc., Warsaw, I		5										
Liebs [25]	2013	Germany	Preservation (R) mobile-bearing prosthesis	Mobile	Depuy		128					Apr-02	Oct-09				
Schelfaut [28]	2013	Belgium	Domed lateral Oxford UKR	Fixed	Zimmer Biomet, Bridgend, UK	Mobile	25	9	16	60	31–86	Jan-09	Apr-11	NS	25	20	12–34

Lustig [98]	2014	France	HLS Uni evolution	Mobile	Tornier, saint-Ismier, France	54	52			72.2 ± 15.2	25–85	Jan-88	Oct-03	44	46	14	10.2–18
Marson [93]	2014	United Kingdom	Domed lateral Oxford UKR	Fixed	Zimmer Biomet, Bridgend, UK	15	NS	NS	NS	58	41–77	Oct07	Aug-11	NS	15	35	16–47
			Zimmer unicompartmental high flex knee system	Fixed	Zimmer, Indiana	12				58	40–84					33	12–71
Smith [17]	2014	United kingdom	AMC Uniglide prosthesis	Mobile	Corin PLC, Cirencester, UK	101	100	32	68	65	36–91	Dec-02	Dec-11	32	33		
Walker [99]	2014	Germany	Domed lateral Oxford UKR	Fixed	Zimmer Biomet, Bridgend, UK		50 (only 22 met matched study criteria)	5	17	62	41–81	Dec-06	Mar-09			22 ± 8	
Kim [18]	2016	South Korea	Zimmer unicompartmental high-flex knee (ZUK) prosthesis	Mobile	Zimmer, Warsaw, IN, USA	30	27	14	13	63	48–80	Jan-11	Feb-14	29	NS	38	24–48
Masud [100]	2018	United Kingdom	Domed lateral Oxford UKR	Mobile	Zimmer Biomet, Bridgend, UK	27		26%	74%			2007	2014				
Newman [19]	2017	United Kingdom	Domed lateral Oxford UKR	Fixed	Zimmer Biomet, Bridgend, UK	64	58	17	41	71	44–92	2005	2009	NS	64	81	24–119
Edmiston [59]	2018	USA	Before 2004: Miller-Galante Unicompartmental Knee Thereafter: cemented Zimmer Unicompartmental Knee	Fixed Mobile	Zimmer, Warsaw, IN		65	22	43	61.3 ± 11.2 SD		2003	2014			82.3 ± 36.8	
Fornell [21]	2018	Spain	Domed lateral Oxford UKR	Fixed	Zimmer Biomet, Bridgend, UK	41	41	10	31	63	38–81	Jun-08	May-15	NS	41	49	25–84
Saragaglia [82]	2018	France	KAPS® prosthesis	Mobile Mobile	X.NOV (Héricourt, France)	17						Mar-05	Mar-10		12		
Walker [20]	2018	Germany	Domed lateral Oxford UKR	Fixed	Zimmer Biomet, Bridgend, UK	3–4	327	90	237	65	36–88	Nov-06	Jan-14	326	344	37	12–93

(continued)

Table 21.4 (continued)

Author	Year	Country of study	Implant	Bearing type	Manufacturing company	Total no. of knees	Total no. of patients	Male	Female	Mean age	Age range	Study start date	Study end date	No. of patients followed up	No. of knees followed up	Mean follow up duration (months)	Follow up range (months)
Deroche [74]	2019	France	HLS Uni evolution	Fixed	Tornier (saint-Ismier, France)	54	52			65.4 ± 11		Jan-88	Oct-03		39	18	15–23
Gill [58]	2019	UK	Physica ZUK	NS	Lima corporate, Udine, Italy	14						Jun-05	2017				
Burger [60]	2020	USA	Metal-backed tibial onlay components	Fixed	NS	171		69	102	63.5 (9.5 SD)		Jun-07	Aug-16		152	58.8 ± 24SD	
Burger [101]	2020	USA	NS	Mobile	NS	168		174	362	30.3 ± 11		2007	2017				
			Domed lateral Oxford UKR	Fixed	Zimmer Biomet, Bridgend, UK	351											
Deroche [26]	2020	France	HLS Uni evolution	Fixed	Tornier (saint-Ismier, France)	91		63	205	68.8 ± 10.5		Jan-88	Sep-14			109.2	60–276
			Alpina Uni®	Fixed	Biomet, France, valence	80											
			ZUK®	Fixed		78											
			Sigma HP®	Fixed		15											
			Uni score®	Fixed		4											
Kagan [68]	2020	USA	Zimmer natural-knee UKA	Mobile	Zimmer Biomet, Warsaw, IN	30		8	22	68	43–86	Jul-00	Dec-10				
Kennedy [22]	2020	United Kingdom	Domed lateral Oxford UKR	Fixed	Zimmer Biomet, Bridgend, UK	325	308	104	204	65	39–90	Sep-04	Dec-15	308	325	84	36–168
Walker [23]	2020	Germany	Oxford fixed lateral prosthesis	Mobile	Biomet Inc., Warsaw, IN, USA	52	51	17	34	67	34–88	Feb-13	Jun-17	51	52	22.8	12–56
Mohammad [102]	2021	United Kingdom	Domed lateral Oxford UKR	Fixed	Zimmer Biomet, Bridgend, UK	992			641	64.5 (12.3 SD)		Jan-05	Dec-17			60 ± 3SD	
Murray [103]	2021	United Kingdom	St Georg sled UKA	Fixed	Waldemar Link, Hamburg, Germany	82	71					1974	1994			177.6 ± 6.6 SD	11–28.3
Xue [104]	2021	China	St Georg sled UKA	Mobile	Waldemar Link, Hamburg, Germany	198		56	142	70.6 ± 8.5		Jan-13	2020			56	15.6–88.9

Appendix B: Registry Information

See Table 21.5.

Table 21.5 Arthroplasty registries from around the world based on those listed in Hughes et al. [128]

Country	Registry report	Dates	English	Included	Notes
Australia [66]	Australian orthopaedic association national joint replacement registry: Annual report 2020	September 1999–December 2019	Yes	Yes	
Belgium [80]	Orthopride Belgian hip and knee arthroplasty registry annual report 2018	2011–2019	Yes	No	Can only find report 6 dated 2018, no implant-specific information.
Canada				No	No lateral implant information and difficult to obtain with cost barrier
Croatia				No	No report found
Denmark		1997		No	Online—No implant specific information
Netherlands [81]	Dutch arthroplasty register (LROI): Online LROI annual report 2020	2010—2019	Yes	Yes	
Egypt	Egyptian community arthroplasty register	2007	N/A	No	No annual report—Publications
Finland	Finnish arthroplasty register	1980	Yes	No	Unclear implant information
France				No	No information found
Germany [79]	German arthroplasty register (EPRD): 2019 annual report	2019	Yes	Yes	
Hungary				No	Access only to certain individuals
Italy [67]	Registro dell'implantologia Protesica Ortopedica: Overall data 2020	2000–2018	Yes	Yes	
New Zealand [78]	New Zealand joint registry: 21-year report	1999–2019	Yes	Yes	
Norway [72]	Norwegian arthroplasty register: Report June 2020	1994–2019	Yes	Yes	
Pakistan			No	No	Website cannot be accessed
Portugal [75]	Portuguese Arthroplasty Register—1st Annual Report 2010	June 2009–May 2010	Yes	Yes	
Romania	Romanian arthroplasty register	2003	Yes	No	Website only has hip report from 2015—Biennial report
Scotland				No	Online report, but no implant-specific information
Slovenia [76]	National arthroplasty registry of Slovenia: 1st Annual Report—Knee Replacement 2020	2020	Yes	Yes	
Slovakia [129]	Slovakian arthroplasty register—Review of the annual report of the Slovakian arthroplasty register	2010	Yes	No	2011 publication, no UKR-specific information
Spain	Catalan arthroplasty registry			No	Site does not work—Not found

Table 21.5 (continued)

Country	Registry report	Dates	English	Included	Notes
Sweden [73]	The Swedish knee arthroplasty register: Annual report 2020	1975–2019	Yes	Yes	
Switzerland [65]	Swiss national hip and knee joint registry (SIRIS): Report 2020	2012–2019	Yes	Yes	
United Kingdom [48]	The national joint registry of England, Wales, Northern Ireland, and the Isle of Man: 17th annual report 2020	2003–2019	Yes	Yes	
USA [77]	American joint replacement registry: The seventh annual report of the AJRR on hip and knee arthroplasty (annual report 2020)	2020	Yes	Yes	

Appendix C: Excluded Registry Listed Implants

See Table 21.6.

Table 21.6 Implants listed as UKR implants, but excluded from summary list

Device	Manufacturer	Registry	Reason for excluding
Duracon	–	Norway [72]	Insufficient information
Persona partial	Biomet	Slovenia [76], Switzerland [65], USA [77], New Zealand [78], UK [48]	Medial only
Journey deuce	Smith & Nephew	Portugal [75]	Bi-compartment (medial and patellofemoral joint)
Profix	Smith & nephew	Portugal [75], Norway [72]	Total
ZUC	Zimmer	Portugal	Not sure which device exactly
Columbus	Aesculap implant systems	USA [77]	TKR
NexGen high-flex	Zimmer Biomet	USA [77], Norway [72]	TKR
Zimmer Uni	Zimmer	New Zealand [78]	Insufficient information
UNIVATION XF	Aesculap	Germany [79]	Medial only
Schlittenprothese	Waldemar Link	Germany [79]	LINK sled device (fixed)
Freedom PKR/active	–	Australia [66]	Insufficient information
GRU	–	Australia [66]	Insufficient information
EFDIOS	Citieffe	Italy [67]	Insufficient information

References

1. Gunther TV, et al. Lateral unicompartmental arthroplasty with the Oxford meniscal knee. Knee. 1996;3:33–9.
2. Saxler G, Temmen D, Bontemps G. Medium-term results of the AMC-unicompartmental knee arthroplasty. Knee. 2004;11(5):349–55.
3. Flandry F, Hommel G. Normal anatomy and biomechanics of the knee. Sports Med Arthrosc Rev. 2011;19(1538–1951)):82–92.
4. Goodfellow J, et al. Unicompartmental arthroplasty with the oxford knee. 2nd ed. Oxford: Goodfellow Publishers Lim; 2015.
5. Szarmach A, et al. Assessment of the relationship between the shape of the lateral meniscus and the risk of extrusion based on MRI examination of the knee joint. PLoS One. 2016;11:1932–6203.
6. Abulhasan J, Grey M. Anatomy and physiology of knee stability. J Functt Morphol Kinesiol. 2017;2(4):34.
7. Ali S, et al. Normal variants of the meniscus; 2013. p. 14.
8. Iwaki H, Pinskerova V, Freeman MA. Tibiofemoral movement 1: the shapes and relative movements of the femur and tibia in the unloaded cadaver knee. J Bone Joint Surg (Br). 2000;82-B(8):1189–95.
9. Victor J, et al. How isometric are the medial patellofemoral, superficial medial collateral, and lateral collateral ligaments of the knee? Am J Sports Med. 2009;37(10):2028–36.
10. Hosseini A, et al. In vivo length change patterns of the medial and lateral collateral ligaments along the flexion path of the knee. Knee Surg Sports Traumatol Arthrosc. 2015;23(10):3055–61.
11. Tokuhara Y, et al. The flexion gap in normal knees. J Bone Joint Surg (Br). 2004;86-B(8):1133–6.
12. Nakagawa S, et al. Tibiofemoral movement 3: full flexion in the living knee studied by MRI. J Bone Joint Surg (Br). 2000;82-B:1199–200.
13. Felson DT. Epidemiology of hip and knee osteoarthritis. Epidemiol Rev. 1988;10(1):1–28.
14. Stoddart JC, et al. The compartmental distribution of knee osteoarthritis - a systematic review and meta-analysis. Osteoarthr Cartil. 2021;29(4):445–55.
15. Scott RD. Lateral unicompartmental replacement: a road less traveled. Orthopedics. 2005;28(9):983–4.
16. Ollivier M, Parratte S, Argenson JN. Results and outcomes of unicompartmental knee arthroplasty. Orthop Clin North Am. 2013;44(3):287–8.
17. Smith JRA, et al. Fixed bearing lateral unicompartmental knee arthroplasty--short to midterm survivorship and knee scores for 101 prostheses. Knee. 2014;21(4):843–7.
18. Kim KT, et al. Clinical results of lateral unicompartmental knee arthroplasty: minimum 2-year follow-up. Clin Orthop Surg. 2016;8(4):386–92.
19. Newman SDS, et al. Up to 10 year follow-up of the Oxford domed lateral partial knee replacement from an independent Centre. Knee. 2017;24(6):1414–21.
20. Walker T, et al. Mid-term results of lateral unicondylar mobile bearing knee arthroplasty - a multicentre study of 363 cases. Bone Joint J. 2018;100-B:42–9.
21. Fornell S, et al. Mid-term outcomes of mobile-bearing lateral unicompartmental knee arthroplasty. Knee. 2018;25(6):1206–13.
22. Kennedy JA, et al. Oxford domed lateral unicompartmental knee arthroplasty ten-year survival and seven-year clinical outcome. Bone Joint J. 2020;102(8):1033–40.
23. Walker T, et al. Minimally invasive lateral unicompartmental knee replacement: early results from an independent center using the Oxford fixed lateral prosthesis. Knee. 2020;27(1):235–41.
24. Ohdera T, Tokunaga J, Kobayashi A. Unicompartmental knee arthroplasty for lateral gonarthrosis: midterm results. J Arthroplast. 2001;16(2):196–200.
25. Liebs TR, Herzberg W. Better quality of life after medial versus lateral unicondylar knee arthroplasty knee. Clin Orthop Relat Res. 2013;471(8):2629–40.
26. Deroche E, et al. Excellent outcomes for lateral unicompartmental knee arthroplasty: multicenter 268-case series at 5 to 23 years' follow-up. Orthop Traumatol Surg Res. 2020;106(5):907–13.
27. Argenson JN, et al. Long-term results with a lateral unicondylar replacement. Clin Orthop Relat Res. 2008;466(11):2686–93.
28. Schelfaut S, et al. The risk of bearing dislocation in lateral unicompartmental knee arthroplasty using a mobile biconcave design. Knee Surg Sports Traumatol Arthrosc. 2013;21(11):2487–94.
29. Derek T, et al. Axial alignment of the lower limband its association with disorders of the knee. Oper Techn Sports Med. 2000;8(2):98–107.
30. Lustig S, et al. Lateral unicompartmental knee arthroplasty relieves pain and improves function in posttraumatic osteoarthritis. Clin Orthop Relat Res. 2012;470(1):69–76.
31. Wolcott M. Osteotomies around the knee for the young athlete with osteoarthritis. Clin Sports Med. 2005;24(1):153–61.
32. Volpi P, et al. Lateral unicompartimental knee arthroplasty: indications, technique and short-medium term results. Knee Surg Sports Traumatol Arthrosc. 2007;15(8):1028–34.
33. Berend KR, et al. Lateral unicompartmental knee arthroplasty through a lateral parapatellar approach has high early survivorship. Clin Orthop Relat Res. 2012;470(1):77–83.
34. Celiker R. Current treatment approaches for osteoarthritis in the elderly. Turkiye Fiziksel Tip ve Rehabilitasyon Dergisi. 2009;55(SUPP.2):75–9.
35. Hangalur G, et al. New adjustable unloader knee brace and its effectiveness. J Med Device. 2018;12(1):015001.

36. Steadman JR, et al. Current state of unloading braces for knee osteoarthritis. Knee Surg Sports Traumatol Arthrosc. 2016;24(1):42–50.

37. Dennis DA, et al. Evaluation of off-loading braces for treatment of unicompartmental knee arthrosis. J Arthroplast. 2006;21(4 Suppl 1):2–8.

38. Mistry DA, Chandratreya A, Lee PYF. An update on unloading knee braces in the treatment of Unicompartmental knee osteoarthritis from the last 10 years: a literature review. Surg J. 2018;4(3):e110–8.

39. Zhang W, et al. OARSI recommendations for the management of hip and knee osteoarthritis, part II: OARSI evidence-based, expert consensus guidelines. Osteoarthr Cartil. 2008;16(2):137–62.

40. Bannuru RR, et al. OARSI guidelines for the non-surgical management of knee, hip, and polyarticular osteoarthritis. Osteoarthr Cartil. 2019;27(11):1578–89.

41. Davis AM, MacKay C. Osteoarthritis year in review: outcome of rehabilitation. Osteoarthr Cartil. 2013;21(10):1414–24.

42. Osteoarthritis: care and management. Clinical guidelines. 2014: National Institute for Health and Care Excellence.

43. O'Rourke MR, et al. The John Insall award: unicompartmental knee replacement: a minimum twenty-one-year followup, end-result study. Clin Orthop Relat Res. 2005;440:27–37.

44. Forster MC, Bauze AJ, Keene GC. Lateral unicompartmental knee replacement: fixed or mobile bearing? Knee Surg Sports Traumatol Arthrosc. 2007;15(9):1107–11.

45. Cao Z, et al. Unicompartmental knee arthroplasty vs. high Tibial osteotomy for knee osteoarthritis: a systematic review and meta-analysis. J Arthroplast. 2018;33(3):952–9.

46. Hoorntje A, et al. Eight respectively nine out of ten patients return to sport and work after distal femoral osteotomy. Knee Surg Sports Traumatol Arthrosc. 2018;27:2345–53.

47. Ryu SM, et al. High Tibial osteotomy versus Unicompartmental knee arthroplasty for medial compartment arthrosis with kissing lesions in relatively young patients. Knee Surg Relat Res. 2018;30(1):17–22.

48. National joint registry 17th annual report 2020. 2020.

49. Smith E, et al. Lateral unicompartmental knee arthroplasty. JBJS Rev. 2020;8(3):e0044.

50. Goodfellow JW, et al. The Oxford knee for unicompartmental osteoarthritis. The first 103 cases. J Bone Joint Surg (Br). 1988;70(5):692–701.

51. Pandit H, et al. Mobile bearing dislocation in lateral unicompartmental knee replacement. Knee. 2010;17(6):392–7.

52. Goodfellow JW, O'Connor J. Clinical results of the Oxford knee. Surface arthroplasty of the tibiofemoral joint with a meniscal bearing prosthesis. Clin Orthop Relat Res. 1986;205:21–42.

53. Argenson J-NA, et al. In vivo determination of knee kinematics for subjects implanted with a unicompartmental arthroplasty. J Arthroplast. 2002;17(8):1049–54.

54. Ho JC, et al. Return to sports activity following UKA and TKA. J Knee Surg. 2016;29(3):254–9.

55. Fiocchi A, et al. Medial vs. lateral unicompartmental knee arthrroplasty: clinical results. Acta Biomed. 2017;88(2S):38–44.

56. Burn E, et al. Ten-year patient-reported outcomes following total and minimally invasive unicompartmental knee arthroplasty: a propensity score-matched cohort analysis. Knee Surg Sports Traumatol Arthrosc. 2018;26(5):1455–64.

57. Davies GS, et al. Changes in patella tendon length over 5 years after different types of knee arthroplasty. Knee Surg Sports Traumatol Arthrosc. 2016;24(9):3029–35.

58. Gill JR, Nicolai P. Clinical results and 12-year survivorship of the Physica ZUK unicompartmental knee replacement. Knee. 2019;26(3):750–8.

59. Edmiston TA, et al. Clinical outcomes and survivorship of lateral Unicompartmental knee arthroplasty: does surgical approach matter? J Arthroplast. 2018;33(2):362–5.

60. Burger JA, et al. Mid-term survivorship and patient-reported outcomes of robotic-arm assisted partial knee arthroplasty. Bone Joint J. 2020;102-B(1):108–16.

61. Heyse TJ, et al. Survivorship of UKA in the middle-aged. Knee. 2012;19(5):585–91.

62. Streit MR, et al. Mobile-bearing lateral unicompartmental knee replacement with the Oxford domed tibial component: an independent series. J Bone Joint Surg (Br). 2012;94 B(10):1356–61.

63. Keblish PA, Briard JL. Mobile-bearing unicompartmental knee arthroplasty: a 2-center study with an 11-year (mean) follow-up. J Arthroplast. 2004;19(7 Suppl 2):87–94.

64. Marmor L. Marmor modular knee in unicompartmental disease. Minimum four-year follow-up. J Bone Joint Surg Am. 1979;61(3):347–53.

65. Swiss national hip and knee joint registry report 2020. 2020.

66. Australian orthopaedic association national joint replacement registry hip, knee and shoulder arthroplasty: annual report 2020. 2020.

67. Report of regional registry of orthopaedic prosthetic implantology: Overall data hip, knee and shoulder arthrplasty in 'Emilia-Romagna Region (Italy). 2020.

68. Kagan R, et al. Ten-year survivorship, patient-reported outcomes, and satisfaction of a fixed-bearing Unicompartmental knee arthroplasty. Arthroplast Today. 2020;6(2):267–73.

69. Lecuire F, Berard JB, Martres S. Minimum 10-year follow-up results of ALPINA cementless hydroxyapatite-coated anatomic unicompartmental knee arthroplasty. Eur J Orthop Surg Traumatol. 2014;24(3):385–94.

70. Scott RD, Santore RF. Unicondylar unicompartmental replacement for osteoarthritis of the knee. J Bone Joint Surg Am. 1981;63(4):536–44.

71. Koskinen E, et al. Unicondylar knee replacement for primary osteoarthritis: a prospective follow-up study of 1,819 patients from the Finnish arthroplasty register. Acta Orthop. 2007;78(1):128–35.

72. Norwegian national advisory unit: Report June 2020. 2020.

73. Swedish knee arthroplasty register annual report 2020. 2020.

74. Deroche E, et al. High survival rate and very low Wear of lateral Unicompartmental arthroplasty at long term: a case series of 54 cases at a mean follow-up of 17 years. J Arthroplast. 2019;34(6):1097–104.

75. Portuguese arthroplasty register: 1st Annual Report June 2009–May 2010. 2010.

76. Levašič, V., D. Savarin, and S. Kovač, The National Arthroplasty Registry of Slovenia (RES) 1st annual report—knee replacement (data from 2019).2020.

77. The seventh annual report of the AJRR on hip and knee arthroplasty: annual report 2020. 2020.

78. The New Zealand joint registry twenty-one year report january 1999–december 2019. 2020.

79. German arthroplasty registry (EPRD) 2019 Annual Report. 2019.

80. Orthopride Belgian hip and knee arthroplasty registry annual report 2018. 2018.

81. Dutch arthroplasty register (LROI): online LROI annual report 2020 - PDF. 2020.

82. Saragaglia D, et al. Results with nine years mean follow up on one hundred and three KAPS uni knee arthroplasties: eighty six medial and seventeen lateral. Int Orthop. 2018;42(5):1061–6.

83. Lewold S, et al. Oxford meniscal bearing knee versus the Marmor knee in unicompartmental arthroplasty for arthrosis. A Swedish multicenter survival study. J Arthroplast. 1995;10(6):722–31.

84. Deshmukh RV, Scott RD. Unicompartmental knee arthroplasty: long-term results. Clin Orthop Relat Res. 2001;392:272–8.

85. Pennington DW, et al. Lateral unicompartmental knee arthroplasty: survivorship and technical considerations at an average follow-up of 12.4 years. J Arthroplast. 2006;21(1):13–7.

86. Streit MR, et al. Mobile-bearing lateral unicompartmental knee replacement with the Oxford domed tibial component: an independent series. J Bone Joint Surg (Br). 2012;94(10):1356–61.

87. Weston-Simons JS, et al. The mid-term outcomes of the Oxford domed lateral unicompartmental knee replacement. Bone Joint J. 2014;96-B(1):59–64.

88. Bergenudd H. Porous-coated anatomic unicompartmental knee arthroplasty in osteoarthritis: a 3- to 9-year follow-up study. J Arthroplast. 1995;10(SUPPL):S8–S13.

89. Walton MJ, Weale AE, Newman JH. The progression of arthritis following lateral unicompartmental knee replacement. Knee. 2006;13(5):374–7.

90. Berend KR, et al. Does preoperative patellofemoral joint state affect medial unicompartmental arthroplasty survival? Orthopedics. 2011;34(9):e494–6.

91. Ashraf T, et al. Lateral unicompartmental knee replacement survivorship and clinical experience over 21 years. J Bone Joint Surg (Br). 2002;84(8):1126–30.

92. Hall MJ, Connell DA, Morris HG. Medium to long-term results of the UNIX uncemented unicompartmental knee replacement. Knee. 2013;20(5):328–31.

93. Marson B, et al. Lateral unicompartmental knee replacements: early results from a district general hospital. Eur J Orthop Surg Traumatol. 2014;24(6):987–91.

94. Sah AP, Scott RD. Lateral unicompartmental knee arthroplasty through a medial approach. Study with an average five-year follow-up. J Bone Joint Surg Am. 2007;89(9):1948–54.

95. John J, Mauffrey C, May P. Unicompartmental knee replacements with miller-Galante prosthesis: two to 16-year follow-up of a single surgeon series. Int Orthop. 2011;35(4):507–13.

96. Lustig S, et al. 5- to 16-year follow-up of 54 consecutive lateral Unicondylar knee arthroplasties with a fixed-all polyethylene bearing. J Arthroplast. 2011;26(8):1318–25.

97. Schiavone Panni A, et al. Unicompartmental knee replacement with ZUK prosthesis: mid-term results. J Orthop Traumatol. 2011;12(SUPPL. 1):S159.

98. Lustig S, et al. Progression of medial osteoarthritis and long term results of lateral unicompartmental arthroplasty: 10 to 18 year follow-up of 54 consecutive implants. Knee. 2014;21(S1):S26–32.

99. Walker T, et al. Total versus unicompartmental knee replacement for isolated lateral osteoarthritis: a matched-pairs study. Int Orthop. 2014;38(11):2259–64.

100. Masud S, et al. Oxford domed lateral Unciompartmental knee arthroplasty: is it as good as Oxford medial Unicompartmental knee arthroplasty? Orthop Proceed. 2017;99-B(SUPP_16)):19.

101. Burger JA, et al. A comprehensive evaluation of lateral Unicompartmental knee arthroplasty short to mid-term survivorship, and the effect of patient and implant characteristics: an analysis of data from the Dutch arthroplasty register. J Arthroplast. 2020;35(7):1813–8.

102. Murray DW, et al. The mid- to long-term outcomes of the lateral domed Oxford Unicompartmental knee replacement: an analysis from the National Joint Registry for England, Wales, Northern Ireland, and the Isle of Man. J Arthroplast. 2021;36(1):107–11.

103. Murray JRD, et al. Fixed bearing, all-polyethylene tibia, lateral unicompartmental arthroplasty - a final outcome study with up to 28 year follow-up of a single implant. Knee. 2021;29:101–9.

104. Xue H, et al. Predictors of satisfactory outcomes with fixed-bearing lateral Unicompartmental knee arthroplasty: up to 7-year follow-up. J Arthroplast. 2021;36(3):910–6.

105. Neufeld ME, et al. A comparison of Mobile and fixed-bearing Unicompartmental knee arthroplasty at a minimum 10-year follow-up. J Arthroplast. 2018;33(6):1713–8.

106. Ko Y-B, Gujarathi MR, Oh K-J. Outcome of Unicompartmental knee arthroplasty: a systematic review of comparative studies between fixed and Mobile bearings focusing on complications. Knee Surg Relat Res. 2015;27(3):141–8.

107. Peersman G, et al. Fixed- versus mobile-bearing UKA: a systematic review and meta-analysis. Knee Surg Sports Traumatol Arthrosc. 2015;23(11):3296–305.

108. Smith TO, et al. Fixed versus mobile bearing unicompartmental knee replacement: a meta-analysis. Orthop Traumatol Surgery Res. 2009;95(8):599–605.

109. Arastu MH, et al. Early failure of a mobile-bearing unicompartmental knee replacement. Knee Surg Sports Traumatol Arthrosc. 2009;17(10):1178–83.

110. van der List JP, Zuiderbaan HA, Pearle AD. Why do lateral Unicompartmental knee arthroplasties fail today? Am J Orthop (Belle Mead, NJ). 2016;45(7):432–62.

111. Yang I, et al. Systematic review and meta-analysis of bearing dislocation in lateral meniscal bearing unicompartmental knee replacement: domed versus flat tibial surface. Knee. 2021;28:214–28.

112. Pandit H, et al. Lateral unicompartmental knee replacement for the treatment of arthritis progression after medial unicompartmental replacement. Knee Surg Sports Traumatol Arthrosc. 2017;25(3):669–74.

113. Cho W-J, et al. Mobile-bearing unicompartmental knee arthroplasty in old-aged patients demonstrates superior short-term clinical outcomes to open-wedge high tibial osteotomy in middle-aged patients with advanced isolated medial osteoarthritis. Int Orthop. 2018;42(10):2357–63.

114. Song SJ, et al. Long-term survival is similar between closed-wedge high tibial osteotomy and unicompartmental knee arthroplasty in patients with similar demographics. Knee Surg Sports Traumatol Arthrosc. 2019;27:1310.

115. Wilson HA, et al. Patient relevant outcomes of unicompartmental versus total knee replacement: systematic review and meta-analysis. BMJ (Clinical research ed). 2019;364:l352.

116. Zhang Q, et al. The learning curve for minimally invasive Oxford phase 3 unicompartmental knee arthroplasty: cumulative summation test for learning curve (LC-CUSUM). J Orthop Surg Res. 2014;9:81.

117. Bare JV, et al. A convex lateral tibial plateau for knee replacement. Knee. 2006;13(2):122–6.

118. Demange MK, et al. Patient-specific implants for lateral unicompartmental knee arthroplasty. Int Orthop. 2015;39(8):1519–26.

119. Robinson BJ, et al. A kinematic study of lateral unicompartmental arthroplasty. Knee. 2002;9(3):237–40.

120. Mohammad HR, et al. Long-term outcomes of over 8,000 medial Oxford phase 3 Unicompartmental knees-a systematic review. Acta Orthop. 2018;89(1):101–7.

121. Weston-Simons JS, et al. The management of mobile bearing dislocation in the Oxford lateral unicompartmental knee replacement. Knee Surg Sports Traumatol Arthrosc. 2011;19(12):2023–6.

122. Robinson BJ, et al. Dislocation of the bearing of the Oxford lateral unicompartmental arthroplasty. A radiological assessment. J Bone Joint Surg (Br). 2002;84(5):653–7.

123. Hamilton TW, et al. The interaction of caseload and usage in determining outcomes of Unicompartmental knee arthroplasty: a meta-analysis. J Arthroplast. 2017;32(10):3228–3237.e2.

124. Diabb Zavala JM, Leija Gutiérrez HM, et al. Manufacture and mechanical properties of knee implants using SWCNTs/UHMWPE composites. J Mech Behav Biomed Mater. 2021;120:104554.

125. Kurtz SM, et al. Advances in the processing, sterilization, and crosslinking of ultra-high molecular weight polyethylene for total joint arthroplasty. Biomaterials. 1999;20(18):1659–88.

126. UHMWPE. Biomaterials for Joint Implants: Structures, Properties and Clinical Performance, vol. 13. Springer Series in Biomaterials Science and Engineering; 2019.

127. van Duren BH, et al. Trans-patella tendon approach for domed lateral unicompartmental knee arthroplasty does not increase the risk of patella tendon shortening. Knee Surg Sports Traumatol Arthrosc. 2014;22(8):1887–94.

128. Hughes RE, Batra A, Hallstrom BR. Arthroplasty registries around the world: valuable sources of hip implant revision risk data. Curr Rev Musculoskelet Med. 2017;10(2):240–52.

129. Necas L., et al., Review of the Annual Report of the Slovakian Arthropasty Register - 2010. 2010.

Index